Small Animal Dermatology
A Color Atlas and Therapeutic Guide

Linda Medleau, DVM, MS, Diplomate ACVD

Professor of Veterinary Dermatology
University of Georgia
College of Veterinary Medicine
Athens, Georgia

Keith A. Hnilica, DVM, MS, Diplomate ACVD

Assistant Professor of Veterinary Dermatology
The University of Tennessee
College of Veterinary Medicine
Knoxville, Tennessee

W.B. SAUNDERS COMPANY

An Imprint of Elsevier Science

Philadelphia • London • New York • St. Louis • Sydney • Toronto

W.B. SAUNDERS COMPANY

An Imprint of Elsevier Science

The Curtis Center
Independence Square West
Philadelphia, Pennsylvania 19106

Library of Congress Cataloging-in-Publication Data

Medleau, Linda.
    Small animal dermatology : a color atlas and therapetic guide / Linda Medleau, Keith A. Hnilica.—1st ed.

      p. cm.

  ISBN 0–7216–8152–2

    1. Dogs—Diseases. 2. Cats—Diseases. 3. Veterinary dermatology. I. Hnilica, Keith A.
II. Title.

SF992.S55 M44 2001
636.7'08965—dc21
                                                 2001020139

SMALL ANIMAL DERMATOLOGY   ISBN 0–7216–8152–2

Printed in the United States of America

Last digit is the print number: 9   8   7   6   5   4   3   2

To my husband, Gil, and children, Rachel and David, for their unwavering love, support, and encouragement.

Linda Medleau

....

To Mae and Sara
Always Forever

Keith A. Hnilica

Preface

This atlas began as a companion text for Muller and Kirk's *Small Animal Dermatology*. We designed the book to be a complete color atlas that included current treatments for each disorder. Great effort has gone into making this book an easy-to-use reference for practicing small animal veterinarians.

Small Animal Dermatology: A Color Atlas and Therapeutic Guide is organized into chapters based on disease etiologies similar to Muller and Kirk's *Small Animal Dermatology*. Since many diseases can present with similar lesions, we devote the first chapter to differential diagnoses for common clinical presentations. This chapter will help the practitioner formulate a workable rule-out list from which a final diagnosis can be obtained.

To make this atlas a complete and useful reference, we incorporate the clinical features, top differentials, diagnostic test findings, and therapies for each disorder. Veterinary dermatology is a specialty that relies greatly on therapies tailored to each patient's needs. This makes listing treatment options for select diseases very difficult; however, we endeavor to provide sufficient guidance so that the practitioner can successfully manage his or her patient's complaints. To help with dispensing treatments, four appendices are included that provide useful product information. In addition, tables are incorporated into select chapters to provide direction for the treatment of certain disorders.

We hope that you will find this color atlas useful during your practice of veterinary dermatology.

Linda Medleau
Keith A. Hnilica

Acknowledgments

My sincerest thanks and appreciation to the many wonderful people of the Helen Keller National Center, the Foundation Fighting Blindness, Guiding Eyes for the Blind, SKI FOR LIGHT, the Office of Disability Services at the University of Georgia, my fellow ACVD diplomats, and my colleagues at the University of Georgia College of Veterinary Medicine who have in various, important ways helped me be a productive member of society in spite of my severe disabilities.

In the writing of this book I gratefully acknowledge the assistance of Dr. Kim Lower, whose help was invaluable. Additionally, I would like to thank Dr. Sherry Sanderson, Kate Averett, Lydia Pryor, Mandy Bliss, Fran Cantrell, and our editors Ray Kersey and Denise LeMelledo.

Linda Medleau

My sincerest appreciation for Donna Angarano and John MacDonald, whose continual mentoring has provided much assistance, great reassurance, and many wonderful opportunities.

My deepest gratitude goes to Michelle Haag, who was largely responsible for getting me through a rather large quagmire.

Much thanks to those who generously allowed us to use photographs from their collections: Donna Angarano, John MacDonald, Anthony Yu, Gail Kunkle, Michaela Austel, Craig Greene, Alice Wolfe, Karen Campbell, Richard Malik, Linda Frank, Lynn Schmeitzel, Patricia White, Dunbar Gram, Jim Noxon, Linda Messinger, Elizabeth Willis, Terese DeManuelle, William Miller, Thomas Manning, Kimberly Boyanowski, Norma White-Weithers, Manon Paradis, Robert Dunstan, Kelly Credille, Pauline Rakich, Charles Martin, Clay Calvert, Sherry Sanderson, Mary Mahaffey, Sue McLaughlin, Edward Roberson, Gary Norsworthy, and Michael Singer.

Thank you all,
Keith A. Hnilica

NOTICE

Veterinary Medicine is an ever-changing field. Standard safety precautions must be followed, but as new research and clinical experience broaden our knowledge, changes in treatment and drug therapy may become necessary or appropriate. Readers are advised to check the most current product information provided by the manufacturer of each drug to be administered to verify the recommended dose, the method and duration of administration, and contraindications. It is the responsibility of the treating veterinarian, relying on experience, and knowledge of the animal, to determine dosages and the best treatment for each individual animal. Neither the Publisher nor the editor assume any liability for any injury and/or damage to animals or property arising from this publication.

The Publisher

Contents

1

Differential Diagnoses

Cellulitis

DOGS

CATS

Pododermatitis

DOGS

CATS

Nodular Diseases

DOGS

CATS

Nodular Diseases (cont.)

CATS (cont.)

Diseases Primarily Limited to the Face

DOGS

CATS

Seborrheic Diseases

DOGS

CATS

Nonpruritic Alopecic Diseases

DOGS

CATS

Vesicular and Pustular Diseases

Nasodigital Hyperkeratosis

Erosive and Ulcerative Diseases

Miliary Dermatitis

Generalized Pruritic Diseases

Diseases of Nasal Depigmentation

2

Bacterial Skin Diseases

- **Skin Fold Dermatitis** (intertrigo, skin fold pyoderma)

- **Mucocutaneous Pyoderma**

- **Pyotraumatic Dermatitis** (acute moist dermatitis, hot spots, moist eczema)

- **Impetigo** (superficial pustular dermatitis)

- **Superficial Pyoderma** (superficial bacterial folliculitis)

- **Chin Pyoderma** (canine acne)

- **Nasal Pyoderma** (nasal folliculitis and furunculosis)

- **Bacterial Pododermatitis** (interdigital pyoderma, pedal folliculitis and furunculosis)

- **Deep Pyoderma**

- **Subcutaneous Abscess** (cat and dog fight/bite abscesses)

- **Botryomycosis** (bacterial pseudomycetoma, cutaneous bacterial granuloma)

- **L-Form Infection**

- **Actinomycosis**

- **Nocardiosis**

- **Opportunistic Mycobacteriosis** (atypical mycobacterial granuloma)

- **Feline Leprosy**

- **Tuberculosis**

- **Plague**

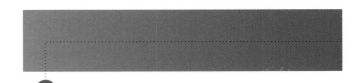

Skin Fold Dermatitis (intertrigo, skin fold pyoderma) (Figs. 2–1 to 2–8)

FEATURES

A bacterial surface skin infection in dogs with excessive skin folds. The infection involves the facial folds of brachycephalic breeds, the lip folds in dogs with large lip flaps, the tail folds of brachycephalic breeds with "corkscrew" tails, the vulvar folds in obese females with small, recessed vulvas, and the body folds of dogs with excessive truncal or leg folds (Chinese shar peis, basset hounds and dachshunds, and obese dogs). Common in dogs.

Facial fold dermatitis • Nonpainful, nonpruritic, erythematous facial folds that may also be malodorous. Concurrent traumatic keratitis or corneal ulceration is common.

Lip fold dermatitis • A fetid breath from saliva accumulating in macerated, erythematous lower lip fold(s) is usually the presenting complaint. Concurrent dental calculi, gingivitis, and excessive salivation may contribute to the halitosis.

Tail fold dermatitis • Skin under the tail is macerated, erythematous, and malodorous.

Vulvar fold dermatitis • Symptoms include erythematous, macerated and malodorous vulvar folds, excessive vulvar licking, and painful urination. A secondary urinary tract infection may be present.

Body fold dermatitis • Erythematous, seborrheic, often malodorous, and sometimes mildly pruritic truncal or leg folds.

TOP DIFFERENTIALS

Superficial pyoderma, demodicosis, dermatophytosis, *Malassezia* dermatitis. Vulvar fold dermatitis also includes urine scald or primary cystitis or vaginitis.

DIAGNOSIS

1. Usually based on signalment, history, clinical findings, and ruling out other differentials.
2. Cytology (skin imprint)—Mixed bacteria are seen. Yeast may also be present.
3. Urinalysis (cystocentesis)—Bacteriuria is seen in dogs with vulvar fold dermatitis that have a secondary urinary tract infection.

TREATMENT AND PROGNOSIS

1. Initiate a weight reduction program if the dog is obese.
2. Surgical excision of excess facial, lip, or vulvar folds or tail amputation for tail fold dermatitis is usually curative.
3. Alternatively, routine topical therapy can be used to control the skin problem. For facial, tail, lip, or vulvar fold dermatitis, cleanse affected area q 1–3 days as needed with an antibacterial shampoo containing chlorhexidine, 2 1/2–3% benzoyl peroxide, or ethyl lactate. Applying an astringent (i.e., aluminum acetate) or benzoyl peroxide gel after cleansing may be helpful.
4. For body fold dermatitis, bathe dog with sulfur, chlorhexidine, benzoyl peroxide, or ethyl lactate-based shampoo q 3–7 days as needed.
5. Topical application of an antibiotic cream, solution, or spray q 24 hours for 5–7 days of therapy may be helpful.
6. Treat any concurrent disease (corneal ulcers, dental disease, gingivitis, urinary tract infection).
7. Prognosis is good, but lifelong topical maintenance therapy may be needed if surgical correction is not performed.

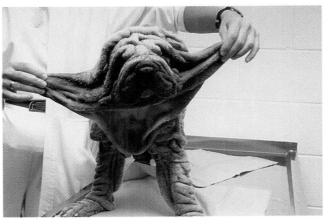

FIGURE 2–1. Skin Fold Dermatitis. A shar pei with its distinctive wrinkles that predispose this breed to skin fold dermatitis.

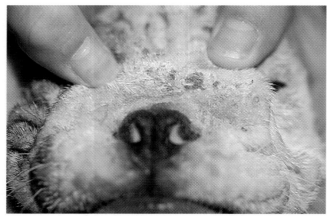

FIGURE 2–2. Skin Fold Dermatitis. Alopecia, erythema, and crusts in the nasal skin fold of a juvenile English bulldog.

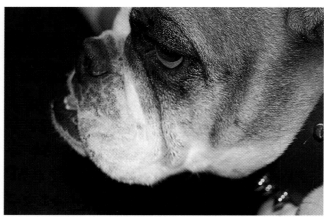

FIGURE 2–5. Skin Fold Dermatitis. A mature boxer with a deep facial skin fold. The dermatitis was not apparent until the skin fold was examined (see Figure 2–6).

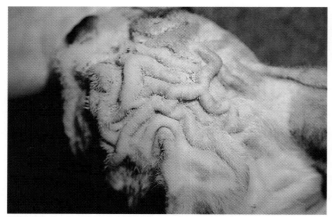

FIGURE 2–3. Skin Fold Dermatitis. Numerous skin folds on the scalp of a juvenile English bulldog. Note the alopecia, erythema, and exudate associated with the folds.

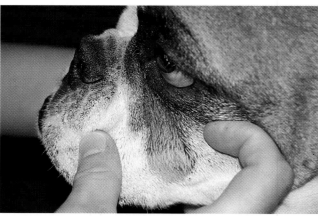

FIGURE 2–6. Skin Fold Dermatitis. Close-up of the dog in Figure 2–5. A mature boxer with a deep facial skin fold. The skin fold was retracted, revealing a moist, erythematous dermatitis.

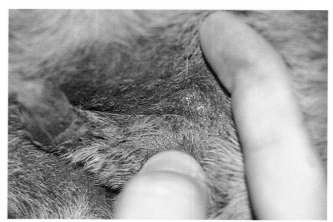

FIGURE 2–4. Skin Fold Dermatitis. A mature English bulldog with tail fold dermatitis. The deep skin folds associated with the tail of this breed are common sites of infection.

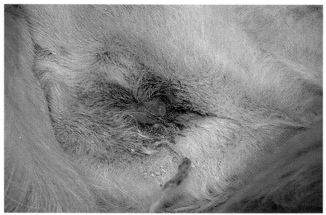

FIGURE 2–7. Skin Fold Dermatitis. A mature golden retriever with vulvar fold dermatitis. The dermatitis was not apparent until the skin fold was retracted (see Figure 2–8).

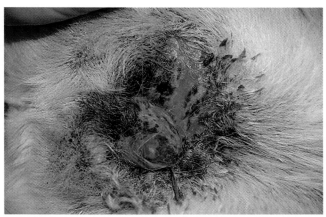

FIGURE 2–8. Skin Fold Dermatitis. Close-up of the dog in Figure 2–7. The skin fold was retracted, revealing a severe moist, erosive dermatitis.

Mucocutaneous Pyoderma
(Figs. 2–9 and 2–10)

FEATURES

A bacterial infection of mucocutaneous junctions. Uncommon in dogs. German shepherd dogs may be predisposed.

Lesions are characterized by mucocutaneous swelling, erythema, and crusting that may be bilaterally symmetrical. Affected areas may be painful or pruritic and self-traumatized, and become exudative, fissured, and depigmented. The margins of the lips, especially at the commissures, are most frequently affected, but the nares, vulva, prepuce, and anus are also sometimes involved.

TOP DIFFERENTIALS

Superficial pyoderma, lip fold dermatitis, demodicosis, dermatophytosis, malasseziasis, candidiasis, autoimmune skin disorders.

DIAGNOSIS

1. Usually based on history, clinical findings, and ruling out other differentials.
2. Cytology (impression smear)—Bacterial cocci and/or rods are seen.
3. Dermatohistopathology—Epidermal hyperplasia, superficial epidermal pustules, crusting, and lichenoid dermatitis with preservation of basement membrane. The dermal infiltrates are often predominantly composed of plasma cells, with lymphocytes and neutrophils.

TREATMENT AND PROGNOSIS

1. For mild to moderate lesions, clip and then clean affected areas with benzoyl peroxide or chlorhexidine-containing shampoo. Apply topical mupirocin ointment or cream q 24 hours for 1 week, then q 3–7 days for maintenance therapy as needed.
2. For severe lesions, in addition to topical therapy give appropriate systemic antibiotics for 3 weeks (Table 2–1).
3. Prognosis is good, but lifelong topical maintenance therapy is often needed.

TABLE 2-1 Oral Antibiotics for Bacterial Skin Infections

Antibiotic	Dose
Cefadroxil	22 mg/kg q 8–12 hours
Cephalexin	22 mg/kg q 8 hours or 30 mg/kg q 12 hours
Cephradine	22 mg/kg q 8 hours
Chloramphenicol	50 mg/kg q 8 hours
Ciprofloxacin	5–15 mg/kg q 12 hours
Clavulanated amoxicillin	22 mg/kg q 8–12 hours
Clindamycin hydrochloride	5.5–11 mg/kg q 12 hours
Enrofloxacin	5–20 mg/kg q 24 hours
Erythromycin	10–15 mg/kg q 8 hours
Marbofloxacin	2.75–5.5 mg/kg q 12 hours
Orbifloxacin	7.5 mg/kg q 24 hours
Ormetoprim/sulfadimethoxine	55 mg/kg once on day 1, then 27.5 mg/kg q 24 hours
Oxacillin	22 mg/kg q 8 hours
Trimethoprim/sulfadiazine	22–30 mg/kg q 12 hours
Trimethoprim/sulfamethoxazole	22–30 mg/kg q 12 hours

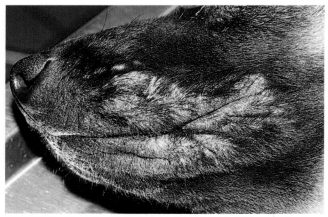

FIGURE 2–10. Mucocutaneous Pyoderma. Alopecia is the principal lesion in this German shepherd with perioral dermatitis.

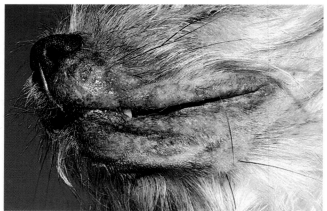

FIGURE 2–9. Mucocutaneous Pyoderma. The acute perioral dermatitis in this terrier was intensely pruritic. Alopecia, erythema, and erosions are visible around the mucocutaneous junction.

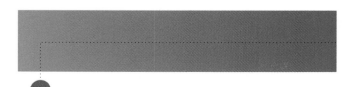

Pyotraumatic Dermatitis (acute moist dermatitis, hot spots, moist eczema) (Figs. 2–11 to 2–16)

FEATURES

An acute and rapidly developing surface bacterial skin infection secondary to self-inflicted trauma. A lesion is created when the animal licks, chews, scratches, or rubs a focal area on its body in response to a pruritic or painful stimulus (Table 2–2). It is usually a seasonal problem when weather is hot and humid. Common in dogs, especially in thick-coated, longhaired breeds. Rare in cats.

Acutely pruritic, rapidly enlarging area of erythema, alopecia, weepy, eroded skin with well-demarcated margins. Lesions are usually single but may be multiple and are often painful. They occur most frequently on the trunk, tail base, lateral thigh, neck, or face.

TOP DIFFERENTIALS

Demodicosis, dermatophytosis, superficial pyoderma.

DIAGNOSIS

1. Usually based on history, clinical findings, and ruling out other differentials.
2. Cytology (skin imprint)—Suppurative inflammation and mixed bacteria are seen.

TREATMENT AND PROGNOSIS

1. Identify and treat the underlying cause.
2. Clip and clean the lesion, under sedation if necessary.
3. Apply a topical drying agent or astringent (i.e., 5% aluminum acetate) q 8–12 hours for 2–7 days. Avoid alcohol-containing products.

4. If pruritus is mild, also apply a topical analgesic (i.e., lidocaine, pramoxine hydrochloride) or corticosteroid-containing cream or solution q 8–12 hours for 5–10 days.
5. If pruritus is severe, give prednisone, 0.5–1.0 mg/kg PO q 24 hours for 5–10 days.
6. If central lesion is surrounded by papules or pustules, systemic antibiotic therapy for 2–4 weeks should also be instituted (Table 2–1).
7. Prognosis is good if the underlying cause can be corrected or controlled.

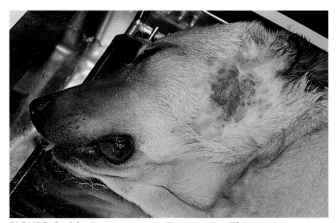

FIGURE 2–11. Pyotraumatic Dermatitis. This moist, erosive lesion at the base of the ear is characteristic of a hot spot.

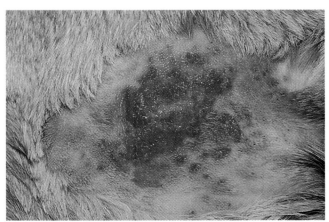

FIGURE 2–12. Pyotraumatic Dermatitis. Close-up of the dog in Figure 2–11. The moist, erosive surface of the lesion is apparent. The papular perimeter suggests an expanding superficial pyoderma.

TABLE 2–2 Causes of Pyotraumatic Dermatitis

Parasites (fleas, pediculosis, cheyletiellosis, scabies)
Hypersensitivity (atopy, food, flea bite)
Anal sac disease
Otitis externa
Folliculitis (bacterial, dermatophytic)
Trauma (minor wounds, foreign body)
Contact dermatitis

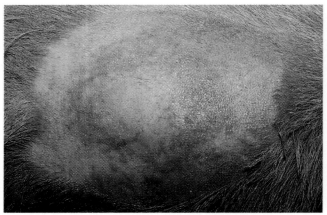

FIGURE 2–13. Pyotraumatic Dermatitis. An early superficial lesion (after clipping) on the lumbar region of a dog with flea allergy dermatitis. The papular perimeter suggests an expanding bacterial folliculitis.

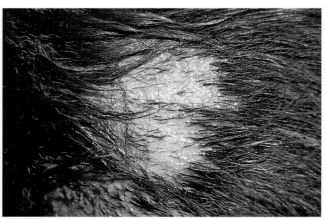

FIGURE 2–15. Pyotraumatic Dermatitis. An early superficial lesion prior to clipping. Note the moist nature of this lesion.

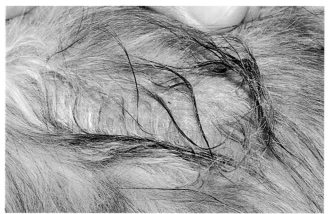

FIGURE 2–14. Pyotraumatic Dermatitis. This moist lesion developed acutely on the dorsum of this flea-allergic cat.

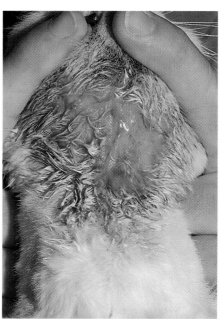

FIGURE 2–16. Pyotraumatic Dermatitis. A severe erosive lesion with a purulent exudate on the ventral neck of a food-allergic cat.

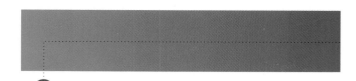

Impetigo (superficial pustular dermatitis) (Figs. 2–17 and 2–18)

FEATURES

A superficial bacterial infection of nonhaired skin that may be associated with a predisposing disease or other underlying factors such as endoparasitism, ectoparasitism, poor nutrition, or a dirty environment. Common in young dogs prior to puberty.

Small, nonfollicular pustules, papules, and crusts that are limited to the inguinal and axillary skin. Lesions are not painful or pruritic.

TOP DIFFERENTIALS

Demodicosis, superficial pyoderma, insect bites, early scabies.

DIAGNOSIS

1. Usually based on signalment, history, clinical findings, and ruling out other differentials.
2. Cytology (pustule)—Neutrophils and bacterial cocci are seen.
3. Dermatohistopathology—Nonfollicular subcorneal pustules containing neutrophils and bacterial cocci.
4. Bacterial culture—*Staphylococcus.*

TREATMENT AND PROGNOSIS

1. Identify and correct any predisposing factors.
2. If lesions are few in number, apply topical mupirocin, neomycin, or chlorhexidine ointment or cream to them q 12 hours for 7–10 days.
3. For widespread lesions, cleanse affected areas q 24–48 hours for 7–10 days with an antibacterial shampoo containing chlorhexidine, ethyl lactate, or benzoyl peroxide.
4. If lesions do not resolve with topical therapy, give appropriate systemic antibiotics for 2–3 weeks, continuing treatment for 1 week beyond complete clinical resolution (Table 2–1).
5. Prognosis is good.

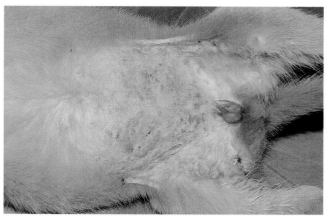

FIGURE 2–17. Impetigo. Numerous superficial pustules and crusts on the abdomen of a puppy.

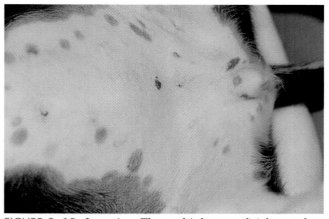

FIGURE 2–18. Impetigo. The multiple superficial pustules on the abdomen of this puppy are typical of impetigo. (Courtesy of D. Angarano)

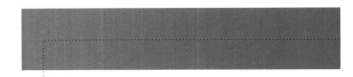

Superficial Pyoderma

(superficial bacterial folliculitis)

(Figs. 2–19 to 2–26)

FEATURES

A superficial bacterial infection involving hair follicles and the adjacent epidermis. The infection is usually secondary to an underlying cause (Table 2–3). Common in dogs and rare in cats.

Focal, multifocal, or generalized areas of papules, pustules, crusts, scales, epidermal collarettes, and/or circumscribed areas of erythema and alopecia that may have hyperpigmented centers. Short-coated dogs often present with a "moth-eaten" patchy alopecia, small tufts of hair standing up, and/or reddish-brown discoloration of white hairs. In long-coated dogs, symptoms may be insidious, with a dull, lusterless haircoat, scales, and excessive shedding. In both short- and long-coated breeds, primary skin lesions are often obscured by remaining hairs but can be readily appreciated if affected area is clipped. Pruritus is variable, ranging from none to intense.

TOP DIFFERENTIALS

Demodicosis, dermatophytosis, pemphigus foliaceus.

DIAGNOSIS

1. Rule out other differentials.
2. Cytology (pustule)—Neutrophils and bacterial cocci are seen.
3. Dermatohistopathology—Epidermal microabscesses, nonspecific superficial dermatitis, perifolliculitis, and folliculitis. Intralesional bacteria may be difficult to find.
4. Bacterial culture—*Staphylococcus*.

TABLE 2–3 Causes of Secondary Superficial and Deep Pyoderma

Foreign body
Trauma or bite wound
Hypersensitivity (atopy, food, flea bite)
Demodicosis, scabies, pelodera
Endocrinopathy (hypothyroidism, hyperadrenocorticism, sex hormone imbalance, alopecia X)
Autoimmune and immune-mediated disorders
Immunosuppressive therapy (glucocorticoids, progestational compounds, cytotoxic drugs)
Poor nutrition

TREATMENT AND PROGNOSIS

1. Identify and correct any underlying cause.
2. Give systemic antibiotics (minimum 3–4 weeks) continued 1 week beyond complete clinical resolution (Table 2–1).
3. Concurrent baths q 2–7 days with an antibacterial shampoo containing chlorhexidine, ethyl lactate, or benzoyl peroxide is helpful.
4. If lesions recur within 7 days of antibiotic discontinuation, the duration of therapy was inadequate and the antibiotics must be reinstituted for a longer time period.
5. If lesions do not completely resolve during antibiotic therapy, or recur weeks to months later, an underlying cause should be sought (Table 2–3).
6. No response to antibiotic therapy suggests antibiotic resistance or a nonbacterial skin disease.
7. If lesions resolve but pruritus persists, underlying ectoparasitism or an allergy is probably present.
8. Prognosis is good if the underlying cause can be identified and corrected or controlled.

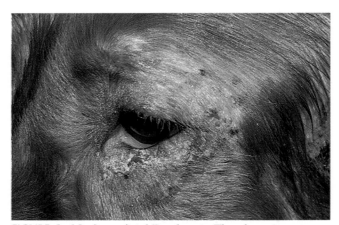

FIGURE 2–19. Superficial Pyoderma. The alopecia, papules, and crusts around the eye of this allergic Irish setter are typical of bacterial folliculitis.

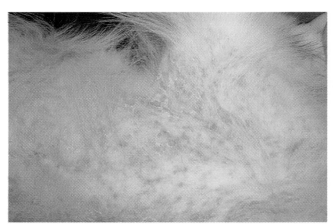

FIGURE 2–20. Superficial Pyoderma. The severe papular rash on the abdomen of this allergic dog was intensely pruritic. Note the early scale formation of epidermal collarettes.

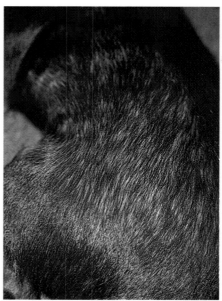

FIGURE 2–21. Superficial Pyoderma. The partial alopecia on the flank of this dog appears as a moth-eaten hair coat.

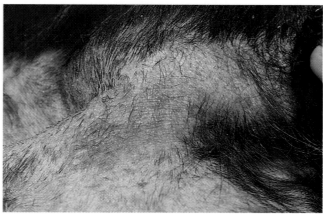

FIGURE 2–24. Superficial Pyoderma. The erythematous papular rash on the inguinal region of this dog was caused by a secondary bacterial folliculitis associated with allergic dermatitis.

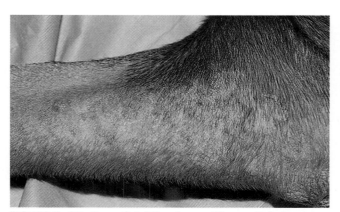

FIGURE 2–22. Superficial Pyoderma. The partial alopecia and mild papular rash on the foreleg of this dog were caused by secondary bacterial folliculitis associated with hypothyroidism.

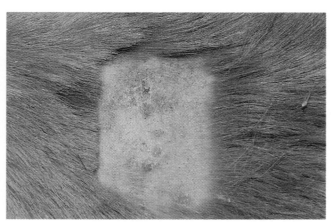

FIGURE 2–25. Superficial Pyoderma. Focal papules and crusts caused by pyoderma can be hidden by a dense fur coat. A window was clipped in the fur coat to reveal these lesions.

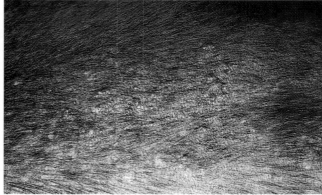

FIGURE 2–23. Superficial Pyoderma. The generalized papules with crust and scale formation on the dorsum of this dog were caused by secondary bacterial folliculitis associated with hypothyroidism.

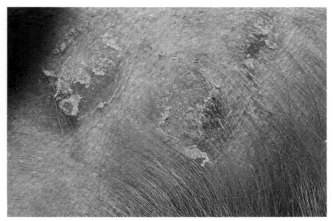

FIGURE 2–26. Superficial Pyoderma. Superficial scaling and epidermal collarettes caused by a chronic infection.

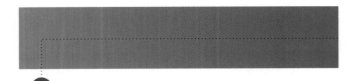

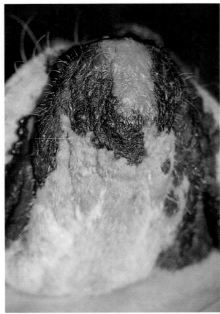

Chin Pyoderma (canine acne)

(Figs. 2–27 to 2–30)

FEATURES

A bacterial infection that is not a true acne. It may be induced by trauma to the chin (e.g., lying on hard floors, friction from chew toys). Common in dogs, especially in young (3–12 months old), large, short-coated breeds.

Nonpainful and nonpruritic comedones, papules, pustules, bullae, and/or ulcerative draining tracts with serosanguineous discharge on the chin or muzzle.

TOP DIFFERENTIALS

Demodicosis, dermatophytosis, early juvenile cellulitis.

DIAGNOSIS

1. Usually based on signalment, history, clinical findings, and ruling out other differentials.
2. Cytology (pustules, exudate)—Suppurative inflammation and bacterial cocci are seen.
3. Dermatohistopathology—Follicular hyperkeratosis, folliculitis, and/or furunculosis. Intralesional bacteria may be difficult to find.
4. Bacterial culture—Primary pathogen is usually *Staphylococcus*. Mixed bacterial infections are possible.

TREATMENT AND PROGNOSIS

1. Minimize trauma to the chin.
2. For mild lesions, cleanse area with benzoyl peroxide shampoo or apply mupirocin ointment or cream or benzoyl peroxide gel q 24 hours until lesions resolve, then q 3–7 days as needed for control.
3. For moderate to severe lesions, in addition to topical treatment, give systemic antibiotics (minimum 4–6 weeks), continued 2 weeks beyond complete clinical resolution (Table 2–1).
4. Prognosis is good. In many dogs, the lesions resolve permanently, but some dogs require lifelong routine topical therapy for control.

FIGURE 2–27. Chin Pyoderma. Erythematous papular lesions with alopecia on the chin of an English bulldog.

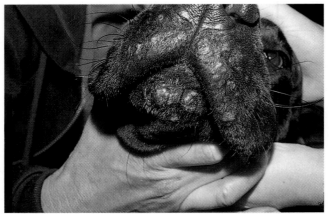

FIGURE 2–28. Chin Pyoderma. These papular to nodular lesions are typical of a deeper infection.

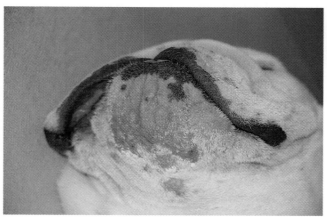

FIGURE 2–29. Chin Pyoderma. Mild erythematous papular lesions with alopecia on the chin of an English bulldog.

Nasal Pyoderma (nasal folliculitis and furunculosis) (Figs. 2–31 and 2–32)

FEATURES

A facial bacterial skin infection that may be secondary to trauma or insect bites. Uncommon in dogs and rare in cats.

Papules, pustules, erythema, alopecia, crusting, swelling, erosions, and/or ulcerative fistulae develop over the bridge of the nose and around the nostrils. Lesions may be painful.

TOP DIFFERENTIALS

Demodicosis, dermatophytosis, autoimmune skin disorders, dermatomyositis, nasal solar dermatitis, eosinophilic furunculosis of the face (dog), mosquito bite hypersensitivity (cat).

DIAGNOSIS

1. Rule out other differentials.
2. Cytology (exudate)—Suppurative inflammation with bacterial cocci and/or rods is seen.
3. Dermatohistopathology—Perifolliculitis, folliculitis, furunculosis, and/or cellulitis. Intralesional bacteria may be difficult to find.
4. Bacterial culture—Primary pathogen is usually *Staphylococcus,* but mixed bacterial infections are also common.

TREATMENT AND PROGNOSIS

1. Use gentle, topical, warm water soaks q 24 hours for 7–10 days to remove crusts.
2. Give systemic antibiotics (minimum 3–4 weeks) continued 2 weeks beyond complete clinical resolution (Table 2–1).
3. Prognosis is good, but scarring may be a permanent sequela in some dogs.

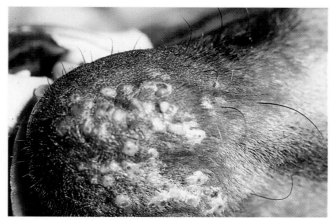

FIGURE 2–30. Chin Pyoderma. Severe papular lesions with purulent exudate caused by a deep infection. The furunculosis can result in permanent alopecia and scarring. (Courtesy of D. Angarano)

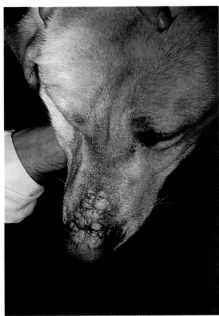

FIGURE 2-31. Nasal Pyoderma. Alopecia, erythema, and papular swelling on the bridge of a dog's nose. (Courtesy of D. Angarano)

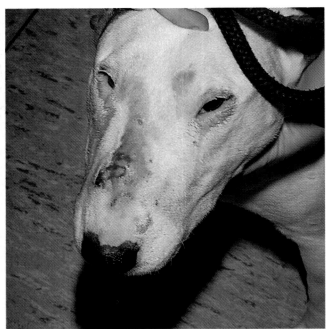

FIGURE 2-32. Nasal Pyoderma. Diffuse erythematous papular rash on the face of a terrier. (Courtesy of D. Angarano)

Bacterial Pododermatitis
(interdigital pyoderma, pedal folliculitis and furunculosis) (Figs. 2-33 to 2-40)

FEATURES

A deep bacterial infection of the feet that is almost always secondary to some underlying factor (Table 2-4). Common in dogs and rare in cats.

One or more feet may be affected with interdigital erythema, pustules, papules, nodules, hemorrhagic bullae, fistulae, ulcers, alopecia, and/or swelling. Pruritus (licking, chewing), pain, and/or lameness may be present. Regional lymphadenomegaly is common. Occasionally pitting edema of the associated metatarsus or metacarpus is seen.

TOP DIFFERENTIALS

Demodicosis, dermatophytosis, actinomycosis, nocardiosis, mycolsactenosis, deep fungal infection, autoimmune skin disorders, neoplasia.

DIAGNOSIS

1. Rule out other differentials.
2. Cytology (exudate)—Suppurative to pyogranulomatous inflammation with bacterial cocci and/or rods is seen.
3. Dermatohistopathology—Suppurative to pyogranulomatous perifolliculitis, folliculitis, furunculosis, and nodular to diffuse pyogranulomatous dermatitis. Intralesional bacteria may be difficult to find.
4. Bacterial culture—The primary pathogen is usually *Staphylococcus.* Mixed gram-positive and gram-negative infections are also common.

TREATMENT AND PROGNOSIS

1. Identify and correct any underlying cause.
2. Give long-term (minimum 8-12 weeks) systemic antibiotics continued 2 weeks beyond complete clinical resolution (Table 2-1). The antibiotic should be selected based on bacterial culture and sensitivity results.
3. Adjunctive topical therapies that may be helpful include daily foot soaks for 10-15 minutes in 0.025% chlorhexidine solution, 0.4% povidone-iodine solution, or magnesium sulfate (30 mg/L water) for 5-7 days. Alternatively, foot scrubs using antibacterial shampoo or surgical scrub every 1-7 days as needed may be used.

4. Minimize foot trauma by having dog confined indoors, leash walked, and kept away from rough surfaces.
5. Fusion podoplasty, whereby all diseased tissue is removed and digits are fused together, is a radical alternative for severe cases.
6. Prognosis is good to guarded, depending on whether the underlying cause can be identified and corrected. In severe and chronic cases, permanent fibrosis and scarring may contribute to future relapses by predisposing feet to traumatic injuries.

TABLE 2–4 Causes of Secondary Bacterial Pododermatitis

Foreign body (plant awn, wood splinter, thorn)
Trauma (stones, stubble, briars, wire floors, burns)
Contact dermatitis (chemicals, fertilizers, weed killers)
Parasite (demodicosis, ticks, pelodera, hookworm dermatitis)
Fungus
Hypersensitivity (food, atopy)
Endocrinopathy (hypothyroidism, hyperadrenocorticism)
Autoimmune and immune-mediated skin disorders

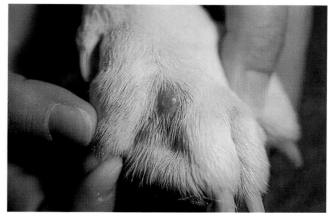

FIGURE 2–34. Bacterial Pododermatitis. Close-up of the dog in Figure 2–33. This bulla was visible only when the interdigital space was closely examined.

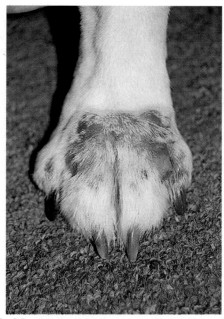

FIGURE 2–35. Bacterial Pododermatitis. Diffuse alopecia, erythema, and swelling affected most of the cutaneous surface. This more severe case also had multiple erosions and draining lesions around the nail bed and in the interdigital spaces (see Figure 2–36).

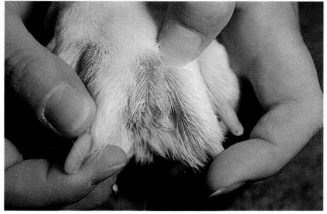

FIGURE 2–33. Bacterial Pododermatitis. Interdigital swelling and erythema are common features of bacterial pododermatitis. This infection was secondary to allergic dermatitis.

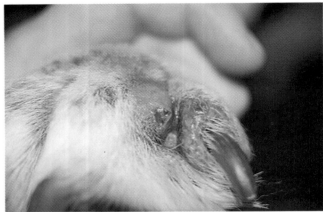

FIGURE 2–36. Bacterial Pododermatitis. Close-up of the dog in Figure 2–35. Multiple erosions and draining lesions around the nail bed and in the interdigital spaces.

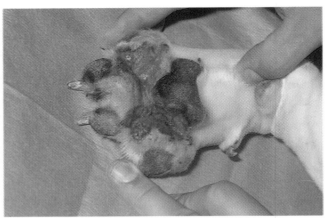

FIGURE 2–39. Bacterial Pododermatitis. Severe erosive, ulcerative lesions in the interdigital spaces caused by chronic bacterial infection. (Courtesy of D. Angarano and A. Yu)

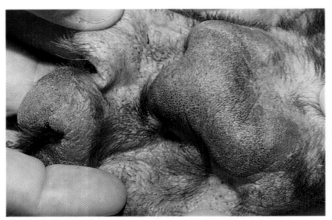

FIGURE 2–37. Bacterial Pododermatitis. Chronic pododermatitis and pruritus caused the diffuse alopecia and erythema between the pads. This infection was secondary to hypothyroidism.

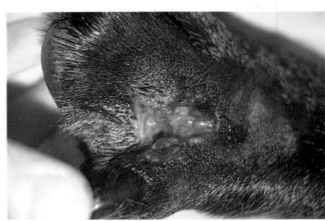

FIGURE 2–40. Bacterial Pododermatitis. This chronic interdigital fistula (draining tract) was caused by a penetrating plant foreign body.

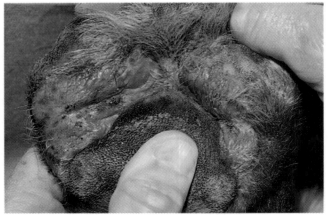

FIGURE 2–38. Bacterial Pododermatitis. Severe swelling with alopecia, erythema, and erosions. The infection was associated with allergic dermatitis.

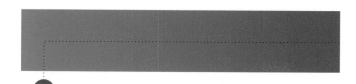

Deep Pyoderma (Figs. 2–41 to 2–46)

FEATURES

A surface or follicular bacterial infection that breaks through hair follicles to produce furunculosis and cellulitis. Its development is often preceded by a history of chronic superficial skin disease and is almost always associated with some predisposing factor (Table 2–3). Common in dogs and rare in cats.

Focal, multifocal, or generalized skin lesions characterized by papules, pustules, cellulitis, tissue discoloration, alopecia, hemorrhagic bullae, erosions, ulcers, crusts, and serosanguineous to purulent draining fistulous tracts. Lesions are often pruritic or painful. They most often involve the trunk and pressure points but can be anywhere on body. Lymphadenomegaly is common. If the animal is septic, symptoms also include fever, anorexia, and depression.

TOP DIFFERENTIALS

Demodicosis, fungal infections, actinomycosis, nocardiosis, mycobacteriosis, neoplasia, autoimmune skin disorders.

DIAGNOSIS

1. Rule out other differentials.
2. Cytology (exudate)—Suppurative to pyogranulomatous inflammation with bacterial cocci and/or rods is seen.
3. Dermatohistopathology—Deep suppurative to pyogranulomatous folliculitis, furunculosis, cellulitis, and panniculitis. Intralesional bacteria may be difficult to find.
4. Bacterial culture—The primary pathogen is usually *Staphylococcus*, but occasionally *Pseudomonas* is isolated. Mixed gram-positive and gram-negative bacterial infections are also common.

TREATMENT AND PROGNOSIS

1. Identify and correct any underlying cause.
2. Clip hairs around lesions. Loosen crusts and remove exudate with daily warm water tub soaks or whirlpool baths containing antiseptic solution (chlorhexidine, povidone-iodine, aluminum acetate). If tub soaks are not possible, shampoo therapy may be effective.
3. Give long-term (minimum 6–8 weeks) systemic antibiotics continued 2 weeks beyond complete clinical resolution (Table 2–1). Antibiotic should be selected based on culture and sensitivity results.
4. Prognosis is good, but in severe or chronic cases, fibrosis, scarring, and alopecia may be permanent sequelae.

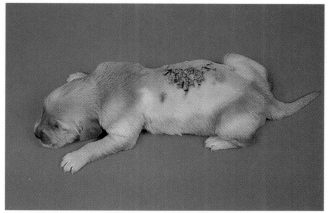

FIGURE 2–41. Deep Pyoderma. Large, well-demarcated area of cellulitis and crusting on the dorsum of a puppy. (Courtesy of D. Angarano)

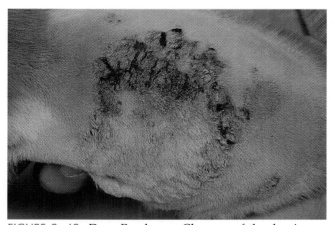

FIGURE 2–42. Deep Pyoderma. Close-up of the dog in Figure 2–41. Draining lesions with superficial crusts. (Courtesy of D. Angarano)

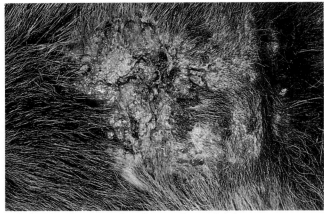

FIGURE 2–43. Deep Pyoderma. Superficial crusts cover the deep exudative lesions. The deep pyoderma was associated with calcinosis cutis caused by iatrogenic Cushing's syndrome.

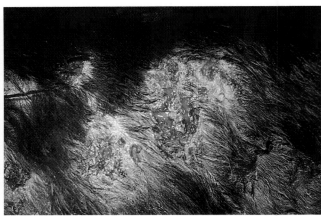

FIGURE 2–45. Deep Pyoderma. These draining lesions with crust formation were associated with a deep bacterial infection subsequent to a severe flea infestation.

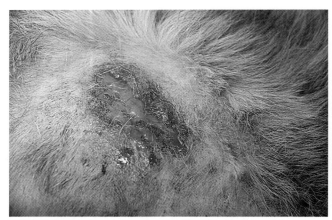

FIGURE 2–44. Deep Pyoderma. Focal cellulitis with superficial erosions.

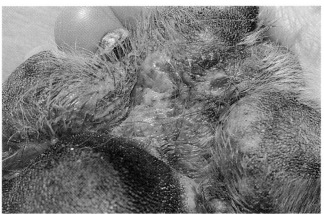

FIGURE 2–46. Deep Pyoderma. Severe tissue swelling, bruising, and draining lesions caused by a chronic bacterial cellulitis of the interdigital space associated with chronic allergy.

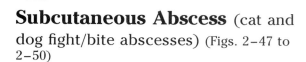

Subcutaneous Abscess (cat and dog fight/bite abscesses) (Figs. 2–47 to 2–50)

FEATURES

Disease occurs when normal oral bacterial microflora are inoculated into skin through puncture wounds. There is usually a history of a recent cat or dog fight. Common in dogs and cats, especially in intact male cats.

Localized, often painful swelling or abscess with crusted-over puncture wound from which a purulent material may drain. Lesions are most commonly found on the tail base, shoulder, neck, face, or leg. Animals may be febrile, anorexic, and depressed and have regional lymphadenomegaly.

TOP DIFFERENTIALS

Abscess caused by foreign body, other bacteria (e.g., actinomycosis, nocardiosis, mycobacteriosis).

DIAGNOSIS

1. Usually based on history and clinical findings.
2. Cytology (exudate)—Suppurative inflammation with a mixed bacterial population.

TREATMENT AND PROGNOSIS

1. Clip, lance, and clean abscess with 0.025% chlorhexidine solution.
2. Give systemic antibiotics for 7–10 days or until lesions completely heal. Effective antibiotics include:

   Amoxicillin, 20 mg/kg PO, SQ, or IM q 8–12 hours.

   Clavulanated amoxicillin, 20 mg/kg PO q 8–12 hours.

   Clindamycin, 10 mg/kg PO or IM q 12 hours.

3. Prognosis is good. Castrating intact male cats is a helpful preventive measure.

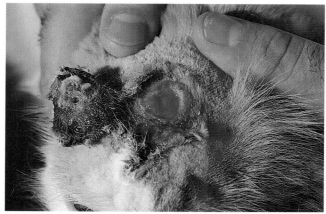

FIGURE 2–47. Subcutaneous Abscess. Chronic abscess on the head of a cat. (Courtesy of D. Angarano)

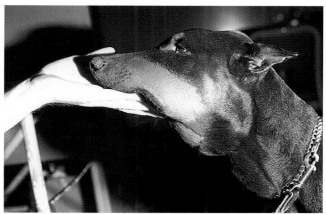

FIGURE 2–48. Subcutaneous Abscess. The submandibular swelling in this Doberman was caused by an extensive subcutaneous abscess. (Courtesy of D. Angarano)

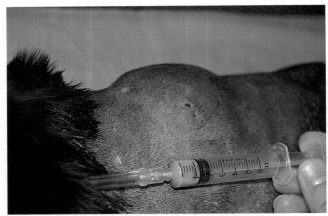

FIGURE 2–49. Subcutaneous Abscess. Feline abscess caused by a cat bite. The syringe contains purulent material aspirated from the abscess.

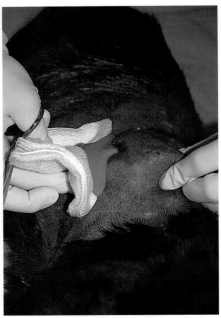

FIGURE 2–50. Subcutaneous Abscess. Purulent material was easily expressed from this abscess.

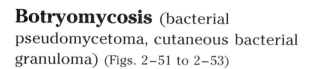

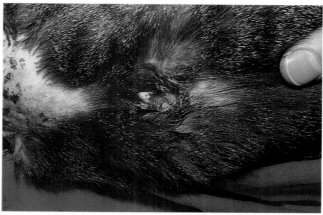

Botryomycosis (bacterial pseudomycetoma, cutaneous bacterial granuloma) (Figs. 2–51 to 2–53)

FEATURES

An unusual type of skin infection in which bacterial organisms form macroscopic or microscopic tissue granules. Infections may be a sequela to a penetrating injury, foreign body reaction, or bite wound. Uncommon in dogs and cats.

Single to multiple nonpainful and usually nonpruritic, firm nodule(s) with draining fistulae. Purulent discharge may contain small, white granules (macroscopic colonies of bacteria). Lesions develop slowly and can be anywhere on the body.

TOP DIFFERENTIALS

Actinomycosis, nocardiosis, mycobacteriosis, deep fungal infections, neoplasia, and foreign body reaction.

DIAGNOSIS

1. Cytology (exudate)—Suppurative inflammation that may contain granules composed of dense bacterial colonies.
2. Dermatohistopathology—Nodular to diffuse (pyo)granulomatous dermatitis and panniculitis with tissue granules composed of bacteria.
3. Bacterial culture—The causative organism is usually *Staphylococcus*, but occasionally other bacteria such as *Pseudomonas* or *Proteus* are isolated.

TREATMENT AND PROGNOSIS

1. Surgically excise nodules(s) and give long-term (mimimum 4 weeks) systemic antibiotics based on culture and sensitivity results. Without surgery, antibiotic therapy alone is rarely effective.
2. Prognosis is good with combined surgical and medical therapy.

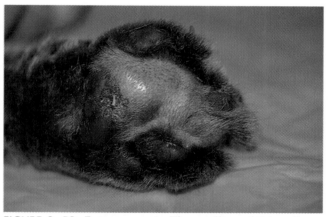

FIGURE 2–51. Botryomycosis. A deep draining lesion with superficial crust formation on the dorsum of a cat.

FIGURE 2–52. Botryomycosis. The swelling of this cat's foot was associated with moderate pain and lameness. The crust was covering a deep tract that periodically drained a purulent exudate.

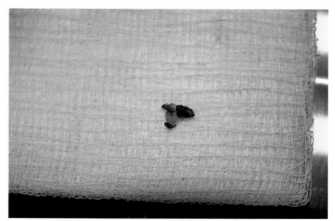

FIGURE 2–53. Botryomycosis. A tissue grain dissected from the foot of the cat shown in Figure 2–52.

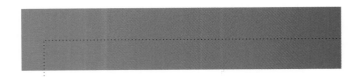

L-Form Infection (Fig. 2–54)

FEATURES

A skin infection caused by cell wall-deficient bacteria that contaminate bite wounds or surgical incisions. Uncommon in cats and rare in dogs.

A persistently spreading and draining cellulitis and synovitis that usually begins on the extremities. Concurrent fever is present. Polyarthritis may also be seen.

TOP DIFFERENTIALS

Other bacterial and deep fungal infections, neoplasia.

DIAGNOSIS

1. Rule out other differentials.
2. Cytology (exudate)—Pyogranulomatous inflammation is seen. L-Forms cannot be visualized, but contaminating bacterial cocci and rods may be present.
3. Dermatohistopathology (nondiagnostic)—Pyogranulomatous dermatitis.
4. Bacterial culture—L-Forms cannot be cultured unless special L-form medium is used. Contaminating bacteria are often isolated.
5. Electron microscopy (biopsy specimens)—Pleomorphic cell wall-deficient organisms are found in phagocytes.

TREATMENT AND PROGNOSIS

1. Antibiotics typically used to treat other bacterial infections are not effective.
2. Give tetracycline, 22 mg/kg PO q 8 hours, or doxycycline, 5–10 mg/kg PO q 12 hours. Continue treatment at least 1 week beyond complete clinical resolution. Improvement should be seen within 2 days.
3. Prognosis is usually good. In severe cases, chronic arthritis may be a permanent sequela.

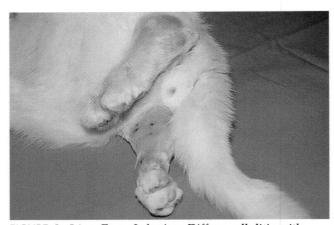

FIGURE 2–54. L-Form Infection. Diffuse cellulitis with multiple draining tracts. Confirming this diagnosis may be difficult and may require special laboratory techniques. (Courtesy of the University of Florida; case material)

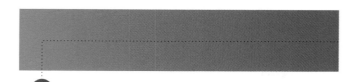

Actinomycosis (Figs. 2–55 and 2–56)

FEATURES

A disease that occurs when *Actinomyces,* a nonpathogenic bacterium found in the oral cavity, is inadvertently inoculated into tissue. There is usually a previous history of bite wound or penetrating injury at site of infection. An uncommon cause of skin disease in cats and dogs, with the highest incidence in outdoor and hunting dogs.

Dogs. Subcutaneous, firm to fluctuant swellings and abscesses that may fistulate or ulcerate. Drainage is serosanguineous to purulent, often malodorous, and may contain yellow-tan granules (macroscopic colonies of *Actinomycetes*). The ventral and lateral cervical, mandibular, and submandibular areas are most often affected. Chronic progressive weight loss and fever suggest concurrent thoracic or abdominal cavity involvement.

Cats. Pyothorax and subcutaneous abscesses containing a malodorous, serosanguineous to purulent exudate are the most common presentations.

TOP DIFFERENTIALS

Other bacterial and deep fungal infections, neoplasia.

DIAGNOSIS

1. Rule out other differentials.
2. Cytology (exudate)—Suppurative to pyogranulomatous inflammation with a mixed population of bacteria that includes *Actinomyces. Actinomyces* appear individually or in aggregates as gram-positive, non-acid-fast, beaded, filamentous organisms with occasional branching.
3. Dermatohistopathology—Nodular to diffuse suppurative or pyogranulomatous dermatitis and panniculitis that may contain tissue grains composed of gram-positive, non-acid-fast, filamentous organisms.
4. Anaerobic bacterial culture (deep percutaneous aspirate or biopsy specimen directly inoculated into anaerobic transport medium; avoid refrigeration). Often a mixed bacterial population is isolated that may not include *Actinomyces* because *Actinomyces* have fastidious growth requirements and are difficult to culture.

TREATMENT AND PROGNOSIS

1. Perform wide surgical excision and tissue debulking to remove as much diseased tissue as possible.
2. Give long-term (several months) systemic antibiotics continued several weeks beyond complete clinical resolution.
3. The antibiotic of choice is penicillin G potassium (PO, SQ, IM, IV) or penicillin V potassium (PO), at least 60,000 U/kg q 8 hours.
4. Alternative drugs that may be effective include:

   Erythromycin, 10 mg/kg PO q 8 hours.

   Clindamycin, 5 mg/kg SQ q 12 hours.

   Minocycline, 5–25 mg/kg IV or PO q 12 hours.

   Amoxicillin, 20–40 mg/kg IM, SQ, or PO q 6 hours.

5. Prognosis for cure is guarded. This disease is not considered contagious to other animals or to humans.

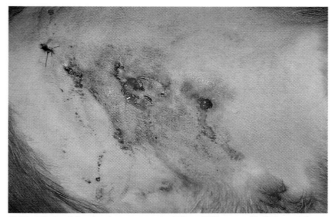

FIGURE 2–55. Actinomycosis. The diffuse cellulitis with multiple draining tracts on the lumbar region of this dog had persisted for several months.

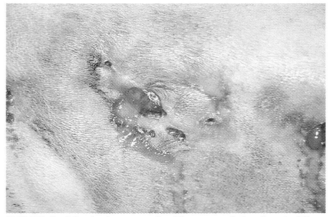

FIGURE 2–56. Actinomycosis. Close-up of the dog in Figure 2–55. Deep draining tracts with tissue discoloration typical of a deep cellulitis.

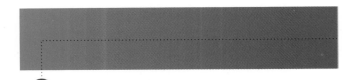

Nocardiosis (Figs. 2–57 and 2–58)

FEATURES

A cutaneous disease that occurs if *Nocardia*, a soil saprophyte, is inadvertently inoculated into a skin puncture wound. Uncommon in dogs and cats.

Localized nodules, cellulitis, and abscesses, with ulcerations and fistulous tracts that drain a serosanguineous discharge. Lesions usually occur on the limbs, feet, or abdomen. Peripheral lymphadenomegaly is common.

TOP DIFFERENTIALS

Other bacterial and deep fungal infections, neoplasia.

DIAGNOSIS

1. Rule out other differentials.
2. Cytology (exudate)—Suppurative to pyogranulomatous inflammation with individual or loose aggregates of gram-positive, partially acid-fast, beaded, branching filamentous organisms.
3. Dermatohistopathology—Nodular to diffuse pyogranulomatous dermatitis and panniculitis with intralesional gram-positive, partially acid-fast, branching, beaded organisms that may form tissue grains.
4. Bacterial culture—*Nocardia*.

TREATMENT AND PROGNOSIS

1. Surgically drain, debulk, and excise as much diseased tissue as possible.
2. Give long-term (weeks to months) systemic antibiotics continued at least 4 weeks beyond complete clinical resolution. Antibiotic selection should be based on culture and sensitivity results if possible.
3. Antibiotics that may be effective empirically include:

   Sulfadiazine, 80 mg/kg PO q 8 hours or 110 mg/kg PO q 12 hours.
   Sulfamethizole, 50 mg/kg PO q 8 hours.
   Sulfisoxazole, 50 mg/kg PO q 8 hours.
   Trimethoprim-sulfadiazine, 15–30 mg/kg PO or SQ q 12 hours.

   Ampicillin, 20–40 mg/kg IV, IM, SQ, or PO q 6 hours.
   Erythromycin, 10 mg/kg PO q 8 hours.
   Minocycline, 5–25 mg/kg PO or IV q 12 hours.

4. Prognosis for cure is guarded. This disease is not contagious to other animals or to humans.

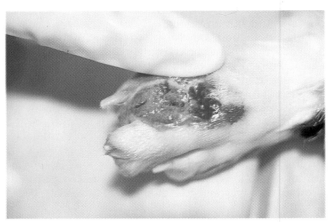

FIGURE 2–57. Nocardiosis. The deep ulcerative lesion on the dorsal surface of this dog's foot developed over several months. Deep tracts with tissue proliferation can be seen with any aggressive bacterial or fungal infection.

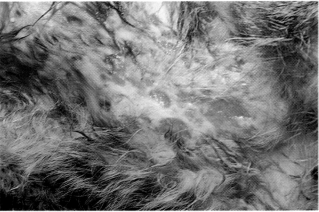

FIGURE 2–58. Nocardiosis. The diffuse area of cellulitis with multiple draining lesions was located on the lateral trunk of this cat.

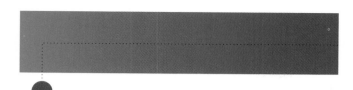

Opportunistic Mycobacteriosis (atypical mycobacterial granuloma) (Figs. 2–59 to 2–62)

FEATURES

An infection that occurs if saprophytic mycobacteria, normally found in soil and water, are inoculated into the skin through puncture wounds. Uncommon in cats and rare in dogs.

Slowly developing, chronic subcutaneous nodules, nonhealing abscesses, and cellulitis with punctate ulcers and fistulae that drain a serosanguineous or purulent discharge. Lesions may be anywhere on the body, but in cats the inguinal, caudal abdominal, or lumbar area is most often involved. Regional lymphadenomegaly may be present.

TOP DIFFERENTIALS

Other bacterial or deep fungal infection, neoplasia.

DIAGNOSIS

1. Rule out other differentials.
2. Cytology (exudate)—Neutrophils and macrophages with intracellular, rod-shaped structures that do not stain with routine stains but stain acid-fast positive. These organisms are often difficult to find.
3. Dermatohistopathology—Nodular to diffuse pyogranulomatous dermatitis and panniculitis. Intralesional acid-fast bacilli may be difficult to find.
4. Mycobacterial culture—Causative organisms include *Mycobacterium fortuitum*, *M. chelonei*, *M. smegmatis*, *M. phlei*, *M. xenopi*, and *M. thermoresistible*.

TREATMENT AND PROGNOSIS

1. Perform wide surgical excision of the lesion if possible.
2. Give long-term (weeks to months) systemic antimicrobial therapy continued at least 4 weeks beyond complete clinical resolution. Antimicrobial selection should be based on culture and sensitivity results, if available.

3. Drugs that may be effective empirically include:

Clarithromycin, 5–10 mg/kg PO q 12 hours.

Enrofloxacin, 5–15 mg/kg PO q 12 hours. (Please note: High doses of enrofloxacin have been reported to cause blindness in cats.)

Doxycycline or minocycline, 5–12.5 mg/kg PO or IV q 12 hours.

Clofazimine, 8 mg/kg PO q 24 hours.

4. Prognosis for cure is guarded, although rare cases of spontaneous resolution have been reported. This disease is not considered contagious to other animals or to humans.

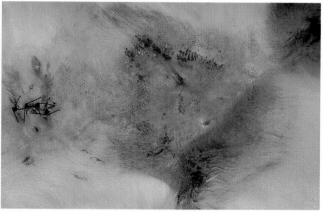

FIGURE 2–59. Opportunistic Mycobacteriosis. The diffuse cellulitis with multiple draining lesions on this cat's ventrum was caused by *Mycobacterium fortuitum*. (Courtesy of the University of Florida; case material)

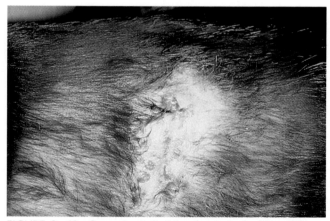

FIGURE 2–60. Opportunistic Mycobacteriosis. The diffuse cellulitis with multiple draining lesions on this cat's trunk was caused by *M. fortuitum*. (Courtesy of the University of Florida; case material)

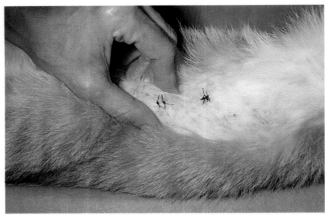

FIGURE 2–61. Opportunistic Mycobacteriosis. Multiple nodules on a cat. A small subcutaneous mass is being palpated. (Courtesy of D. Angarano)

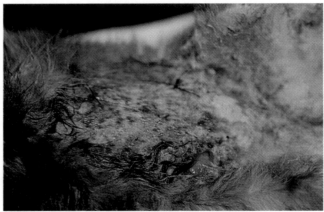

FIGURE 2–62. Opportunistic Mycobacteriosis. Extensive alopecia, erythema, and erosions on the ventral abdomen of a cat. (Courtesy of L. Frank)

Feline Leprosy (Figs. 2–63 and 2–64)

FEATURES

This disease is thought to be caused by *Mycobacterium lepraemurium*, the agent of rat leprosy. Presumably the organism is transmitted to cats through bites or contact with infected rats. Uncommon in cats, with reports limited to seaside cities in the western United States, the Netherlands, Australia, New Zealand, and Great Britain.

Chronic, single to multiple, nonpainful, nonhealing cutaneous and subcutaneous nodule(s) that usually ulcerate. Lesions are most common on the face, trunk, and forelimbs. Regional lymphadenomegaly may be present. There are no systemic signs of illness.

TOP DIFFERENTIALS

Other bacterial and deep fungal infections, neoplasia.

DIAGNOSIS

1. Rule out other differentials.
2. Cytology (aspirate, tissue imprint)—Neutrophils and macrophages, some with intracellular, rod-shaped structures that do not stain with routine stains, but stain acid-fast positive.
3. Dermatohistopathology—Diffuse granulomatous dermatitis and panniculitis with intracellular and extracellular acid-fast bacilli.
4. Mycobacterial culture—Usually negative because *M. lepraemurium* is extremely difficult to culture.

TREATMENT AND PROGNOSIS

1. Complete surgical excision of all nodules is the treatment of choice.
2. If complete excision is not possible, long-term (months) medical therapy is sometimes effective. Continue therapy for 6–12 weeks beyond complete clinical resolution. Either clofazimine, 8 mg/kg PO q 24 hours, or dapsone, 1 mg/kg PO q 12 hours, may be effective. Dapsone is potentially toxic to cats.
3. Prognosis is best if lesions can be excised. Feline leprosy is not considered a public health risk.

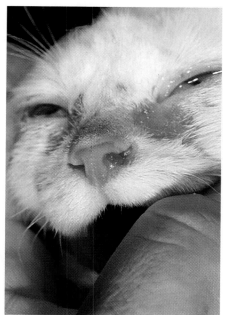

FIGURE 2–63. Feline Leprosy. Erosive lesions on the face of a cat infected with *Mycobacterium lepraemurium*. (Courtesy of A. Yu)

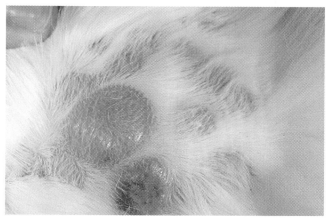

FIGURE 2–64. Feline Leprosy. Multiple alopecic, erythematous lesions on the body of a cat infected with *M. lepraemurium*. (Courtesy of A. Yu)

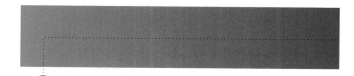

Tuberculosis

FEATURES

Tuberculous mycobacteria are transmitted to pets through close contact with infected owners or through consumption of contaminated milk or meat. Rare in dogs and cats, with highest incidence in areas of endemic tuberculosis.

Single or multiple dermal nodules, plaques, abscesses, and nonhealing ulcers that drain a thick, purulent exudate. Lesions are found on the head, neck, and limbs. Concurrent symptoms of systemic involvement (fever, anorexia, depression, weight loss, lymphademomegaly, cough, dyspnea, vomiting, and/or diarrhea) are usually present.

TOP DIFFERENTIALS

Other bacterial and deep fungal infections, neoplasia.

DIAGNOSIS

1. Rule out other differentials.
2. Cytology (exudate)—Neutrophils and macrophages, some containing rod-shaped structures that do not stain with routine stains but stain acid-fast positive.
3. Dermatohistopathology—Nodular to diffuse pyogranulomatous dermatitis with few to many intracellular acid-fast bacilli.
4. Mycobacterial culture—Causative organisms include *Mycobacterium tuberculosis*, *M. bovis*, *M. tuberculosis-M. bovis* variant, and *M. avium* complex.

TREATMENT AND PROGNOSIS

1. Notify public health officials. Affected animals should be euthanized because tuberculosis is contagious to humans.
2. If owner refuses euthanasia, long-term (6–12 months) chemotherapy may be effective in some animals.
3. For *M. tuberculosis*, therapies that may be effective include:

   Dogs and cats: combination isoniazid, 10–20 mg/kg PO q 24 hours, plus ethambutol, 15 mg/kg PO q 24 hours.
   Dogs: combination pyrazinamide, 15–40 mg/kg PO q 24 hours, plus rifampin, 10–20 mg/kg PO q 12–24 hours.

4. For *M. bovis* (cats), surgically excise localized lesions and give rifampin, 4 mg/kg PO q 24 hours.

5. For *M. tuberculosis-M. bovis* variant (cats), give combination rifampin, 10–20 mg/kg PO q 24 hours, plus enrofloxacin, 5–10 mg/kg PO q 12–24 hours, plus clarithromycin, 5–10 mg/kg PO q 12 hours.
6. For *M. avium complex* (dogs and cats), give combination doxycycline, 10 mg/kg PO q 12 hours, or clofazimine, 4 mg/kg PO q 24 hours, plus enrofloxacin, 5–10 mg/kg PO q 12–24 hours, plus clarithromycin, 5 mg/kg PO q 12 hours.
7. Prognosis is guarded. Tuberculosis is contagious to other animals and to humans.

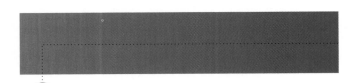

Plague

FEATURES

A zoonotic bacterial disease caused by *Yersinia pestis*. Dogs appear to be resistant, but cats are susceptible. Plague develops when cats eat infected rodents (natural reservoir) or are bitten by infected rodent fleas (vectors). Uncommon in cats, with highest incidence in endemic areas of the southwestern and western United States.

Acute and often fatal disease characterized by fever, dehydration, lymphadenomegaly, and lymph node abscessation (bubo). The bubo may fistulate and drain a thick, purulent exudate. The submandibular, retropharyngeal, and cervical lymph nodes are most often affected.

TOP DIFFERENTIALS

Subcutaneous abscesses caused by other bacteria.

DIAGNOSIS

1. Cytology (exudate, lymph node aspirate)—Suppurative inflammation with small gram-negative, bipolar coccobacilli.
2. Serology—Fourfold increase in the antibody titer against *Y. pestis* in serial serum samples taken 10–14 days apart.
3. Direct fluorescent antibody or polymerase chain reaction test (exudate, lymph node aspirate)—Detection of *Y. pestis* antigen.
4. Bacterial culture—*Y. pestis* is isolated.

TREATMENT AND PROGNOSIS

1. Maintain strict sanitation because infected pus, saliva, tissue, and airborne respiratory droplets are highly contagious to humans and other animals. If possible, cage suspected animals in an isolation room. When handling suspected animals and specimens, wear gloves, gown, and surgical mask. Use routine disinfectants to clean tables and cages, and double plastic bag and incinerate all contaminated materials (e.g., gauze pads).
2. Initiate antibiotic therapy immediately in all suspected cases. To minimize likelihood of contracting infection, parenteral, not oral, administration is recommended. Treatment (minimum 3 weeks) should be continued well beyond complete clinical recovery.
3. The antibiotic of choice is gentamycin, 2–4 mg/kg IV or IM or SQ q 12–24 hours.
4. Alternative antibiotics that may be effective include:

   Chloramphenicol, 15 mg/kg SQ q 12 hours.
   Trimethoprim-sulfadiazine, 15 mg/kg IM or IV q 12 hours.

5. Treat animal with topical flea spray to kill and prevent fleas (vectors).
6. Lance and flush abscesses with 0.025% chlorhexidine solution.
7. Prophylactically treat asymptomatic, exposed animals with tetracycline, 20 mg/kg PO q 8 hours for 7 days.
8. Prognosis is poor unless antibiotic therapy is initiated early in the course of the disease. Plague is contagious to other animals and to humans.

Suggested Readings

Bacterial Diseases, Section II, pp. 179–343. In Green CE (ed). 1998. Infectious Diseases of the Dog and Cat. Ed. 2. W.B. Saunders, Philadelphia, PA.

Bacterial Skin Diseases, pp. 279–328. In Scott DW, Miller WH Jr, and Griffin CE. 1995. Muller & Kirk's Small Animal Dermatology. Ed. 5. W.B. Saunders, Philadelphia, PA.

Carlotti D, Guaguere E, Pin D, Jasmin P, Thomas E, and Guiral V. 1999. Therapy for difficult cases of canine pyoderma with marbofloxacin: a report of 39 dogs. J Small Anim Pract. 40(6): 265–270.

DeBoer DJ. 1995. Management of Chronic and Recurrent Pyoderma in the Dog, pp. 611–617. In Bonagura JD (ed). Kirk's Current Veterinary Therapy, XII, Small Animal Practice. W.B. Saunders, Philadelphia, PA.

Fritz C. 1999. Feline Plague in California. Calif Vet. 53(3): 16–19.

Gerds-Grogan S and Dayrell-Hart B. 1997. Feline Cryptococcosis: A Retrospective Evaluation. JAAHA. 33: 118–122.

Ihrke PJ and Gross TL. 1995. Canine Mucocutaneous Pyoderma. pp 618–622. In Bonagura JD (ed). Kirk's Current Veterinary Therapy, XII, Small Animal Practice. W.B. Saunders, Philadelphia, PA.

Malik R, Love DN, Wigney DI, and Martin P. 1998. Mycobacterial Nodular Granulomas Affecting the Subcutis and Skin of Dogs (Canine Leprosy-Like Syndrome). Aust. Vet. J. 76(6):403–407, 398.

Mundall AC. 1995. Mycobacterial Skin Diseases in Small Animals, pp. 622–624. In Bonagura JD (ed). Kirk's Current Veterinary Therapy, XII, Small Animal Practice. W.B. Saunders, Philadelphia, PA.

Plumb DC. 1999. Veterinary Drug Handbook. Ed. 3. Iowa State University Press, Ames, IA.

3

Fungal Skin Diseases

- **Dermatophytosis** (ringworm)

- **Malasseziasis** (*Malassezia* dermatitis)

- **Candidiasis** (candidosis, thrush)

- **Dermatophytic Granuloma and Pseudomycetoma** (Majocchi's granuloma)

- **Eumycotic Mycetoma** (maduromycosis)

- **Phaeohyphomycosis** (chromomycosis)

- **Protothecosis**

- **Pythiosis**

- **Zygomycosis** (mucormycosis, entomophthoromycosis)

- **Sporotrichosis**

- **Blastomycosis**

- **Coccidioidomycosis**

- **Cryptococcosis**

- **Histoplasmosis**

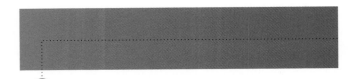

Dermatophytosis (ringworm) (Figs. 3-1 to 3-20)

FEATURES

An infection of hair shafts and stratum corneum caused by keratinophilic fungi. Common in dogs and cats, with the highest incidence in kittens, puppies, immunocompromised animals, and long-haired cats. It is endemic in many Persian catteries.

Skin involvement may be localized, multifocal, or generalized. Pruritus, if present, is usually minimal to mild but occasionally may be intense. Lesions usually include areas of circular, irregular, or diffuse alopecia with variable scaling. Remaining hairs may appear stubbled or broken off. Other symptoms in dogs and cats include erythema, papules, crusts, seborrhea, and paronychia or onychodystrophy of one or more digits. Rarely, cats present with miliary dermatitis or dermal nodules (see Dermatophytic Granuloma and Pseudomycetoma). Other cutaneous manifestations in dogs include facial folliculitis and furunculosis resembling nasal pyoderma, kerions (acutely developing alopecic and exudative nodules) on the limb or face, and truncal dermal nodules (see Dermatophytic Granuloma and Pseudomycetoma). Asymptomatic carrier states (subclinical infection) are common in cats, especially long-haired cats. Asymptomatic disease, although rare in dogs, has been reported in Yorkshire terriers.

TOP DIFFERENTIALS

Dogs. Demodicosis, superficial pyoderma. If nodular, include neoplasia and acral lick dermatitis.

Cats. Parasitic, allergic, and feline psychogenic alopecia.

DIAGNOSIS

1. Rule out other differentials.
2. Ultraviolet (Wood's lamp) exam—Hairs fluoresce yellow-green with some *Microsporum canis* strains. This is an easy screening test, but false-negative and false-positive results are common.
3. Microscopy (hairs or scales in potassium hydroxide preparation)—Look for hair shafts infiltrated with hyphae and arthrospores. Fungal elements are often difficult to find.
4. Dermatohistopathology—Variable findings may include perifolliculitis, folliculitis, furunculosis, superficial perivascular or interstitial dermatitis, epidermal and follicular ortho- or parakeratosis,

and/or suppurative epidermitis. Fungal hyphae and arthrospores in stratum corneum or hair shafts may be difficult to find without special fungal stains.
5. Fungal culture—*Microsporum* or *Trichophyton* spp.

TREATMENT AND PROGNOSIS

1. If lesion is focal, clip a wide margin around it and apply topical antifungal medication q 12 hours until lesion resolves. Effective topicals for localized treatment include:

   1% Chlorhexidine ointment.
   1% Clotrimazole cream, lotion, or solution.
   2% Enilconazole cream.
   2% Ketoconazole cream.
   1-2% Miconazole cream, spray, or lotion.
   4% Thiabendazole solution.
   1% Terbinafine cream.

2. If response to localized treatment is poor, treat animal for generalized dermatophytosis.
3. For animals with multifocal or generalized lesions, clip entire haircoat if animal is medium- to long-haired. Apply topical antifungal rinse or dip to the entire body one or two times per week (minimum 4-6 weeks) until follow-up fungal cultures are negative. Dogs with generalized dermatophytosis may be cured with topical therapy alone, whereas cats almost always require concurrent systemic therapy. Effective topical antifungal solutions include:

   Chlorhexidine 0.05% solution.
   Enilconazole 0.2% solution.
   Lime sulfur 2% solution.
   Povidone-iodine 0.4% solution.

4. For cats with generalized dermatophytosis and dogs unresponsive to topical therapy alone, combine topical therapy for generalized infection with long-term (minimum 4-6 weeks) systemic antifungal therapy continued for 3-4 weeks beyond negative follow-up fungal culture results. Effective systemic antifungal drugs include:

   Microsize griseofulvin, at least 50 mg/kg/day PO with fat-containing meal.
   Ultramicrosize griseofulvin, 5-10 mg/kg/day PO with fat-containing meal.
   Ketoconazole, 10 mg/kg PO q 24 hours with food.
   Itraconazole, 10 mg/kg PO q 24 hours with food (capsules), or on an empty stomach (suspension).
   Terbinafine, 10-20 mg/kg PO q 24 hours.

5. Recent reports suggest that treatment with a single dose of lufenuron 60 mg/kg PO with food may be effective in some cases.

6. *M. canis* killed vaccine may be a useful adjunctive therapy in cats but is rarely effective when used alone.

7. Identify and treat all infected animals, including asymptomatic carriers.

8. Prophylactically treat exposed, noninfected cats and dogs with weekly topical antifungal rinse or dip for the duration of the infected animals' treatment.

9. Thoroughly vacuum and disinfect the environment.

10. Prognosis is generally good except for endemically infected multi-cat households and catteries. Animals with underlying immunosuppressive diseases also have a poorer prognosis for cure. Dermatophytosis is contagious to other animals and to humans.

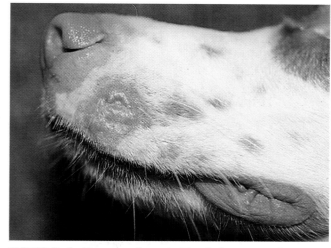

FIGURE 3–3. Dermatophytosis. Focal alopecia and erythema on the muzzle of a Brittany spaniel.

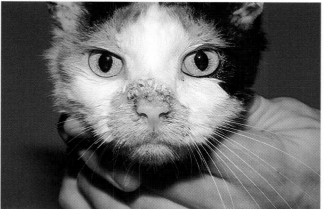

FIGURE 3–1. Dermatophytosis. Focal alopecia and crusting on the muzzle of a cat caused by *M. canis*. (Courtesy of J. MacDonald)

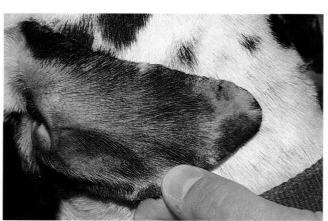

FIGURE 3–4. Dermatophytosis. Alopecia and erythema on the distal ear pinnae caused by *M. canis*. Note the similarity to lesions caused by *Sarcoptes* infections; however, this dalmatian was not pruritic.

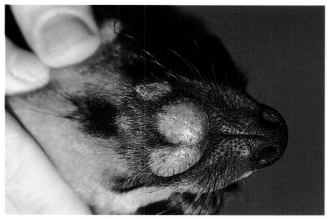

FIGURE 3–2. Dermatophytosis. Multifocal areas of alopecia and erythema. The intense inflammatory reaction caused tissue swelling similar to that of a kerion. (Courtesy of J. MacDonald)

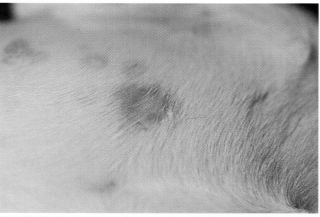

FIGURE 3–5. Dermatophytosis. Focal alopecia and erythema in a classic circular pattern often associated with dermatophytic infections.

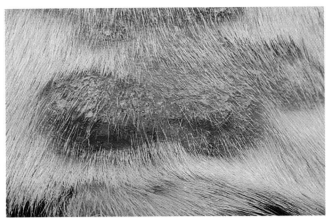

FIGURE 3–6. Dermatophytosis. Alopecia and erythema caused by *M. canis*.

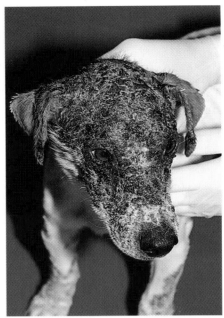

FIGURE 3–9. Dermatophytosis. The severe crusting on the entire head of this Jack Russell terrier was caused by a *Trichophyton* infection. The furunculosis resulted in a severe cellulitis with subsequent scarring. (Courtesy of J. MacDonald)

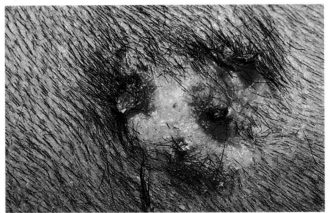

FIGURE 3–7. Dermatophytosis. A focal nodule with alopecia and crusting caused by *T. mentagrophytes*.

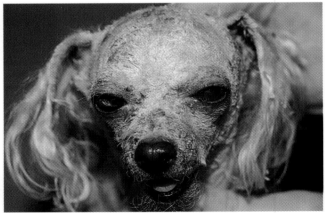

FIGURE 3–10. Dermatophytosis. Generalized alopecia, scale, and crust formation in a toy poodle.

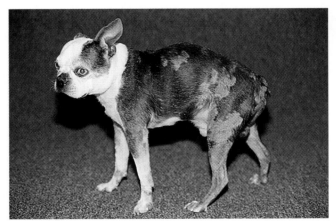

FIGURE 3–8. Dermatophytosis. Generalized alopecia and erythema in a Boston terrier.

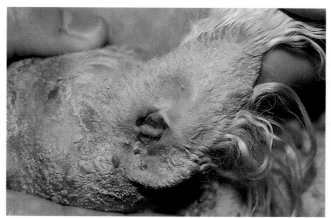

FIGURE 3–11. Dermatophytosis. Same dog as in Figure 3–10. Alopecia, scale, and crusting on the ear pinnae and base.

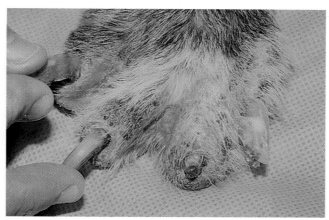

FIGURE 3–13. Dermatophytosis. Pododermatitis and onychomycosis caused by a dermatophyte. The nail is dystrophic and fractured. The cutaneous lesion consists of alopecia, scale, and crusting. (Courtesy of D. Angarano)

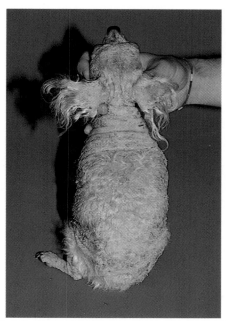

FIGURE 3–12. Dermatophytosis. Same dog as in Figures 3–10 and 3–11. Generalized alopecia and crusting on the entire dorsal cutaneous surface.

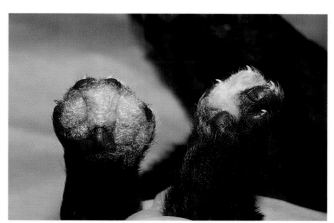

FIGURE 3–14. Dermatophytosis. Pododermatitis in a puppy caused by *T. mentagrophytes*. The feet are swollen, alopecic, and crusting. (Courtesy of J. MacDonald)

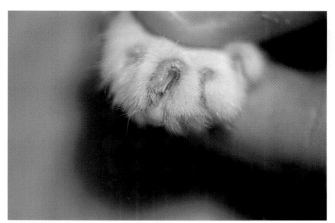

FIGURE 3–15. Dermatophytosis. Paronychia in a cat caused by *M. canis*. The nail bed is erythematous and alopecic.

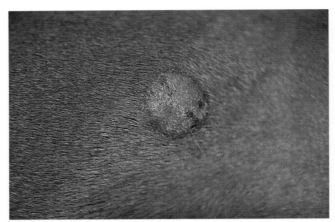

FIGURE 3–16. Dermatophytosis. This alopecic, erythematous nodule (kerion) on the flank of a boxer was caused by *M. canis.*

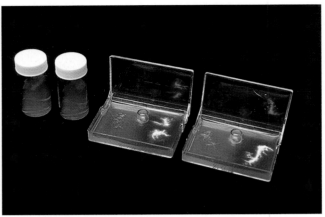

FIGURE 3–19. Dermatophytosis. *M. canis* growing on several commercially available dermatophyte media. The white colony growth and red color change of the culture media are suggestive of a dermatophyte.

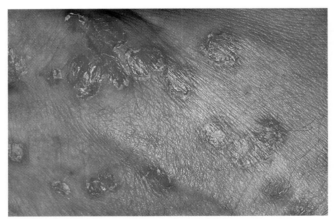

FIGURE 3–17. Dermatophytosis. Multiple erythematous lesions on a human hand infected with *M. canis.*

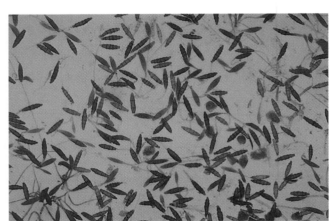

FIGURE 3–20. Dermatophytosis. The microscopic examination of the fungal organisms from culture stained with methylene blue clearly shows the *Microsporum gypseum* macroconidia.

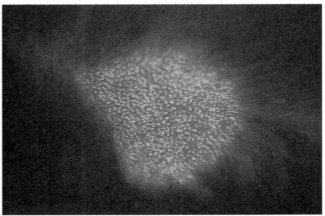

FIGURE 3–18. Dermatophytosis. Positive Woods' lamp examination of a cat with *M. canis.* Note the apple green glow.

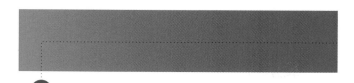

Malasseziasis (*Malassezia dermatitis*) (Figs. 3–21 to 3–28)

FEATURES

Malassezia pachydermatis is a yeast normally found in low numbers in the external ear canals, periorally, perianally, and moist skin folds. Skin disease occurs when there is a hypersensitivity reaction to the organisms or a cutaneous overgrowth. An overgrowth is almost always associated with an underlying cause such as atopy, food allergy, endocrinopathy, keratinization disorder, or prolonged antibiotic therapy. Common in dogs and rare in cats.

Dogs. Moderate to intense pruritus with regional or generalized alopecia, excoriations, erythema, and seborrhea. With chronicity, affected skin may become lichenified, hyperpigmented, and hyperkeratotic. An unpleasant body odor is usually present. Lesions may involve the interdigital spaces, ventral neck, axillae, perineal region, and/or leg folds. Paronychia with a dark brown nail bed discharge may be present. Concurrent yeast otitis externa is common.

Cats. Symptoms include black, waxy otitis externa, chronic chin acne, alopecia, and/or multifocal to generalized erythema and seborrhea.

TOP DIFFERENTIALS

Other causes of pruritus and seborrhea such as demodicosis, superficial pyoderma, dermatophytosis, ectoparasites, and allergies.

DIAGNOSIS

1. Rule out other differentials.
2. Cytology (tape preparation, skin imprint)—Yeast overgrowth is confirmed by finding more than two round to oval budding yeasts per high power field (100×). In yeast hypersensitivity, organisms may be difficult to find.
3. Dermatohistopathology—Superficial perivascular to interstitial lymphohistiocytic dermatitis with yeasts and occasionally pseudohyphae in keratin. Organisms may be few in number and difficult to find.
4. Fungal culture—*M. pachydermatis.*

TREATMENT AND PROGNOSIS

1. Identify and correct any underlying cause.
2. For mild cases, topical therapy alone is often effective. Bathe with shampoo containing 2% keto-conazole (dogs only), 2% miconazole, 2–4% chlorhexidine, or 1% selenium sulfide (dogs only) q 2–3 days. For added effect, baths can be followed with an application of 2% lime sulfur dip, 0.2% enilconazole dip, or a 1:1 dilution of white vinegar in water. Continue treatment until lesions resolve and follow-up skin cytology reveals no organisms (approximately 2–4 weeks).
3. Treatment of choice for moderate to severe cases is ketoconazole, 5–10 mg/kg PO with food q 12–24 hours, or itraconazole, 5–10 mg/kg PO with food q 24 hours. Concurrent shampoo therapy is helpful. Continue treatment until lesions resolve and follow-up skin cytology reveals no organisms (approximately 2–4 weeks).
4. Prognosis is good if the underlying cause can be identified and corrected. Otherwise, regular once or twice weekly antifungal shampoo baths may be needed to prevent relapses. This disease is not considered contagious to other animals or to humans, except to immunocompromised individuals.

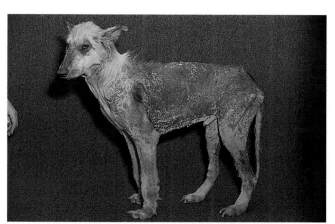

FIGURE 3–21. Malasseziasis. Generalized alopecia and lichenification in an adult collie. The yeast infection was secondary to allergic dermatitis.

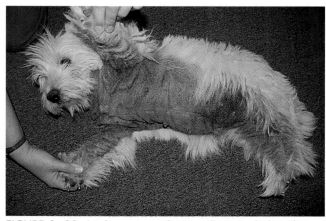

FIGURE 3–22. Malasseziasis. Severe alopecia, lichenification, and hyperpigmentation on the entire ventrum of a West Highland white terrier. The yeast infection was secondary to allergic dermatitis.

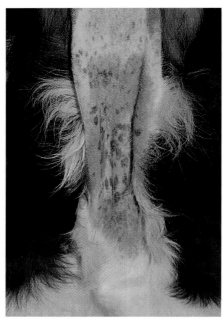

FIGURE 3–23. Malasseziasis. Alopecia, erythema, and lichenification on the ventral neck of an allergic dog.

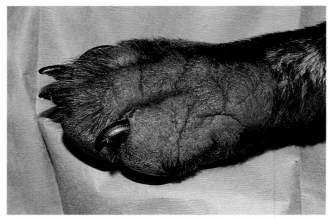

FIGURE 3–25. Malasseziasis. Alopecia, hyperpigmentation, and lichenification on the entire dorsal cutaneous surface of a foot. This secondary yeast dermatitis was associated with hypothyroidism.

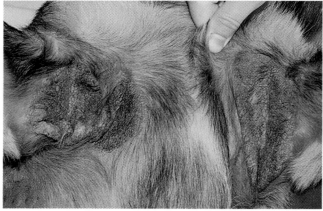

FIGURE 3–24. Malasseziasis. Alopecia, hyperpigmentation, and lichenification on the axillary skin caused by secondary yeast dermatitis. The dog was atopic and food allergic.

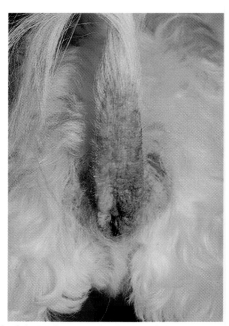

FIGURE 3–26. Malasseziasis. Perianal dermatitis caused by a secondary yeast infection in a food-allergic dog. The alopecia, erythema, and lichenification are characteristic of *Malassezia* dermatitis.

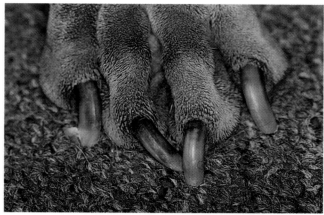

FIGURE 3–27. Malasseziasis. The brown discoloration of the nail is caused by a secondary yeast infection in the nail fold associated with allergic dermatitis.

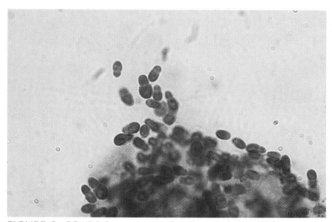

FIGURE 3–28. Malasseziasis. Cytology of the *Malassezia* organisms as viewed with the 100× objective.

Candidiasis (candidosis, thrush)
(Figs. 3–29 and 3–30)

FEATURES

An opportunistic cutaneous infection from overgrowth of *Candida,* a dimorphic fungus that is a normal mucosal inhabitant. Cutaneous overgrowth is usually facilitated by an underlying factor, such as skin damage from chronic trauma or moisture, an immunosuppressive disease, or long-term use of cytotoxic drugs or broad-spectrum antibiotics. Rare in dogs and cats.

Mucosal involvement is characterized by eroded or shallowly ulcerated mucocutaneous junctions, or single to multiple nonhealing mucosal ulcers covered by grayish-white plaques with erythematous margins. Cutaneous involvement is characterized by nonhealing, erythematous, moist, eroded, exudative, and crusty skin or nail bed lesions.

TOP DIFFERENTIALS

Demodicosis, pyotraumatic dermatitis, superficial pyoderma, mucocutaneous pyoderma, other fungal infections, autoimmune disorders, cutaneous lymphoma.

DIAGNOSIS

1. Rule out other differentials.
2. Cytology (exudate)—Suppurative inflammation with numerous budding yeasts and rare pseudohyphae.
3. Dermatohistopathology—Superficial epidermitis, parakeratotic hyperkeratosis, budding yeasts, and occasional pseudohyphae or true hyphae in keratin.
4. Fungal culture—*Candida* spp. Because *Candida* is a normal mucosal inhabitant, positive fungal culture results should be confirmed histologically.

TREATMENT AND PROGNOSIS

1. Identify and correct any underlying cause.
2. For localized cutaneous or mucocutaneous lesions, clip, clean, and dry affected area with a topical astringent. Apply a topical antifungal product until lesions have healed (approximately 1–4 weeks). Effective topical therapies include:

   Nystatin, 100,000 U/g cream or ointment q 8–12 hours.

   3% Amphotericin B cream, lotion, or ointment q 6–8 hours.

   1–2% Miconazole cream, spray, or lotion q 12–24 hours.

   1% Clotrimazole cream, lotion, or solution q 6–8 hours.

   2% Ketoconazole cream q 12 hours.

3. For oral or generalized lesions, give systemic antifungal medications (minimum 4 weeks) continued at least 1 week beyond complete clinical resolution. Effective therapies include:

   Ketoconazole, 5–10 mg/kg PO with food q 12 hours.

   Itraconazole, 5–10 mg/kg PO with food q 12–24 hours.

   Fluconazole, 5 mg/kg PO or IV q 12 hours.

4. Prognosis is good to fair, depending on whether the underlying cause can be corrected. Candidiasis is not contagious to other animals or to humans.

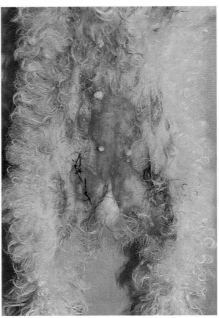

FIGURE 3–29. Candidiasis. Superficial moist, erosive lesions on the ventrum of a dog. (Courtesy of A. Yu)

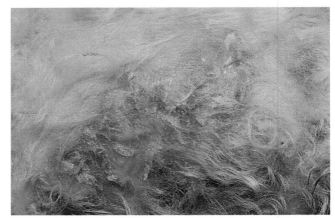

FIGURE 3–30. Candidiasis. Close-up of the dog in Figure 3–29. Erythema and crusting on the abdomen. (Courtesy of A. Yu)

Dermatophytic Granuloma and Pseudomycetoma

(Majocchi's granulomas) (Figs. 3–31 to 3–34)

FEATURES

An unusual form of dermatophytosis in which dermatophilic fungi form hyphae in dermal and subcutaneous tissue. Uncommon in cats, with reports limited to Persian cats. Rare in dogs.

Nonpainful, nonpruritic, firm dermal or subcutaneous nodules and masses that may ulcerate and form draining tracts. Lesions are most frequently found on the trunk, flanks, or tail. Concurrent superficial dermatophytosis is common. Peripheral lymphadenomegaly may be present.

TOP DIFFERENTIALS

Other fungal and bacterial infections, foreign body reaction, neoplasia.

DIAGNOSIS

1. Cytology (exudate, aspirate)—(Pyo)granulomatous inflammation and fungal elements are seen.
2. Dermatohistopathology—Nodular to diffuse (pyo)granulomatous dermatitis and panniculitis with broad, hyaline, septate hyphae, chain-like pseudohyphae and chlamydospore-like cells (pseudomycetoma), or fungal hyphae scattered diffusely throughout the tissue (granuloma).
3. Fungal culture (exudate, aspirate, biopsy specimen)—Only *M. canis* has been isolated from cats. *M. canis* and *Trichophyton mentagrophytes* have been isolated from dogs.

TREATMENT AND PROGNOSIS

1. Surgically excise lesions if possible.
2. Give long-term (weeks to months) systemic antifungal therapy continued at least 1 month beyond complete clinical resolution.
3. The drug of choice is itraconazole, 10 mg/kg PO with food q 24 hours.
4. Alternative drugs that may be effective include:

   Microsize griseofulvin, at least 50 mg/kg/day PO with fat-containing meal.

   Ketoconazole, 10 mg/kg PO with food q 24 hours.

5. Combination surgical excision plus systemic antifungal therapy is more effective than either used alone.
6. Prognosis is fair to poor, with drug resistance and relapses common. Affected animals are potentially contagious and can cause superficial dermatophytosis in other animals and in humans.

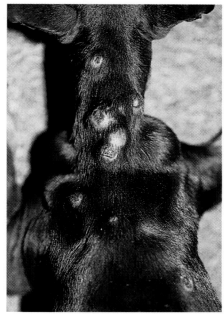

FIGURE 3–31. Dermatophyte Granuloma and Pseudomycetoma. Multiple nodules with draining tracts on the dorsum of a dog infected with *T. mentagrophytes*.

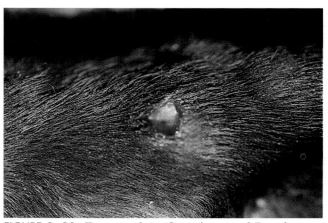

FIGURE 3–32. Dermatophyte Granuloma and Pseudomycetoma. Close-up of the dog in Figure 3–31. This nodular granuloma with a central ulcer periodically drained a purulent exudate.

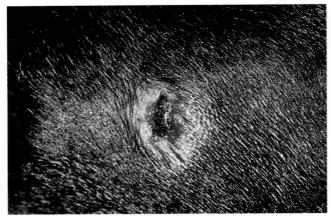

FIGURE 3-33. Dermatophyte Granuloma and Pseudomycetoma. This focal alopecic, crusting, ulcerative nodule was caused by *M. canis*. (Courtesy of A. Yu)

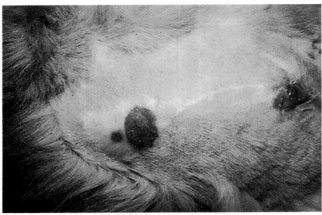

FIGURE 3-34. Dermatophyte Granuloma and Pseudomycetoma. Nodular granulomas on the ventrum of a cat infected with *M. canis*.

Eumycotic Mycetoma
(maduromycosis)

FEATURES

A skin infection that can be caused by a variety of saprophytic environmental and pathogenic plant fungi. After inoculation into the skin, these fungi form dermal and subcutaneous grains or granules. Uncommon to rare in dogs and cats.

Usually a solitary nodule that is relatively poorly circumscribed, often painful, with fistulous tracts. Draining exudate is serous, hemorrhagic, or purulent and contains grains or granules (macroscopic fungal colonies). These grains may be dark-colored (black grain mycetoma), or light-colored (white grain mycetoma), depending on the causative organism. The lesion is usually on the head or limb.

TOP DIFFERENTIALS

Other fungal and bacterial infections, foreign body reaction, neoplasia.

DIAGNOSIS

1. Cytology (exudate)—(Pyo)granulomatous inflammation and occasional fungal elements.
2. Dermatohistopathology—Nodular to diffuse (pyo)-granulomatous dermatitis and panniculitis with irregularly shaped tissue grains composed of broad, septate, branching, pigmented or nonpigmented fungal hyphae.
3. Fungal culture—White grain mycetomas are most commonly caused by *Pseudoallescheria* or *Acremonium* spp. In black grain mycetomas, *Curvularia* or *Madurella* spp. are usually isolated. Because these organisms are environmental contaminants, positive fungal culture results should be confirmed histologically.

TREATMENT AND PROGNOSIS

1. Radical surgical excision or amputation of the affected limb is the treatment of choice.
2. Medical treatment is usually ineffective. If complete surgical excision is not possible, select systemic antifungal therapy based on culture and sensitivity results. Continue treatment 2-3 months beyond complete clinical resolution.
3. Prognosis is poor if complete surgical excision is not possible. Eumycotic mycetomas are not contagious to other animals or to humans.

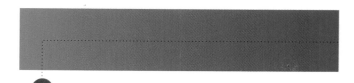

Phaeohyphomycosis

(chromomycosis) (Figs. 3–35 and 3–36)

FEATURES

Cutaneous lesions are caused by a variety of ubiquitous saprophytic fungi that, if introduced into the skin, form pigmented hyphae without granules in tissue. Uncommon in cats and rare in dogs.

Cats. Usually a solitary, firm to fluctuant, subcutaneous nodule, abscess, or cyst-like lesion that may ulcerate and drain. Lesion is most common on distal extremities or the face. Dissemination is rare.

Dogs. Single to multiple poorly circumscribed subcutaneous nodules that are often ulcerated and sometimes necrotic. Lesions are most common on the extremities and are often associated with underlying osteomyelitis. Dissemination may occur.

TOP DIFFERENTIALS

Other fungal and bacterial infections, foreign body reaction, neoplasia.

DIAGNOSIS

1. Cytology (exudate)—(Pyo)granulomatous inflammation. Pigmented fungal hyphae may be difficult to find.
2. Dermatohistopathology—Nodular to diffuse (pyo)granulomatous dermatitis and panniculitis with thick-walled, pigmented, septate, branched or nonbranched hyphae of varying diameters with yeast-like swellings.
3. Fungal culture—Causative organisms include *Alternaria, Bipolaris, Cladosporium (Xylohypha), Curvularia, Exophiala, Moniliella, Ochroconis, Phialemonium, Phialophora, Pseudomicrodochium, Scolecobasidium,* and *Stemphilium* spp. Because these fungi are common environmental contaminants, positive fungal culture results should be confirmed histologically.

TREATMENT AND PROGNOSIS

1. Perform wide surgical excision if possible.
2. Give long-term (weeks to months) systemic antifungal therapy continued at least 1 month beyond complete clinical resolution. Select antifungal medication based on culture/sensitivity results. Ketoconazole, itraconazole, amphotericin B, and flucytosine are variably effective.
3. Prognosis is poor, especially if disease is widespread or disseminated. It is not contagious to other animals or to humans.

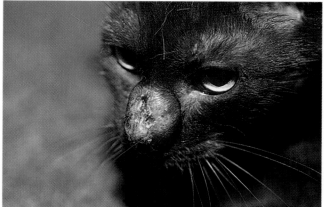

FIGURE 3–35. Phaeohyphomycosis. The swelling, alopecia, crusting, and purulent exudate on the nose of this cat was caused by a pigmented fungus.

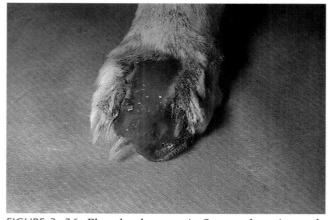

FIGURE 3–36. Phaeohyphomycosis. Severe ulceration and tissue destruction of a cat's foot. (Courtesy of D. Angarano)

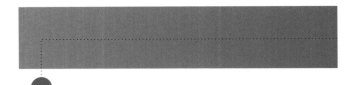

Protothecosis (Figs. 3–37 and 3–38)

FEATURES

Prototheca spp. are saprophytic, achlorophyllous algae found primarily in Europe, Asia, and North America (especially in the southeastern United States). *Prototheca* spp. may cause infection via the gastrointestinal tract or through contact with injured skin or mucosae. Rare in dogs and cats, with highest incidence in immunosuppressed animals.

Cats. Large, firm, cutaneous nodules that are most commonly found on the distal extremities, the head, or the base of the tail.

Dogs. Usually a disseminated disease with multiorgan involvement. Signs may include protracted, bloody diarrhea, weight loss, central nervous system (CNS) signs, ocular lesions, and chronic nodules, draining ulcers, and crusty exudates on the trunk, on the extremities, and at mucocutaneous junctions.

TOP DIFFERENTIALS

Other fungal and bacterial infections, neoplasia.

DIAGNOSIS

1. Cytology (exudate, tissue aspirates)—(Pyo)granulomatous inflammation with numerous intracellular *Prototheca* organisms (round, oval, and polyhedral spherules that vary in size and often contain endospores).
2. Dermatohistopathology—Nodular to diffuse (pyo)granulomatous dermatitis and panniculitis with large numbers of *Prototheca* organisms.
3. Fungal culture—*Prototheca* spp.

TREATMENT AND PROGNOSIS

1. Wide surgical excision of localized lesions is the treatment of choice.
2. Systemic antifungal therapy is usually ineffective; however, the following protocols have been proposed:

   Combination amphotericin B, 0.25–0.5 mg/kg (dogs) or 0.25 mg/kg (cats) IV, three times per week until a cumulative dose of 8 mg/kg (dogs) or 4 mg/kg (cats) is reached, plus tetracycline, 22 mg/kg PO q 8 hours.

   Ketoconazole, 10–15 mg/kg PO with food q 12–24 hours.

   Itraconazole, 5–10 mg/kg PO with food q 12 hours.

   Fluconazole, 2.5–5.0 mg/kg PO or IV q 12 hours.

3. Prognosis is poor if the disease is disseminated or the lesions are not surgically resectable. It is not contagious to other animals or to humans.

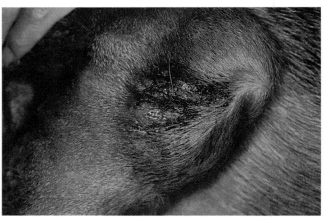

FIGURE 3–37. Protothecosis. Focal ulcerated draining lesions on the elbow of a mixed-breed dog. (Courtesy of K. Boyanowski)

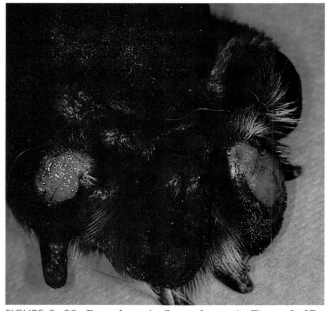

FIGURE 3–38. Protothecosis. Same dog as in Figure 3–37. Ulcerated footpads. (Courtesy of K. Boyanowski)

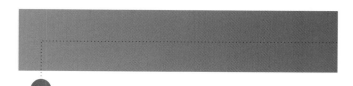

Pythiosis (Figs. 3–39 to 3–42)

FEATURES

Pythium insidiosum is a protozoan with fungus-like features in tissue. This pathogenic aquatic organism causes disease when it enters damaged skin or mucosae. It is found in subtropical and tropical swamps of Asia, Australia, Japan, and parts of Central America and South America. In the United States it is found primarily along the Gulf of Mexico in Alabama, Florida, Louisiana, and Texas. Uncommon in dogs, with the highest incidence in large-breed male dogs, especially hunting dogs and German shepherds. Rare in cats.

Dogs. Can be a cutaneous or gastrointestinal disease. Skin lesions are variably pruritic nodule(s) that converge to form large, spongy, proliferative, often rapidly expanding, fistulating, ulcerated mass(es). Draining exudate is serosanguineous or purulent. Lesions may be anywhere on the body but are most common on the limbs, perineum, tail, and head. Gastrointestinal disease is characterized by progressive weight loss, vomiting, regurgitation, or diarrhea from infiltrative granulomatous gastritis, esophagitis, or enteritis.

Cats. Only a cutaneous disease, as described above for dogs, is seen.

TOP DIFFERENTIALS

Foreign body reaction, neoplasia, other fungal and bacterial infections.

DIAGNOSIS

1. Cytology (exudate)—Granulomatous inflammation that may contain eosinophils, but fungal elements are often not found.
2. Dermatohistopathology—Nodular to diffuse granulomatous dermatitis and panniculitis with foci of necrosis and accumulated eosinophils. Special fungal stains are often needed in order to visualize wide, occasionally septate, irregularly branching hyphae.
3. Fungal culture—*P. insidiosum.*

TREATMENT AND PROGNOSIS

1. Complete, wide surgical excision or amputation of affected limb is the treatment of choice.
2. Long-term systemic antifungal therapy based on culture and sensitivity results can be attempted, but treatments with ketoconazole, itraconazole, and amphotericin B are usually ineffective.
3. Vaccine therapy has not been shown to be effective in dogs.
4. Prognosis is poor if complete surgical excision is not possible. Pythiosis is not contagious to other animals or to humans.

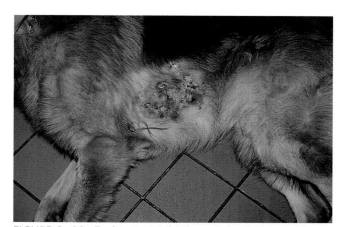

FIGURE 3–39. Pythiosis. Multiple nodular lesions with draining tracts on the lateral thorax of an adult Belgian Tervuren. (Courtesy of D. Angarano.)

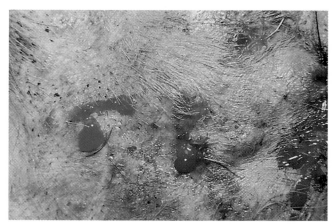

FIGURE 3–40. Pythiosis. Close-up of the dog in Figure 3–39. The draining nodular lesions are typical of infectious cellulitis. (Courtesy of D. Angarano.)

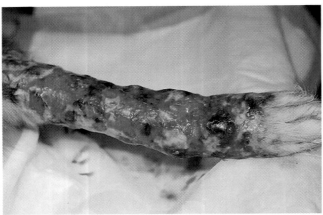

FIGURE 3–41. Pythiosis. Severe ulceration and cellulitis with multiple draining tracts on the entire distal limb of a dog. The infection had gradually progressed up the limb over several weeks. (Courtesy of M. Singer)

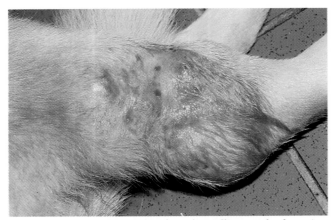

FIGURE 3–42. Pythiosis. Profound swelling with alopecia, papules, nodules, and multiple draining tracts on the proximal rear limb of a dog. (Courtesy of D. Angarano)

Zygomycosis (mucormycosis, entomophthoromycosis) (Figs. 3–43 and 3–44)

FEATURES

Zycomycetes are ubiquitous saprophytic environmental fungi. Organisms may enter the body through the respiratory or gastrointestinal (GI) tract or through wound inoculation. Rare in dogs and cats.

This is often a fatal gastrointestinal, respiratory, or disseminated disease. Skin lesions are characterized by ulcerated, draining nodules or nonhealing wounds.

TOP DIFFERENTIALS

Other fungal and bacterial infections, foreign body reaction, neoplasia.

DIAGNOSIS

1. Cytology (exudate)—(Pyo)granulomatous inflammation with fungal elements.
2. Dermatohistopathology—Nodular to diffuse (pyo)granulomatous dermatitis and panniculitis with numerous broad, occasionally septate, irregularly branching hyphae that have nonparallel sides.
3. Fungal culture—Causative organisms include *Absidia*, *Basidiobolus*, *Conidiobolus*, *Mortierella*, *Mucor*, and *Rhizopus* spp. Because these fungi are common environmental contaminants, positive fungal culture results should be confirmed histologically.

TREATMENT AND PROGNOSIS

1. Wide surgical excision or debulking is indicated.
2. Give long-term (weeks to months) systemic antifungal therapy continued at least 1 month beyond complete clinical resolution. Select antifungal medication based on culture and sensitivity results.
3. Pending sensitivity results, begin treatment with amphotericin B, 0.5 mg/kg (dogs) or 0.25 mg/kg (cats) IV three times per week until a cumulative dose of 8–12 mg/kg (dogs) or 4–6 mg/kg (cats) is given.
4. Treatment with itraconazole or ketoconazole is usually ineffective.
5. Prognosis is poor if complete surgical excision is not possible. This disease is not contagious to other animals or to humans.

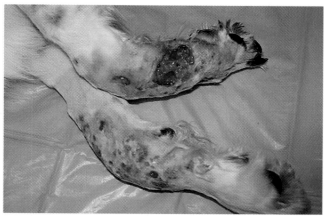

FIGURE 3–43. Zygomycoses. Severe swelling and ulceration with multiple draining lesions on the distal limbs of a dog infected with *Basidiobolus*.

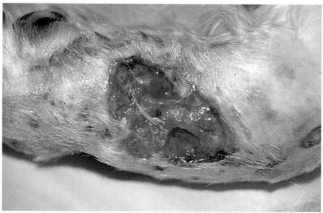

FIGURE 3–44. Zygomycoses. Close-up of the dog in Figure 3–43. Severe tissue destruction on the dorsal carpus.

Sporotrichosis (Figs. 3–45 to 3–48)

FEATURES

Sporothrix schenkii is a dimorphic fungus and environmental saprophyte found worldwide. Infection occurs when the organisms are inoculated into tissue through puncture wounds. Uncommon to rare in dogs and cats, with the highest incidence in hunting dogs and intact male outdoor cats.

Dogs. Skin lesions are characterized by multiple nonpainful, nonpruritic, firm nodules that may ulcerate, drain purulent exudate, and crust over. Lesions are most commonly found on the head, trunk, or distal extremities. Nodules on distal limbs may spread up ascending lymphatic vessels to form more ulcerated, draining nodules. Regional lymphadenomegaly is common. Dissemination is rare.

Cats. Skin lesions may include nonhealing puncture wounds, abscesses, cellulitis, crusted nodules, ulcerations, purulent draining tracts, and sometimes tissue necrosis. Lesions usually involve the head, distal limbs, or tail base. Concurrent lethargy, depression, anorexia, and fever may be present. Dissemination is common.

TOP DIFFERENTIALS

Other fungal and bacterial infections, foreign body reaction, neoplasia.

DIAGNOSIS

1. Cytology (exudate, tissue aspirate)—Suppurative or (pyo)granulomatous inflammation. Intracellular and extracellular round, oval, and cigar-shaped yeasts are usually easy to find in cats but are difficult to find in dogs.
2. Dermatohistopathology—Nodular to diffuse suppurative or (pyo)granulomatous dermatitis. Yeasts that may resemble cryptococcal organisms are easily found in cats but rarely found in dogs.
3. Immunofluorescent testing—Detection of *Sporothrix* antigen in tissue or exudate.
4. Fungal culture—*S. schenckii* is easy to culture from infected cats but may be difficult to isolate from infected dogs.

TREATMENT AND PROGNOSIS

1. Give long-term (weeks to months) systemic antifungal therapy continued at least 1 month beyond complete clinical resolution.
2. In dogs the traditional treatment is supersaturated potassium iodide, 40 mg/kg PO with food q 8 hours.
3. Alternative treatments in dogs include:

   Ketoconazole, 5–15 mg/kg PO with food q 12 hours.

   Itraconazole, 5–10 mg/kg PO with food q 12–24 hours.

4. In cats the drug of choice is itraconazole, 5–10 mg/kg PO with food q 12–24 hours.
5. Alternative treatments in cats include:

   Ketoconazole, 5–10 mg/kg PO with food q 12 hours.

   Supersaturated potassium iodide, 20 mg/kg PO with food q 12 hours.

6. Wear disposable gloves, and scrub hands and arms after handling possibly contaminated animals.
7. Prognosis is fair to good, but relapses can occur. There are no reports of disease transmission from dogs to humans, but infected cats are highly contagious to people.

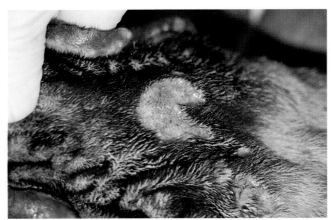

FIGURE 3–46. Sporotrichosis. Same dog as in Figure 3–45. Erosive lesion with purulent drainage on the ventral neck.

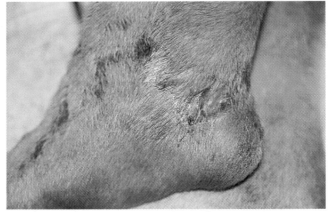

FIGURE 3–47. Sporotrichosis. Same dog as in Figures 3–45 and 3–46. These lesions on the hock periodically drained a purulent exudate.

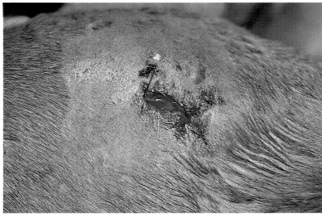

FIGURE 3–45. Sporotrichosis. Draining lesions with crusting on the swollen stifle of a dog.

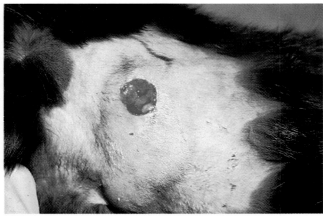

FIGURE 3–48. Sporotrichosis. A large, fluctuant mass with a central ulcerative lesion on the lateral thorax of a cat. (Courtesy of D. Angarano)

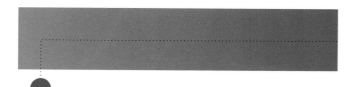

Blastomycosis (Figs. 3–49 to 3–52)

FEATURES

Disease is caused by inhaling the conidia of *Blastomyces dermatitis,* a dimorphic fungus and environmental saprophyte. After inhalation, a lung infection is established which disseminates to lymph nodes, eyes, skin, bones, and other organs. Occasionally, direct inoculation may result in localized skin disease. *B. dermatitis* is found in moist, acidic, or sandy soil primarily in North America along the Ohio, Mississippi, Missouri, St. Lawrence, and Tennessee Rivers, in southern Mid-Atlantic states, and in the southern Great Lakes region. Rare in cats and uncommon in dogs, with the highest incidence in young male large-breed outdoor dogs, especially hounds and sporting breeds.

Cutaneous lesions may include firm, granulomatous to proliferative masses, subcutaneous abscesses, ulcerations, and fistulous tracts that drain a serosanguineous to purulent exudate. Lesions may be found anywhere on the body but are most common on the head and extremities. Nonspecific symptoms include anorexia, weight loss, and fever. Other symptoms, depending on the organ systems involved, may include exercise intolerance, cough, dyspnea, lymphadenomegaly, uveitis, retinal detachment, glaucoma, lameness, and CNS signs.

TOP DIFFERENTIALS

Other fungal and bacterial infections, neoplasia, foreign body reaction.

DIAGNOSIS

1. Cytology (exudate, tissue aspirate)—Suppurative or (pyo)granulomatous inflammation with numerous large, round, broad-based budding yeasts that have thick, refractile, double-contoured cell walls.
2. Dermatohistopathology—Nodular to diffuse suppurative to (pyo)granulomatous dermatitis with large, thick, double-walled, broad-based budding yeasts.
3. Serology—Detection of antibodies against *B. dermatitis* by agar-gel immunodiffusion. In early infections, test results may be negative.
4. Fungal culture (not needed to confirm diagnosis unless cytology and histopathology fail to reveal organisms; submit to diagnostic laboratory)—*B. dermatitis.*

5. Radiography—Pulmonary changes if lungs are involved. Osteolytic lesions if long bones are involved.

TREATMENT AND PROGNOSIS

1. Give long-term (minimum 2–3 months) systemic antifungal therapy continued 1 month beyond complete clinical resolution.
2. The drug of choice is itraconazole. For cats, give 5 mg/kg PO with food q 12 hours. For dogs, give 5 mg/kg PO with food q 12 hours for 5 days, then give 5 mg/kg PO with food q 24 hours.
3. Alternative therapies include:

   Fluconazole, 2.5–5.0 mg/kg PO or IV q 24 hours.

   Amphotericin B, 0.5 mg/kg (dogs) or 0.25 mg/kg (cats) IV three times per week until a cumulative dose of 8–12 mg/kg (dogs) or 4–6 mg/kg (cats) is given.

   Amphotericin B lipid complex (dogs), 1.0 mg/kg IV three times per week until a cumulative dose of 12 mg/kg is given.

4. Prognosis is good unless brain or severe lung involvement is present. Infected animals (yeast form) are not considered contagious to other animals or to humans, but fungal cultures (mycelial form) are highly infectious.

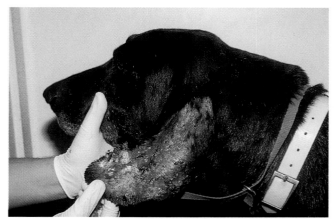

FIGURE 3–49. Blastomycosis. Multiple draining lesions on the ear pinnae of a dog. (Courtesy of D. Angarano)

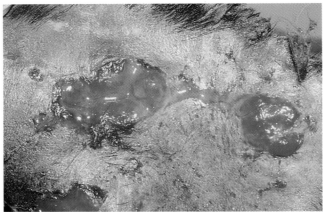

FIGURE 3–50. Blastomycosis. Close-up of the dog in Figure 3–49. Cellulitis with draining tracts affecting the entire ear pinnae. (Courtesy of D. Angarano)

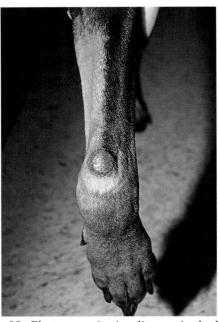

FIGURE 3–52. Blastomycosis. A solitary raised, alopecic, erosive lesion on the carpus of an adult doberman pincher. Note the similarity to an acral lick granuloma. (Courtesy of D. Angarano)

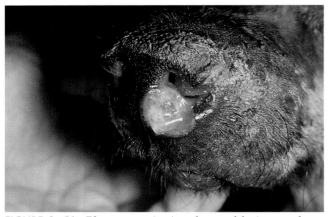

FIGURE 3–51. Blastomycosis. An ulcerated lesion on the nasal planum of a dog. (Courtesy of D. Angarano)

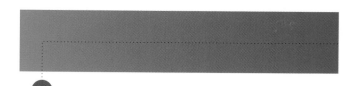

Coccidioidomycosis (Figs. 3–53 and 3–54)

FEATURES

Coccidioides immitis is a dimorphic fungus and soil saprophyte endemic to desert areas in the southwestern United States, Mexico, Central America, and parts of South America. The organisms are inhaled, and a lung infection is established which may disseminate to lymph nodes, eyes, skin, bones, and other organs. Rare in cats and uncommon in dogs, with the highest incidence in young, medium to large-breed outdoor dogs.

Skin lesions in dogs include nodules, abscesses, and draining tracts over sites of long bone infection. Regional lymphadenomegaly is common. In cats, subcutaneous masses, abscesses, and draining lesions occur without underlying bone involvement. Regional lymphadenomegaly may be seen.

Other signs in dogs and cats include anorexia, weight loss, fever, and depression. Depending on the organs infected, cough, dyspnea, tachypnea, lameness from painful bone swellings, and ocular disease may be seen.

TOP DIFFERENTIALS

Other fungal and bacterial infections, foreign body reaction, neoplasia.

DIAGNOSIS

1. Cytology (exudate, tissue aspirate)—Suppurative to (pyo)granulomatous inflammation, but fungal organisms are seldom found.
2. Dermatohistopathology—Nodular to diffuse suppurative or (pyo)granulomatous dermatitis and panniculitis, with few to several large, round, double-walled structures (spherules) containing endospores.
3. Serology—Detection of antibodies against *C. immitis* by precipitin, complement fixation, latex agglutination, or enzyme-linked immunosorbent assay (ELISA) testing.
4. Fungal culture (submit to diagnostic laboratory)—*C. immitis*.
5. Radiography—Pulmonary changes are common. There are osteolytic lesions if bone is involved.

TREATMENT AND PROGNOSIS

1. Give long-term (minimum 1 year if disseminated) systemic antifungal therapy continued at least 2 months beyond complete clinical and radiographic resolution of the lesions. Ideally, treatment should also be continued until follow-up *C. immitis* antibody titers are negative.
2. Effective therapies include:

   Ketoconazole (dogs), 5–10 mg/kg PO with food q 12 hours.

   Ketoconazole (cats), 5 mg/kg PO with food q 12 hours or 10 mg/kg PO with food q 24 hours.

   Itraconazole, 5–10 mg/kg PO with food q 12 hours.

   Fluconazole, 5 mg/kg PO q 12 hours.

3. In preliminary studies, lufenuron, 10 mg/kg PO q 24 hours for 16 weeks, was effective in controlling clinical signs in dogs, although serology was still positive.
4. Prognosis is unpredictable and relapses are common. If relapse occurs, reinstituting treatment until lesions resolve, followed by chronic low-dose therapy, may be needed to maintain remission. Infected animals (yeast form) are not considered contagious to other animals or to humans, but fungal cultures (mycelial form) are highly infectious.

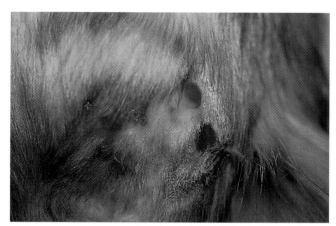

FIGURE 3–53. Coccidioidomycosis. Multiple draining tracts on the ischium of an infected cat. (Courtesy of A. Wolf)

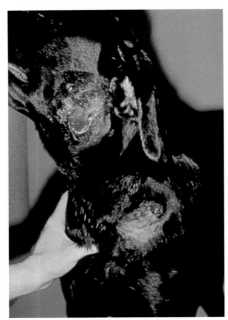

FIGURE 3–54. Coccidioidomycosis. Multiple ulcerated draining tracts on the head and neck of an infected dog. (Courtesy of A. Wolf)

Cryptococcosis (Figs. 3–55 to 3–58)

FEATURES

Cryptococcus neoformans is an environmental saprophytic yeast-like fungus found worldwide. The disease occurs if inhaled organisms establish an infection in the nasal cavity, paranasal sinuses, or lungs. Dissemination to skin, eyes, CNS, and other organs may follow. Uncommon in cats. Rare in dogs, with the highest incidence in young adults.

Cats. The upper respiratory tract is most commonly involved, with sneezing, snuffling, nasal discharge, nasal mass, and/or a firm, subcutaneous swelling over the bridge of the nose. Skin involvement is characterized by multiple nonpainful papules and nodules that may ulcerate. Regional lymphadomegaly is common. Signs of CNS (variable neurologic signs) and ocular disease (fixed, dilated pupils, blindness) are also often seen.

Dogs. A neurologic and/or ophthalmic disease usually occurs. The upper respiratory tract is also frequently involved. Occasionally cutaneous ulcers occur, especially on the nose and lips, in the oral cavity, or around the nailbeds.

TOP DIFFERENTIALS

Other fungal and bacterial infections, neoplasia.

DIAGNOSIS

1. Cytology (exudate, tissue aspirates)—(Pyo)-granulomatous inflammation with narrow-based budding, thin-walled yeasts surrounded by variably sized, clear, refractile capsules.
2. Dermatohistopathology—Nodular to diffuse (pyo)-granulomatous dermatitis and panniculitis with numerous yeast-like organisms or vacuolated-appearing dermis and subcutis due to large numbers of organisms without inflammation.
3. Serology—Detection of cryptococcal capsular antigen by latex agglutination or ELISA testing. In localized infections, test results may be negative.
4. Fungal culture—*C. neoformans.*

TREATMENT AND PROGNOSIS

1. Surgically excise cutaneous lesions if possible.
2. Give long-term (several months) systemic antifungal therapy continued at least 1 month beyond complete clinical resolution. Ideally, treatment should also be continued until follow-up cryptococcal antigen titers are negative.

3. Give itraconazole, 5–10 mg/kg PO with food q 12–24 hours, or fluconazole, 5–15 mg/kg PO q 12–24 hours.

4. Alternative therapies that may be effective include:

Ketoconazole (cats), 5–10 mg/kg PO with food q 12–24 hours.

Amphotericin B, 0.5–0.8 mg/kg (added to 0.45% saline/2.5% dextrose—400 ml for cats, 500 ml for dogs <20 kg, and 1000 ml for dogs >20 kg) SQ two or three times per week until a cumulative dose of 8–26 mg/kg is given. Concentrations of amphotericin B >20 mg/L cause local irritation.

5. Prognosis for cats is fair to good unless the CNS is involved. Prognosis for cats with CNS involvement and for dogs in general is poor. Infected animals and cultures are not considered contagious to other animals or to humans.

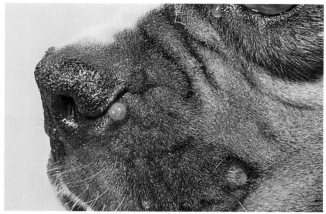

FIGURE 3–57. Cryptococcosis. This focal ulcerated nodule was caused by *Cryptococcus*. (Courtesy of D. Angarano)

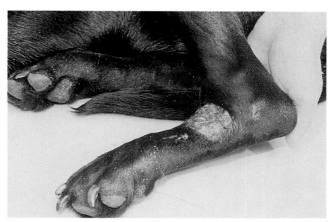

FIGURE 3–58. Cryptococcosis. The alopecic, crusting plaque on the rear leg of this dog was associated with a systemic infection. (Courtesy of D. Angarano)

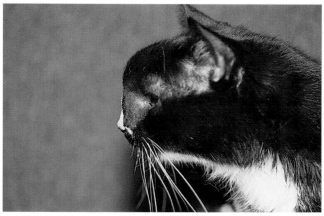

FIGURE 3–55. Cryptococcosis. The dramatic swelling of the bridge of the nose of this adult cat is typical of cryptococcal infections.

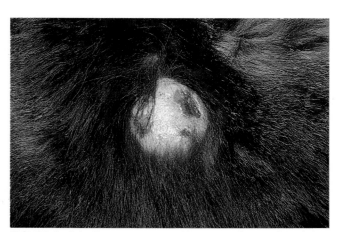

FIGURE 3–56. Cryptococcosis. Alopecic, ulcerated nodule on the head of an adult cat.

Histoplasmosis (Figs. 3–59 and 3–60)

FEATURES

A systemic disease caused by *Histoplasma capsulatum*, a dimorphic fungus and soil saprophyte. After conidia are inhaled or ingested, an infection is established in the lungs or gastrointestinal tract that then disseminates elsewhere. *H. capsulatum* is found in most temperate and subtropical areas. In the United States, the disease occurs most commonly along the Mississippi, Missouri, and Ohio Rivers. Rare in dogs and uncommon in cats, with the highest incidence in young adult animals.

Skin involvement is rare, but multiple small nodules that ulcerate and drain or crust over have been reported. Nonspecific symptoms such as anorexia, depression, weight loss, and fever are more typical. Other symptoms in dogs and cats may include dyspnea, tachypnea, and ocular disease. Lameness in cats and cough, diarrhea, icterus, and ascites in dogs may be seen.

TOP DIFFERENTIALS

Other fungal and bacterial infections, neoplasia.

DIAGNOSIS

1. Cytology (tissue aspirates)—(Pyo)granulomatous inflammation with numerous intracellular small yeasts that have basophilic centers.
2. Dermatohistopathology—Nodular to diffuse (pyo)-granulomatous dermatitis with numerous intracellular yeasts. Special fungal stains may be needed in order to visualize organisms.
3. Radiography—Pulmonary lesions are often seen.
4. Fungal culture (not needed to confirm the diagnosis unless cytology and histopathology fail to reveal organisms; submit to diagnostic laboratory)—*H. capsulatum*.

TREATMENT AND PROGNOSIS

1. Give long-term (minimum 4–6 months) systemic antifungal therapy continued 2 months beyond complete clinical resolution.
2. The drug of choice is itraconazole, 10 mg/kg PO with food q 12–24 hours.
3. Alternatively, fluconazole, 2.5–5 mg/kg PO q 12–24 hours, may be effective.
4. For severe cases, a quicker response may be achieved by combining itraconazole or flucona-zole with amphotericin B, 0.25 mg/kg (cats) or 0.5 mg/kg (dogs) IV three times per week, until a cumulative dose of 4–8 mg/kg (cats) or 5–10 mg/kg (dogs) is given.
5. Prognosis is fair to good for most cats. Prognosis is poor for severely debilitated cats and for dogs with GI or severe signs of disseminated disease. Infected animals (yeast form) are not considered contagious to other animals or to humans, but fungal cultures (mycelial form) are highly infectious.

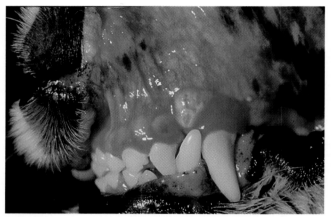

FIGURE 3–59. Histoplasmosis. An erosive lesion on the gingiva of an adult dog. (Courtesy of L. Schmeitzel)

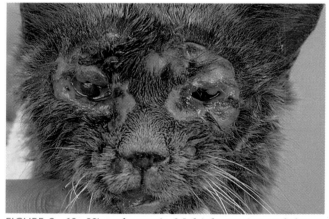

FIGURE 3–60. Histoplasmosis. Multiple erosive nodules and draining tracts on the face of an 11-year-old cat. (Courtesy of P. White)

Suggested Readings

Akerstedt J and Vollset I. 1995. *Malassezia* Pachydermatis with Special Reference to Canine Skin Disease. Br Vet J. 152: 269–281.

Ben-Ziong Y and Avzi B. 2000. Use of lufenuron for treating fungal infections in dogs and cats: 297 cases (1997–1999). J Am Vet Med Assoc. 217(10):1510–1513.

de Jaham C, Paradis M, and Papich MG. 2000. Traditional Antifungal Dermatolic Agents. Compend Cont Edu Pract Vet. 22: 461–469.

de Jaham C, Paradis M, and Papich MG. 2000. Antifungal Dermatologic Agents: Azoles and Allyamines. Compend Cont Edu Pract Vet. 22: 548–561.

Fungal Diseases, pp. 329–391. In Scott DW, Miller WH Jr, and Griffin CE 1995. Muller & Kirk's Small Animal Dermatology. Ed. 5. W.B. Saunders, Philadelphia, PA.

Fungal Diseases, Section III, pp. 349–430. In Green CE (ed). 1998. Infectious Diseases of the Dog and Cat. Ed. 2. W.B. Saunders, Philadelphia, PA.

Greene R and Troy G. 1995. Coccidiomycosis in 48 Cats: A Retrospective Study (1984–1993). J Vet Int Med. 9(2): 86–91.

Martin S. 1999. Pharm Profile: Itraconazole. Compend Cont Edu Pract Vet. 21: 145–147.

Moriello KA and DeBoer DJ. 1995. Feline Dermatophytosis: Recent Advances and Recommendations for therapy. Vet Clin North Am Sm Ani Pract. 25: 901–921.

Outerbridge C, Myers S, and Summerbell R. 1995. Phaeohyphomycosis in a Cat. Can Vet J. 36: 629–630.

Plumb DC. 1999. Veterinary Drug Handbook. Ed. 3. Iowa State University Press, Ames, IA.

Werner A and Werner B. 1993. Feline Sporotrichosis. Compend Cont Edu Pract Vet. 15(9): 1189–1197.

4

Parasitic Skin Disorders

- **Ixodid Ticks** (hard ticks)

- **Spinous Ear Tick** (*Otobius megnini*)

- **Canine Localized Demodicosis**

- **Canine Generalized Demodicosis**

- **Feline Demodicosis**

- **Canine Scabies** (sarcoptic mange)

- **Feline Scabies** (notoedric mange)

- **Cheyletiellosis** (walking dandruff)

- **Ear Mites** (*Otodectes cynotis*)

- **Trombiculiasis** (chigger mites, harvest mites)

- **Cat Fur Mite** (*Lynxacarus radosky*)

- **Fleas**

- **Pediculosis**

- **Cuterebra**
- **Fly Bite Dermatitis**
- **Myiasis**
- **Hookworm Dermatitis** (ancylostomiasis and uncinariasis)
- **Pelodera Dermatitis** (rhabditic dermatitis)
- **Dracunculiasis**

Ixodid Ticks (hard ticks) (Figs. 4–1 and 4–2)

FEATURES

Ixodid ticks include the genera *Rhipicephalus* (i.e., brown dog tick), *Dermacentor* (i.e., American dog tick, Rocky Mountain wood tick, Pacific or West Coast tick), *Ixodes* (i.e., shoulder tick of North America, deer tick, British dog tick [Europe]), *Amblyomma* (i.e., black-legged tick, Lone Star tick), and *Haemophysalis* (yellow dog tick [Africa and Asia]). Ixodid ticks are more commonly found on dogs than on cats.

Symptoms of tick infestation include none (asymptomatic), an inflamed nodule at the site of tick attachment, signs of tick-borne diseases, and/or tick paralysis. Ticks are most commonly found on the ears or interdigitally but can be anywhere on the body.

DIAGNOSIS

1. Direct visualization of tick(s) on body.

TREATMENT AND PROGNOSIS

1. If infestation is mild, carefully remove ticks manually.
2. For severe infestations, spray with or dip animal in topical insecticide labeled for use against ticks.
3. Treat concurrent tick-borne disease if present.
4. Periodic premise treatment with appropriately labeled insecticides may be needed in homes and kennels infested with *R. sanguineous* (brown dog tick).
5. Spraying grassed and shrubbed areas every spring and midsummer with appropriately labeled pesticides may be helpful in controlling ticks.
6. Regular applications of fipronil spray or solution on dogs and cats, or using 9% amitraz collars (dogs only) as instructed on label, may help prevent reinfestations.
7. Prognosis is good. Infected animals are sources of tick transmission to other animals and to humans.

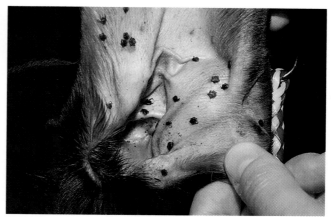

FIGURE 4–1. Ixodid Ticks. Multiple ticks attached to the inner ear pinnae. (Courtesy of D. Angarano)

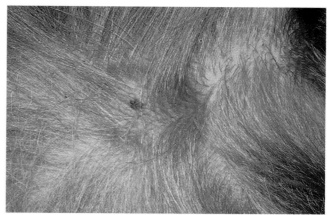

FIGURE 4–2. Ixodid Ticks. This erythematous lesion developed at the site of tick attachment. (Courtesy of D. Gram)

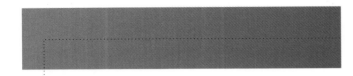

Spinous Ear Tick (*Otobius megnini*)

FEATURES

A soft (argasid) tick primarily found in arid areas of North and South America, India, and southern Africa. Adult ticks are not parasitic, but larvae and nymphs infest external ear canals of animals. Uncommon in dogs and rare in cats.

Acute onset of otitis externa with severe inflammation and waxy exudate, vigorous head shaking, and ear scratching.

TOP DIFFERENTIALS

Other causes of otitis externa.

DIAGNOSIS

1. Otoscopy—Visualization of larval, nymph, and immature adult spinous ear ticks.

TREATMENT AND PROGNOSIS

1. Manually remove ticks with forceps.
2. Spray on or dip animal in topical insecticide labeled for use against ticks.
3. Treat any secondary ear infection with appropriate topical medication.
4. Adult ticks infest the animal's premises, so environmental treatment with insecticidal sprays is important.
5. Prognosis is good, but reinfestation can occur if adult ticks are not eliminated from the environment. Although these ticks are primarily parasitic on animals, they can also infest humans.

Canine Localized Demodicosis (Fig. 4–3)

FEATURES

Skin lesions occur when there is a localized overpopulation of *Demodex canis*, a normal commensal inhabitant of canine skin. Demodectic overgrowth is often associated with a predisposing factor such as endoparasitism, poor nutrition, immunosuppressive drug therapy, or transient stress (estrus, pregnancy, surgery, boarding). Common in dogs with highest incidence in puppies 3–6 months old.

One to five localized areas of alopecia with variable erythema, hyperpigmentation, and scaling. Lesions are most common on the face but can be anywhere on the body. Lesions are not usually pruritic unless they are secondarily infected.

TOP DIFFERENTIALS

Superficial pyoderma, dermatophytosis, trauma.

DIAGNOSIS

1. Microscopy (deep skin scrapes)—Many demodectic adults, nymphs, larvae, and/or ova.
2. Dermatohistopathology—Intrafollicular demodectic mites with varying degrees of perifolliculitis, folliculitis, and/or furunculosis.

TREATMENT AND PROGNOSIS

1. Identify and treat any predisposing factors.
2. Treat lesions topically with 2.5–3% benzoyl peroxide shampoo, lotion, cream, or gel q 24 hours.
3. Miticidal treatment may not be necessary because many cases resolve spontaneously.
4. Rotenone-containing products or benzyl benzoate lotion may be miticidal when applied to lesions q 24 hours.
5. Alternatively, 0.03–0.05% amitraz solution (0.7 ml Mitaban, 1 ml Taktic, or 2.5 ml Ectodex in 240 ml water, mixed fresh daily) applied to lesions q 24 hours is often effective.
6. Topical therapy is continued until follow-up skin scrapings are negative and lesions have resolved.
7. Prognosis is good. Most cases resolve within 4–8 weeks, but a few may progress to generalized demodicosis. *D. canis* is not considered contagious to other dogs (except for newborn puppies), to cats, or to humans.

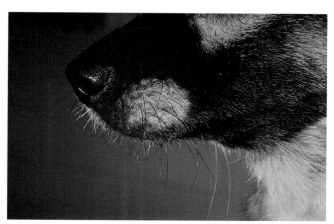

FIGURE 4–3. Canine Localized Demodicosis. A focal area of alopecia on the muzzle of a young dog. (Courtesy of D. Angarano)

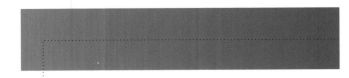

Canine Generalized Demodicosis (Figs. 4–4 to 4–14)

FEATURES

A generalized skin disease that can be caused by two different species of demodectic mites—*D. canis* (a normal commensal of dog skin) and an unnamed *Demodex* mite (normal habitat unknown). Depending on the dog's age at onset, generalized demodicosis is classified as juvenile-onset or adult-onset. Both forms are common in dogs. Juvenile-onset generalized demodicosis occurs in young dogs, usually between 3 and 18 months old, with the highest incidence in medium-sized and large purebred dogs. Adult-onset generalized demodicosis occurs in dogs >18 months old, with the highest incidence in middle-aged to older dogs that are immunocompromised due to an underlying condition such as endogenous or iatrogenic hyperadrenocorticism, hypothyroidism, immunosuppressive drug therapy, diabetes mellitus, or neoplasia.

Clinical signs are variable. The disease often begins as localized lesions that spread. Usually there is patchy, regional, multifocal, or diffuse alopecia with variable erythema, silvery-grayish scaling, papules, and/or pruritus. The affected skin may become lichenified, hyperpigmented, pustular, eroded, crusted, and/or ulcerated from secondary superficial or deep pyoderma. Lesions can be anywhere on the body, including the feet. Pododemodicosis is characterized by any combination of interdigital pruritus, pain, erythema, alopecia, hyperpigmentation, lichenification, scaling, swelling, crusts, pustules, bullae, and draining tracts. Peripheral lymphadenomegaly is common. Systemic signs (fever, depression, anorexia) may be seen if secondary bacterial sepsis develops.

TOP DIFFERENTIALS

Pyoderma (superficial or deep), dermatophytosis, hypersensitivity (flea bite, food, atopy), autoimmune skin disorders.

DIAGNOSIS

1. Microscopy (deep skin scrapes)—Many demodectic adults, nymphs, larvae, and/or ova (mites may be difficult to find in fibrotic lesions and in feet).
2. Dermatohistopathology—Intrafollicular demodectic mites with varying degrees of perifolliculitis, folliculitis, and/or furunculosis.

TREATMENT

1. Identify and correct any underlying conditions.
2. Neuter intact dogs, especially females, because estrus or pregnancy may trigger relapse.
3. Treat any secondary pyoderma with appropriate long-term (minimum 3–4 weeks) systemic antibiotics continued at least 1 week beyond clinical resolution of the pyoderma.
4. Traditional miticidal treatment entails:

   Total body haircoat clip if dog is medium- to long-coated.

   Weekly bath with 2.5–3% benzoyl peroxide shampoo followed by a total body application of 0.025–0.05% amitraz solution (5.3 ml Mitaban/gal water, 50 ml Ectodex/5 L water, or 13 ml Taktic/5 L water). The cure rate ranges from 50% to 86%.

5. For demodectic pododermatitis, in addition to weekly amitraz dips, perform foot soaks in 0.125% amitraz solution (0.7 ml Mitaban, 2.5 ml Ectodex, or 1.0 ml Taktic per 100 ml water) q 1–3 days.
6. Alternatively, treatment with ivermectin, 0.6 mg/kg PO q 24 hours, is often effective against generalized demodicosis. Initially, ivermectin, 0.1 mg/kg PO, is given on day 1, then 0.2 mg/kg PO is given on day 2, continuing oral daily increments by 0.1 mg/kg until 0.6 mg/kg/day is being given, assuming that no signs of toxicity develop. If the dog cannot tolerate a 0.6 mg/kg/day dosage, treatment with 0.4 mg/kg/day can be attempted. The cure rate with 0.6 mg/kg/day ivermectin is 85–90%, and with 0.4 mg/kg/day it is 45–50%.
7. Another effective alternative therapy is milbemycin oxime, 2 mg/kg PO q 24 hours. The cure rate is 85–90%.
8. For dogs that are poorly responsive and/or have unacceptable side effects with traditional amitraz, ivermectin, and milbemycin therapy, daily half-body applications of a concentrated amitraz solution may be effective. The treatment protocol includes a total body haircoat clip if the dog is medium- to long-coated and weekly baths with 2.5–3% benzoyl peroxide shampoo. A 0.125% amitraz solution (1 ml Taktic, 2.5 ml Ectodex, or 0.7 ml Mitaban per 100 ml water used) is applied with a sponge to half of the body each day, alternating the body half treated. The cure rate is 75–80%.
9. Regardless of the miticidal treatment chosen, therapy is long-term (weeks to months). Continue treatments at least 1 month beyond the time when follow-up skin scrapings become negative for mites.
10. Prognosis is good to fair. Relapses may occur, requiring periodic or lifelong treatment in some dogs. The use of glucocorticosteroids in any dog that has been diagnosed with demodicosis

should be avoided. Because of its hereditary predisposition, neither female nor male dogs with juvenile-onset generalized demodicosis should be bred. *D. canis* is not considered contagious to other dogs (except for newborn puppies), to cats, or to humans. The mode of transmission for the unnamed *Demodex* mite is unknown.

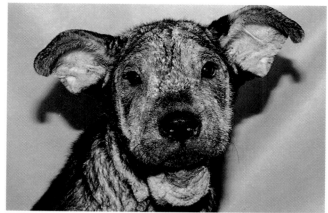

FIGURE 4–6. Generalized Demodicosis. Generalized alopecia and papules with crusts and scales on the head and neck of a juvenile dog.

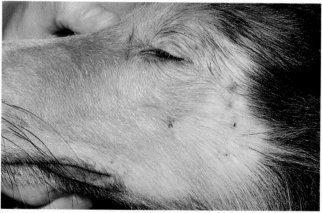

FIGURE 4–4. Canine Demodicosis. Multiple alopecic, papular lesions on the face of an adult shetland sheep dog. (Courtesy of D. Angarano)

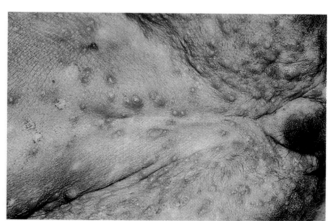

FIGURE 4–7. Canine Generalized Demodicosis. Close-up of the dog in Figure 4–6. Multiple pustules on the ventral abdomen.

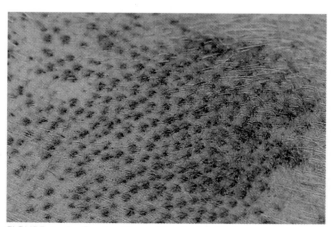

FIGURE 4–5. Canine Demodicosis. Multiple comedones on the ventral abdomen of a dog. (Courtesy of D. Angarano)

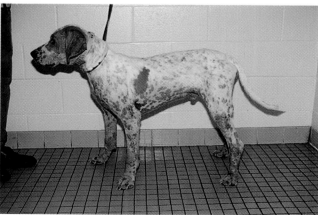

FIGURE 4–8. Canine Generalized Demodicosis. Generalized alopecia, erythema, and crusting papules on the body of a young adult dog.

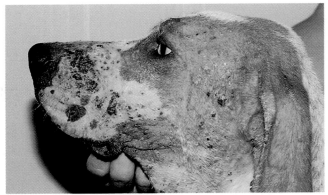

FIGURE 4–9. Canine Generalized Demodicosis. Close-up of the dog in Figure 4–8. Diffuse alopecic, erythematous, crusting, papular lesions affecting the entire head and neck.

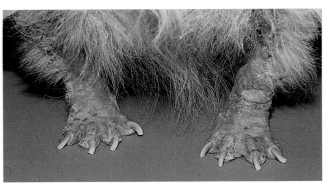

FIGURE 4–12. Canine Generalized Demodicosis. Diffuse alopecia and erythema on the distal extremities of a dog caused by adult-onset demodicosis secondary to iatrogenic Cushing's disease.

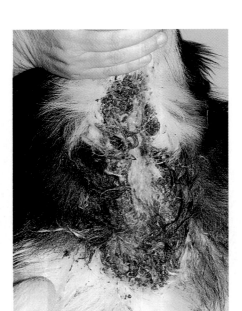

FIGURE 4–10. Canine Generalized Demodicosis. The severe cellulitis and crusting on the ventral neck of this shetland sheep dog were caused by demodicosis and secondary deep pyoderma. (Courtesy of D. Angarano)

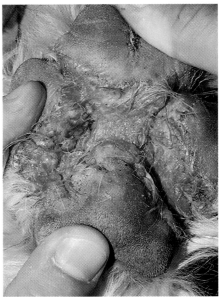

FIGURE 4–13. Canine Generalized Demodicosis. Severe pododermatitis caused by a *Demodex* and bacterial infection. Cutaneous biopsies may be necessary to identify the mites in severe cases of pododermatitis.

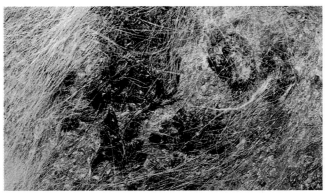

FIGURE 4–11. Canine Generalized Demodicosis. Alopecia, crusting, and papular lesions typical of folliculitis and furunculosis caused by *Demodex*.

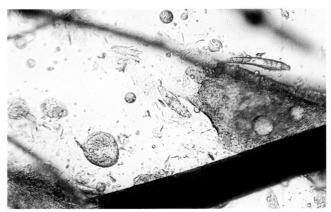

FIGURE 4–14. Canine Demodicosis. *Demodex* mites from a deep skin scraping.

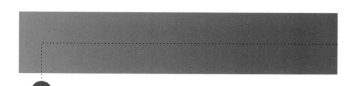

Feline Demodicosis (Figs. 4–15 to 4–20)

FEATURES

A skin disease that can be caused by two different species of demodectic mites—*Demodex cati* (a normal commensal of cat skin) and *D. gatoi* (normal habitat unknown). Skin disease may be localized or generalized. Generalized demodicosis is often associated with an underlying immunosuppressive or metabolic disease such as feline immunodeficiency virus (FIV), feline leukemia virus (FELV), toxoplasmosis, systemic lupus erythematosus, or diabetes mellitus. Localized and generalized demodicosis are rare in cats.

Localized disease is characterized by either a variably pruritic ceruminous otitis externa or by focal patchy alopecia and erythema that may be scaly or crusty. Localized skin lesions are most common around the eyes, on the head, or on the neck.

Generalized disease is characterized by variably pruritic, multifocal, patchy, regional, or symmetric alopecia, with or without erythema, scaling, crusts, macules, and hyperpigmentation. Lesions usually involve the head, neck, limbs, flanks, and/or ventrum. Ceruminous otitis externa and secondary pyoderma may be present.

TOP DIFFERENTIALS

Dermatophytosis, other ectoparasite (*Cheyletiella*, notoedres, ear mites), hypersensitivity (flea bite, food, atopy), psychogenic alopecia, and other causes of otitis externa.

DIAGNOSIS

1. Microscopy (deep and superficial skin scrapings, ear swabs)—Demonstration of demodectic adults, nymphs, larvae, and/or ova.
2. Dermatohistopathology—Minimal to mild suppurative perivascular dermatitis with mites in stratum corneum or intrafollicular mites with varying degrees of perifolliculitis and folliculitis.

TREATMENT AND PROGNOSIS

1. Identify and correct any predisposing conditions.
2. Localized lesions may resolve spontaneously without treatment.
3. For localized lesions, topical therapies that may be effective when applied q 24 hours include:

    Rotenone (Canex).

    0.025% Amitraz solution (0.66 ml Mitaban or 2.5 ml Ectodex in 240 ml water mixed fresh daily).

4. For generalized lesions, treatments that may be effective include:

    2% Lime sulfur solution applied to the entire body q 7 days.

    0.015–0.025% Amitraz solution (2.5 ml Mitaban/gal water or 25 ml Ectodex/5 L water) applied to entire body q 1–2 weeks. Note: do not use amitraz on diabetic cats.

5. For both localized and generalized disease, continue treatments until lesions have resolved and follow-up skin scrapings are negative for mites (approximately 3–4 weeks).
6. Prognosis for localized demodicosis is good. Prognosis for generalized demodicosis is good to guarded, depending on the underlying cause. *D. cati* is not considered contagious to other cats (except for newborn kittens), to dogs, or to humans. The mode of transmission for *D. gatoi* is unknown, but reports of unrelated household cats being simultaneously affected suggest that it may be contagious from cat to cat.

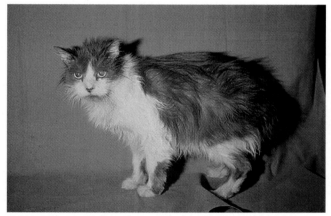

FIGURE 4–15. Feline Demodicosis. Generalized alopecic dermatitis caused the unkempt appearance of this cat's fur coat. (Courtesy of J. MacDonald)

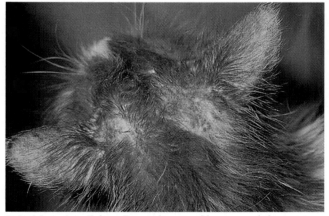

FIGURE 4–16. Feline Demodicosis. Close-up of the cat in Figure 4–15. Generalized alopecic, erythematous lesions on the head. (Courtesy of J. MacDonald)

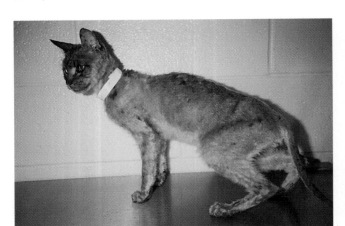

FIGURE 4–17. Feline Demodicosis. An adult cat with generalized alopecic dermatitis.

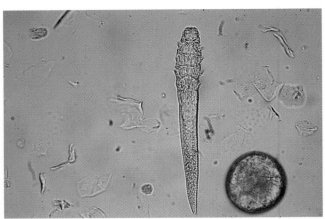

FIGURE 4–19. Feline Demodicosis. *D. cati* mite from a skin scraping. (Courtesy of J. MacDonald)

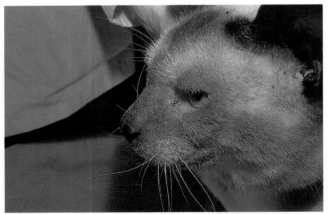

FIGURE 4–18. Feline Demodicosis. Close-up of the cat in Figure 4–17. Alopecia, erythema, and papular lesions on the face and head.

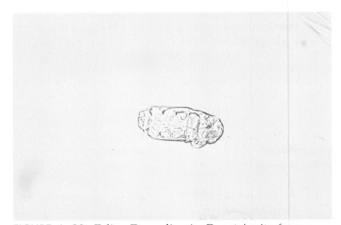

FIGURE 4–20. Feline Demodicosis. *D. gatoi* mite from a skin scraping.

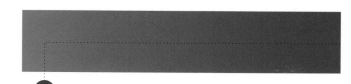

Canine Scabies (sarcoptic mange)
(Figs. 4–21 to 4–28)

FEATURES

A disease that is caused by *Sarcoptes scabiei* var. *canis,* a superficial burrowing skin mite. Mites secrete allergenic substances that elicit an intensely pruritic hypersensitivity reaction in sensitized dogs. Common in dogs. Affected dogs often have a previous history of being in an animal shelter, having contact with stray dogs, or visiting a grooming or boarding facility. In multiple-dog households, more than one dog is usually affected.

Nonseasonal intense pruritus that responds poorly to corticosteroids. Lesions include papules, alopecia, erythema, crusts, and excoriations. Initially, less hairy skin is involved—hocks, elbows, pinnal margins, and the ventral abdomen and chest. With chronicity, lesions may spread over the body, but the dorsum of the trunk is usually spared. Peripheral lymphadenomegaly is often present. Secondary weight loss and debility may occur. Heavily infested dogs may develop severe scaling and crusting. Some dogs may present with intense pruritus but no or minimal skin lesions. Although uncommon, asymptomatic carrier states are possible in dogs.

TOP DIFFERENTIALS

Hypersensitivity (flea bite, food, contact, atopy), pyoderma, *Malassezia* dermatitis.

DIAGNOSIS

1. Usually based on history, clinical findings, and response to scabicidal treatment.
2. Pinnal-pedal reflex—Rubbing ear margin between thumb and forefinger may elicit a scratch reflex. This reflex is highly suggestive but not pathognomonic for scabies.
3. Microscopy (superficial skin scrapings)—Detection of sarcoptic mites, nymphs, larvae, and/or ova. False-negative results are common because mites are extremely difficult to find.
4. Serology—Detection of antibodies against *Sarcoptes* antigens; at this writing, not available in the United States.
5. Dermatohistopathology (usually nondiagnostic)—Varying degrees of epidermal hyperplasia and superficial perivascular dermatitis with lymphocytes, mast cells, and eosinophils. Mite segments within stratum corneum are rarely found.

TREATMENT AND PROGNOSIS

1. Treat affected and all in-contact dogs with a scabicide.
2. Traditional therapy is to bathe dogs with an antiseborrheic shampoo to remove crusts, followed by a total body application of a topical scabicide q 7 days for at least 5 weeks. Effective topical products include:

   2–3% Lime sulfur solution.

   Organochlorines (gmma HCL, bromocyclen).

   Organophosphates (malathion, phosmet, mercaptomethyl phtalimide).

3. Alternative treatments include:

   Selamectin, 6–12 mg/kg, applied topically once or twice 1 month apart.

   0.025–0.03% Amitraz solution (5.3 ml Mitaban/gal water, 50 ml Ectodex/5 L water, or 13 ml Taktic/5 L water) applied to entire body three times at 2-week intervals.

   Fipronil spray, 6 ml/kg, applied to entire body three times at 2-week intervals.

   Ivermectin, 0.2–0.4 mg/kg SC, two or three times at 2-week intervals, or PO once weekly for 3–4 treatments.

   Milbemycin oxime, 0.75 mg/kg PO q 24 hours for 30 days or 2 mg/kg q 7 days for 21 days.

4. If animal is severely pruritic, prednisone, 0.5–1.0 mg/kg PO q 24 hours for the first 2–5 days of treatment, may be helpful.
5. For secondary pyoderma give appropriate systemic antibiotics for 3–4 weeks.
6. In kennel situations, dispose of beddings, and thoroughly clean and treat environment with parasiticidal sprays.
7. Prognosis is good. *S. scabei* is a highly contagious parasite of dogs that can also transiently infest humans and, rarely, cats.

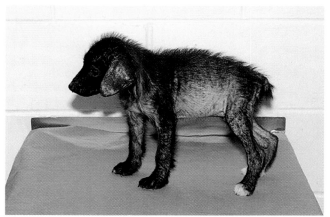

FIGURE 4–21. Canine Scabies. Generalized alopecia and crusts affecting a pruritic puppy. The alopecic ear pinnae is characteristic of scabies.

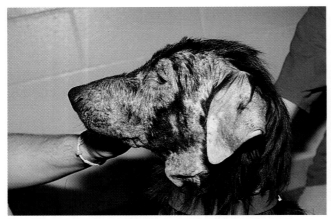

FIGURE 4–22. Canine Scabies. Generalized alopecia with a crusting papular dermatitis affecting the head and neck of a young adult dog. Note that the ear margins are severely affected.

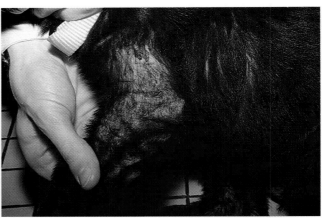

FIGURE 4–24. Canine Scabies. Alopecia and crusting papular dermatitis on the elbow are typical of scabies.

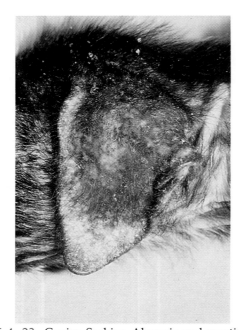

FIGURE 4–23. Canine Scabies. Alopecia and crusting dermatitis on the ear pinnae margin of this dog are characteristic of scabies.

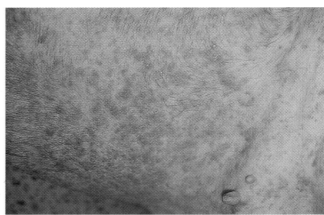

FIGURE 4–25. Canine Scabies. Generalized papular dermatitis affected almost the entire cutaneous surface of this dog.

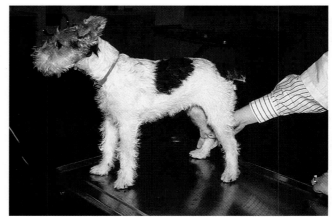

FIGURE 4–26. Canine Scabies. This pruritic 9-month-old fox terrier had no cutaneous lesions other than diffuse erythema.

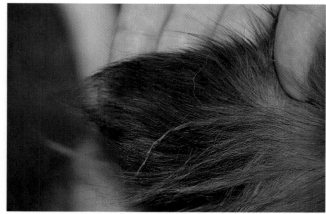

FIGURE 4–27. Canine Scabies. Focal alopecia on the ear margin of a diffusely pruritic dog.

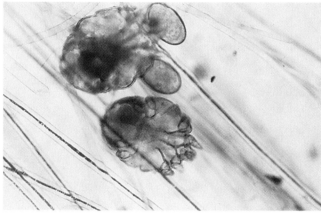

FIGURE 4–28. Canine Scabies. *Sarcoptes* mites and eggs from a skin scraping.

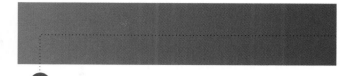

Feline Scabies (notoedric mange)
(Figs. 4–29 to 4–32)

FEATURES

A disease caused by *Notoedres cati*, a sarcoptic mite that burrows superficially in skin. In multiple-cat households and catteries, more than one cat is usually affected. Rare in cats.

Intensely pruritic, dry, crusted lesions usually first appear on the medial edges of ear pinnae and then spread rapidly over the ears, head, face, and neck. Lesions may subsequently spread to the feet and perineum. Infested skin becomes thickened, lichenified, alopecic, crusted, and/or excoriated. Peripheral lymphadenomegaly is common. If untreated, lesions may spread over large areas of the body, and anorexia, emaciation, and death may occur.

TOP DIFFERENTIALS

Ear mites, dermatophytosis, demodicosis, hypersensitivity (flea bite, food, atopy), autoimmune skin disorders.

DIAGNOSIS

1. Microscopy (superficial skin scrapings)—Detection of notoedric mites, nymphs, larvae, and/or ova.
2. Dermatohistopathology—Superficial perivascular or interstitial dermatitis with varying numbers of eosinophils and pronounced focal parakeratosis. Mite segments may be found in the superficial epidermis.

TREATMENT AND PROGNOSIS

1. Treat affected and all in-contact cats with a scabicide.
2. Traditional therapy is to clip hairs and then bathe with a mild antiseborrheic shampoo to loosen crusts, followed by a total body application of 2–3% lime sulfur solution q 7 days until follow-up skin scrapings are negative for mites and lesions have resolved (approximately 4–8 weeks).
3. Alternative therapies include:

   Doramectin, 0.2–0.3 mg/kg SC once.

   Ivermectin, 0.2–0.3 mg/kg PO or SC twice 2 weeks apart.

   0.015–0.025% Amitraz solution (2.5 ml Mitaban/gal water or 25 ml Ectodex/5 L water) applied to entire body q 7 days for 7–21 days.

4. Prognosis is good. *N. cati* is a highly contagious parasite of cats that can also transiently infest dogs, rabbits, and humans.

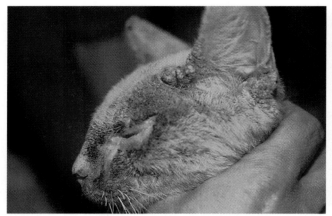

FIGURE 4–29. Feline Scabies. Severe alopecic, crusting, papular dermatitis affecting the entire head and neck of this adult cat. (Courtesy of G. Norsworthy)

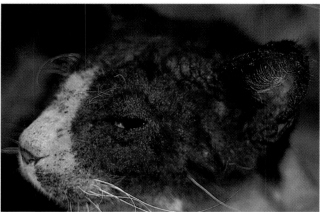

FIGURE 4–31. Feline Scabies. Generalized alopecia and crusting papular dermatitis on the head of an adult cat.

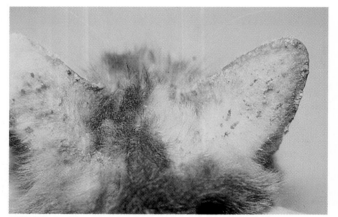

FIGURE 4–30. Feline Scabies. Close-up of the cat in Figure 4–29. Alopecia and crusting lesions on the head and ear pinnae. (Courtesy of G. Norsworthy)

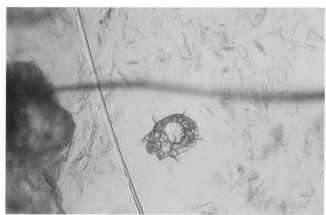

FIGURE 4–32. Feline Scabies. *N. cati* mite from a skin scraping. (Courtesy of G. Norsworthy)

Cheyletiellosis (walking dandruff)
(Figs. 4–33 to 4–36)

FEATURES

A skin disease that is caused by *Cheyletiella* mites which live on hair and fur, visiting the skin only to feed. All stages (larvae, nymphs, and adults) are parasitic. In a multiple-pet household, more than one animal is usually affected. Uncommon in dogs and cats. The most common symptom is excessive scaling (dandruff, scurf) which gives the haircoat a powdery or mealy appearance, especially over the dorsal midline of the back. Pruritus is usually minimal. Papular, crusting eruptions (cats) or scabies-like lesions (dogs) are present. Other adult pets (dogs, cats, rabbits) in the household may be asymptomatic carriers.

TOP DIFFERENTIALS

Other ectoparasites (pediculosis, scabies, demodicosis, hypersensitivities [atopy, food, flea bite]), and other causes of miliary dermatitis in cats.

DIAGNOSIS

1. Rule out other differentials.
2. Direct visualization of mites—Part haircoat along back over sacrum, comb out dandruff onto dark paper, and observe for movement of mites in debris (may be difficult to find).
3. Microscopy (superficial skin scrapings, acetate tape impressions, flea combed hairs and scales)—Detection of *Cheyletiella* mites, nymphs, larvae, and/or ova (may be difficult to find).
4. Dermatohistopathology (usually nondiagnostic)—Varying degrees of superficial perivascular dermatitis with few to many eosinophils. Mite segments in stratum corneum are rarely seen.

TREATMENT AND PROGNOSIS

1. Treat all affected and in-contact animals once weekly for 4 weeks with a topical parasiticidal dip, powder, spray, or shampoo.
2. Effective topical products for dogs include those containing 2–3% lime sulfur, pyrethrin, pyrethroid, carbamate, or an organophosphate.
3. Effective products for cats include those containing 2–3% lime sulfur or a pyrethrin.
4. Alternative treatments include:
   Ivermectin, 0.2–0.3 mg/kg PO or SC twice, 2–3 weeks apart.
   Fipronil spray, 6 ml/kg, or fipronil spot on, applied topically twice, one month apart.
5. Clean and treat environment with a flea insecticide.
6. Prognosis is good. *Cheyletiella* mites are highly contagious to cats, dogs, rabbits, and humans.

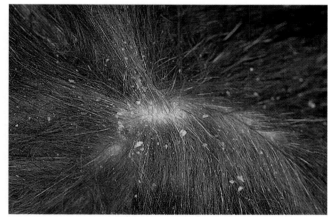

FIGURE 4–33. Cheyletiellosis. An unkempt fur coat in an adult cat.

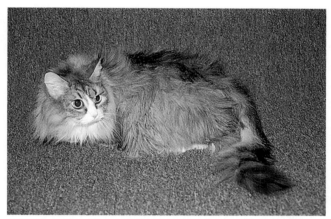

FIGURE 4–34. Cheyletiellosis. Close-up of the cat in Figure 4–33. Diffuse scaling and erythema are apparent upon close examination.

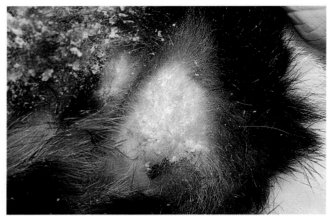

FIGURE 4–35. Cheyletiellosis. Alopecia with scale and crust.

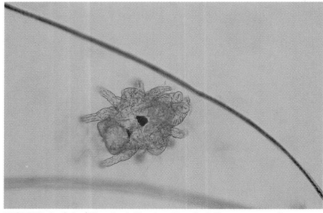

FIGURE 4–36. Cheyletiellosis. *Cheyletiella* sp. mite from a skin scraping. Note the hooked mouthparts used for piercing the skin.

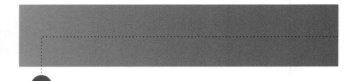

Ear Mites (*Otodectes cynotis*) (Figs. 4–37 to 4–40)

FEATURES

A disease that is caused by infestation with *Otodectes cynotis*, a psoroptic mite that lives on the surface of skin and in ear canals. Common in dogs and cats, with the highest incidence in kittens. Adult cats are often asymptomatic carriers.

Typically, there is a mild to marked accumulation of dark brown to black waxy or crusty exudate in the ear canals. The otic discharge becomes purulent if a secondary bacterial otitis develops. The ears are usually intensely pruritic, and scratching results in secondary alopecia and excoriations on the ears and head. Head shaking may result in aural hematomas. Occasionally ectopic mites may cause a pruritic, papular, crusting skin eruption, especially on the neck, rump, or tail (otodectic acariasis).

TOP DIFFERENTIALS

Other causes of otitis externa.

DIAGNOSIS

1. Otoscopy—Direct visualization of mites (moving white specks).
2. Positive pinnal-pedal reflex (cats)—Cat scratches with ipsilateral hind limb when ear canal is swabbed.
3. Microscopy (ear swabs, superficial skin scrapings)—Detection of *O. cynotis* mites, nymphs, larvae, and/or ova.

TREATMENT AND PROGNOSIS

1. Clean the ear canals of affected animals to remove accumulated debris.
2. Treat affected animals and all in-contact dogs and cats.
3. Traditional treatment is to instill a parasiticidal otic preparation at the dosage, frequency, and duration indicated on label instructions.
4. Other treatments effective against *Otodectes* include:

   Selamectin, 6–12 mg/kg, applied topically once or twice 1 month apart for cats and twice at a 1-month interval for dogs.

   Neomycin-thiabendazole-dexamethasone (Tresaderm), 0.125–0.25 ml AU q 12 hours for 2–3 weeks.

Gentamycin-clotrimazole-dexamethasone (Otomax), 0.125–0.25 ml AU q 12 hours for 2–3 weeks.

Fipronil (Frontline Flea Spray), 0.1–0.15 ml AU q 14 days for two or three treatments (based on anecdotal reports).

Ivermectin, 0.3 mg/kg PO q 7 days for three or four treatments or 0.3 mg/kg SC q 10–14 days for two or three treatments.

5. When otic treatments are used, they should be combined with body treatments to eliminate any ectopic mites. Apply to body a pyrethrin spray, powder, or dip once weekly for 4 weeks or use fipronil spray or spot on twice 2 weeks apart.

6. Prognosis is good. Ear mites are highly contagious to other cats and dogs. Rarely, humans may become transiently infested.

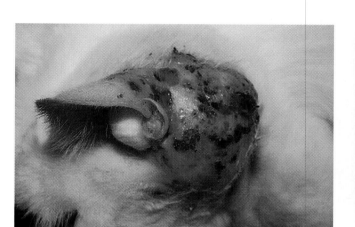

FIGURE 4–37. Ear Mites. Severe erosive, crusting lesions on a cat's ear caused by intense pruritus associated with an ear mite infection.

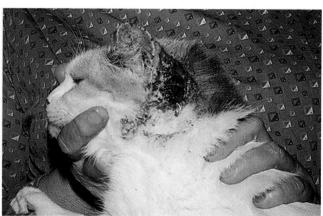

FIGURE 4–39. Ear Mites. Severe erosive, crusting dermatitis on the ears, neck, and head of a cat.

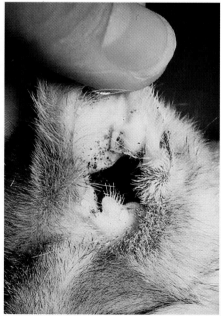

FIGURE 4–38. Ear Mites. Dark black otic exudate typical of an *Otodectes* infection. (Courtesy of E. Roberson)

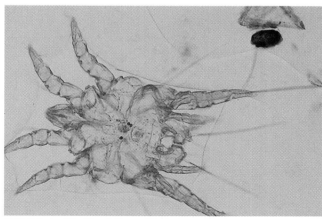

FIGURE 4–40. Ear Mites. *Otodectes* mite from an ear swab.

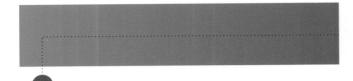

Trombiculiasis (chigger mites, harvest mites) (Figs. 4–41 to 4–44)

FEATURES

Adults and nymphs of the genera *Neotrombicula* (harvest mites) and *Eutrombicula* (chiggers) are found in habitats ranging from semidesert to swamp. They are free-living mites and are not parasitic. However, the larvae hatch from eggs laid in the soil and crawl up vegetation to attack avian and mammalian hosts that pass by. The skin disease they cause is seasonal (summer-fall) in temperate climates and year-round in warm regions. Rare to uncommon in dogs and cats.

Typically, intensely pruritic wheals, papules, and vesicles develop on skin that contacts ground (limbs, feet, head, ears, ventrum). Occasionally lesions are nonpruritic. Secondary scaling and alopecia may be present.

TOP DIFFERENTIALS

Superficial pyoderma, other ectoparasites (insect stings/bites, scabies, demodicosis, pelodera, hookworm dermatitis), contact dermatitis.

DIAGNOSIS

1. Microscopy (skin scrapings)—Intensely bright orange, ovoid trombiculid larvae (about 0.6 mm long). Sometimes only the mouthparts (stylostomes) are present (the rest of the mite having been removed by the animal's scratching).
2. Dermatohistopathology (usually nondiagnostic)— Superficial perivascular dermatitis with numerous eosinophils. Occasionally, mite stylostomes may be seen.

TREATMENT AND PROGNOSIS

1. Treat affected animal with one or two weekly applications of a parasiticidal dip and/or otic preparation. In dogs, Fipronil spray 6 ml/kg q 2–4 weeks may also be effective.
2. If pruritus is severe, give prednisone, 0.5 mg/kg (dogs) or 1.0 mg/kg (cats) PO q 12 hours for 2–3 days.
3. Give appropriate systemic antibiotics for 2–4 weeks if secondary pyoderma is present.
4. Keep pets away from areas known to harbor large numbers of mites.
5. Prognosis is good. Infested areas are a potential source of infection for other dogs, for cats, and for humans.

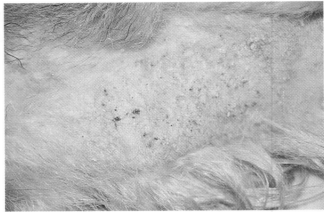

FIGURE 4–41. Trombiculiasis. Crusting papular lesions on the ventrum of an adult dog infected with chiggers.

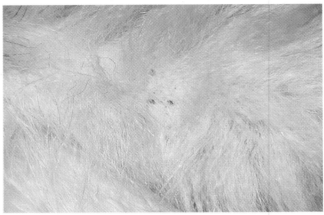

FIGURE 4–42. Trombiculiasis. Close-up of the dog in Figure 4–41. Multiple papular lesions on the ventrum.

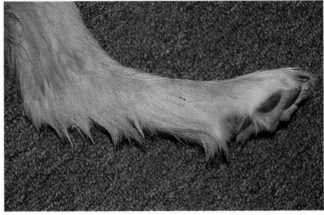

FIGURE 4–43. Trombiculiasis. Close-up of the dog in Figures 4–41 and 4–42. Alopecia and erythema on the distal rear leg.

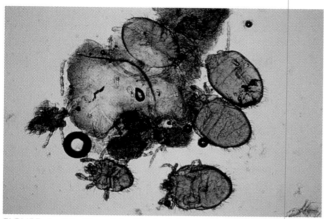

FIGURE 4–44. Trombiculiasis. Mites form a deep skin scrape. (Courtesy of R. Malik)

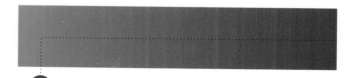

Cat Fur Mite (*Lynxacarus radosky*)
(Fig. 4–45)

FEATURES

A hair-clasping mite of cats primarily reported in Australia, Fiji, Hawaii, Puerto Rico, and Florida. Rare in cats.

Hordes of mites on hairs give the coat a salt and pepper or scurfy appearance, especially over the dorsum of the back. Widespread papular crusting eruptions may also be present. There is minimal pruritus.

TOP DIFFERENTIALS

Pediculosis, cheyletiellosis.

DIAGNOSIS

1. Microscopy (skin scrapings, acetate tape impressions)—fur mites are clasped to hairs.

TREATMENT AND PROGNOSIS

1. Treat all affected cats with pyrethrin dips or sprays or with 2% lime sulfur solution once a week for 4 weeks.
2. Alternative treatment is ivermectin, 0.3 mg/kg SQ twice 2 weeks apart.
3. Prognosis is good. The cat fur mite is moderately contagious to other cats and is not considered contagious to dogs, but it can cause a papular rash in humans.

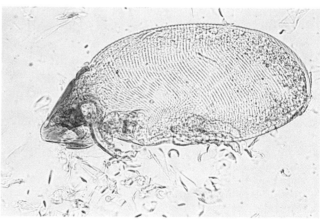

FIGURE 4–45. Cat Fur Mite. *L. radosky* mite from a skin scraping. (Courtesy of L. Messinger)

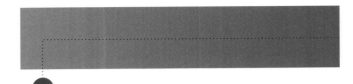

Fleas (Figs. 4–46 to 4–52)

FEATURES

Fleas are small, wingless, blood-sucking insects. Although more than 2000 species and subspecies exist worldwide, *Ctenocephalides felis* is the species most commonly associated with dogs and cats. In temperate climates, problems with fleas are usually restricted to warm weather months. In warmer climates, flea problems may be year round. Fleas are a common cause of skin disease in dogs and cats.

Dogs. Non-flea-allergic dogs may have no symptoms (asymptomatic carriers), be anemic, have tapeworms, show mild skin irritation, develop pyotraumatic dermatitis, and/or create acral lick dermatitis lesions. Flea-allergic dogs have pruritic, papular, crusting eruptions with secondary seborrhea, alopecia, excoriations, pyoderma, hyperpigmentation, and/or lichenification. The distribution of the lesions usually involves the caudodorsal lumbosacral area, dorsal tailhead, caudomedial thighs, abdomen, and/or flanks.

Cats. Non-flea-allergic cats may have no symptoms (asymptomatic carriers), be anemic, have tapeworms, or develop mild skin irritation. Flea-allergic cats often present with pruritic miliary dermatitis with variable secondary excoriations, crusting, and alopecia. The distribution of the lesions usually involves the head, neck, dorsal lumbosacral area, caudomedial thighs, and/or ventral abdomen. Other symptoms of fleas include a symmetrical alopecia that is secondary to excessive grooming and eosinophilic granuloma complex lesions.

TOP DIFFERENTIALS

Atopy, food hypersensitivity, scabies, cheyletiellosis, pyoderma, dermatophytosis, demodicosis, *Malassezia* dermatitis.

DIAGNOSIS

1. Usually based on history and clinical findings.
2. Visualization of fleas or flea excreta on body (may be difficult to find in flea-allergic animals).
3. Visualization of tapeworm segments (*Dipylidium* spp.) on body or in fecal flotation.
4. Allergy testing (intradermal, serologic)—Positive skin test reaction to flea antigen or positive serum IgE anti-flea antibody titer is highly suggestive of flea-allergic dermatitis, but false-negative results are possible.
5. Dermatohistopathology (nondiagnostic)—Varying degrees of superficial or deep perivascular to interstitial dermatitis, with eosinophils often predominating.
6. Response to flea treatment—Symptoms resolve.

TREATMENT AND PROGNOSIS

1. Strict flea eradication is the only effective treatment.
2. Treat affected and all in-contact dogs and cats with adulticidal flea sprays, spot-on solutions, or dips q 7–30 days, as instructed on label. Products containing fipronil or imidocloprid are especially efficacious when used every 3–4 weeks.
3. Insect growth regulators (lufenuron, pyriproxifen, methoprene) may be effective alone or in combination with adulticidal therapy.
4. Continue flea control therapy from spring until first snowfall in temperate areas and year round in warm climates.
5. In heavily flea-infested environments, treat areas where pets spend the most time. Treat indoor premises with an insecticide and an insect growth regulator (methoprene, pyriproxifen). Treat outdoor environment with insecticidal or biologic products designed for such use.
6. If pruritus is severe, give prednisone, 0.5 mg/kg (dogs) or 1.0 mg/kg (cats) q 12 hours for 3–7 days, then q 24 hours for 3–7 days, and then q 48 hours for 3–7 days. Or give cats methyprednisolone acetate, 20 mg/cat or 4 mg/kg SC once or twice 2–3 weeks apart.
7. For secondary pyoderma, give appropriate systemic antibiotics for at least 3–4 weeks.
8. Prognosis is good if strict flea control is practiced. Fleas are contagious to other animals and to humans.

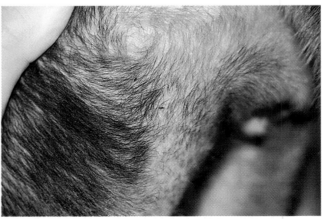

FIGURE 4–46. Fleas. Fleas on the caudal aspect of the rear leg of a dog.

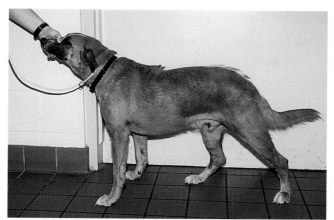

FIGURE 4–47. Fleas. Alopecia and hyperpigmentation on the lumbar region of a dog with flea allergy dermatitis.

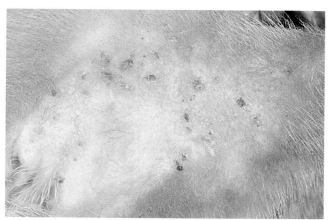

FIGURE 4–50. Fleas. Generalized alopecia with crusting papular lesions (miliary dermatitis) on the body of a flea-allergic cat.

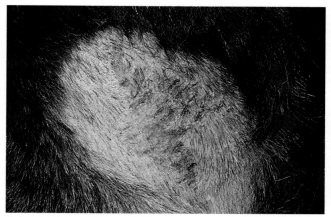

FIGURE 4–48. Fleas. Alopecia, erythema, and crusting associated with a healing hot spot (pyotraumatic dermatitis) caused by fleas.

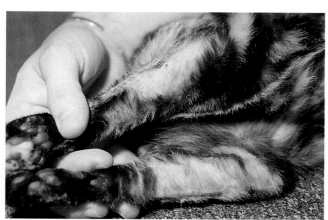

FIGURE 4–51. Fleas. Alopecia on the distal extremities of a flea-allergic cat.

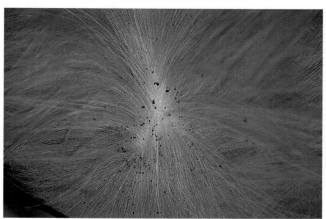

FIGURE 4–49. Fleas. Flea dirt (feces) on the skin of a cat.

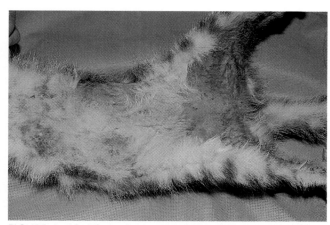

FIGURE 4–52. Fleas. An eosinophilic plaque on the abdomen of a flea-allergic cat. Note the similarity to food allergy and atopy.

Pediculosis (Figs. 4–53 to 4–56)

FEATURES

An infestation with host-specific sucking (*Linognathus setosus*—dog) or biting (*Trichodectes canis*—dog, *Felicola subrostratus*—cat) lice. Uncommon in dogs and cats, with the highest incidence in young, neglected, underfed animals.

Symptoms usually include restlessness and pruritus, with secondary seborrhea, alopecia, and/or excoriations. Thickly matted hairs, small papules and crusts, and, in severe infestations, anemia and debilitation may be present.

TOP DIFFERENTIALS

Fleas, scabies, cheyletiellosis, hypersensitivity (flea bite, food, atopy).

DIAGNOSIS

1. Direct visualization of lice (flea combing).
2. Microscopy (acetate tape impressions, hairs)—Detection of lice and nits (ova).

TREATMENT AND PROGNOSIS

1. Treat affected and all in-contact same-species animals.
2. Clip away matted hairs.
3. Treat entire body with 2% lime sulfur, pyrethrin, pyrethroid (dogs only), carbaryl, or organophosphate (dogs only) shampoo, powder, spray or dip twice, 2 weeks apart.

4. An alternative treatment is to give ivermectin, 0.2 mg/kg SC twice, 2 weeks apart. Alternatively, fipronil spray 6 ml/kg, fipronil spot on, or imidocloprid spot on are usually effective when used once or twice at one month intervals.
5. Severely anemic animals may require blood transfusions and good nursing care.
6. Clean bedding, grooming tools, and environment at least once.
7. Prophylactically using insecticidal flea collars may prevent exposed animals from infestation.
8. Prognosis is good. Lice are highly contagious from dog to dog and from cat to cat but are not considered contagious from dogs or cats to humans.

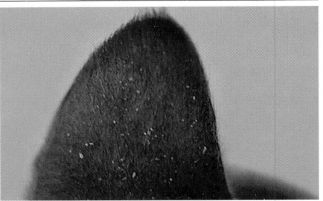

FIGURE 4–54. Pediculosis. Nits attached to the hair on the ear pinnae associated with a *T. canis* infection.

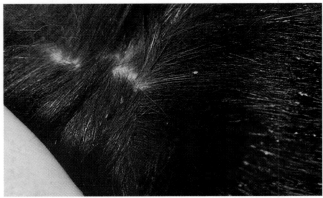

FIGURE 4–55. Pediculosis. The lice are more clearly visible on the black fur. (Courtesy of D. Angarano)

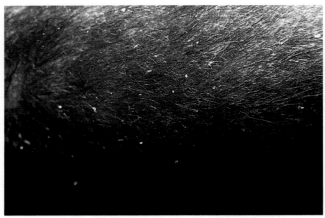

FIGURE 4–53. Pediculosis. These white specks on the trunk of this dog are a combination of scale, lice, and nits associated with a *T. canis* infection.

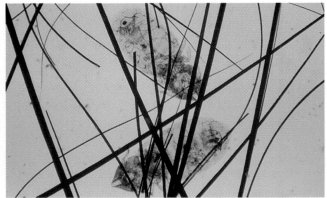

FIGURE 4–56. Pediculosis. Biting lice. (Courtesy of D. Angarano)

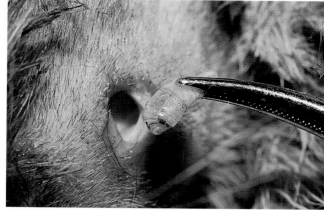

FIGURE 4–58. Cuterebra. Close-up of the cat in Figure 4–57. The cuterebra has been removed with hemostats. The lesion consists of a fibrosed tunnel with a purulent exudate.

Cuterebra (Figs. 4–57 to 4–60)

FEATURES

Cuterebra flies lay their eggs near rabbit runs and rodent burrows. Hatched larvae crawl into the fur of a mammalian host, enter the host through a natural body opening, and migrate to a subcutaneous site. The normal hosts are rabbits, squirrels, chipmunks, and mice. Uncommon in dogs and cats, with the highest incidence of disease during late summer and fall.

A solitary, 1 cm diameter, nonpainful subcutaneous swelling that fistulates (larva's breathing hole). The lesion is usually located on the head, neck, or trunk. Rarely, larvae migrate aberrantly to the brain, pharynx, nostrils, or other atypical sites.

TOP DIFFERENTIALS

Subcutaneous abscess, dracunculiasis.

DIAGNOSIS

1. Direct visualization of *Cuterebra* larva within lesion—a white, cream, brown, or black larva with stout black spines covering its body.

TREATMENT AND PROGNOSIS

1. Gently enlarge breathing hole and carefully extract larva with forceps.
2. Perform daily routine wound care.
3. If secondary bacterial infection is suspected, give appropriate systemic antibiotics for 10–14 days.
4. Prognosis is good, but wound tends to heal slowly. It is not contagious from dogs or cats to other animals or to humans.

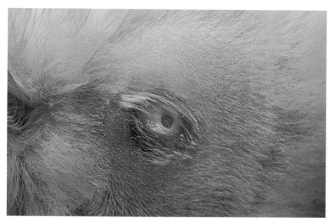

FIGURE 4–59. Cuterebra. Erythema and fibrosis surround the cuterebra's breathing hole on the body of this young cat.

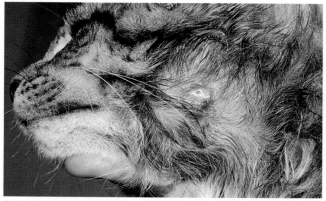

FIGURE 4–57. Cuterebra. Erythema and fibrosis surround the cuterebra's breathing hole on the neck of this adult cat. A purulent exudate is common.

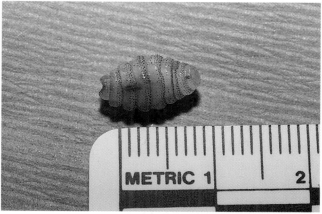

FIGURE 4–60. Cuterebra. The cuterebra has been removed and placed on a centimeter ruler.

Fly Bite Dermatitis (Figs. 4–61 to 4–64)

FEATURES

Lesions are caused by biting flies. Common in dogs housed outdoors. Lesions include erythema and hemorrhagic crusts overlying erosions or ulcers at or near the ear tips. Similar lesions may occasionally occur on the face. Lesions are mildly to intensely pruritic.

TOP DIFFERENTIALS

Scabies, vasculitis, autoimmune skin disorders.

DIAGNOSIS

1. Usually based on history, clinical findings, and ruling out other differentials.
2. Response to treatment—Lesions resolve with fly control.

TREATMENT AND PROGNOSIS

1. Apply topical antibiotic-steroid cream or ointment to lesions q 12 hours, and keep dog indoors until lesions have healed.
2. Apply fly repellant, fly spray, or flea spray daily to affected skin as a preventive measure.
3. Identify the sources of flies and spray these areas with insecticide.
4. Prognosis is good if repeated attacks by flies can be prevented.

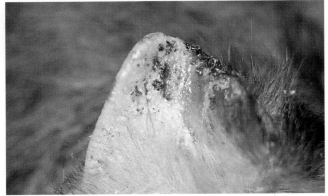

FIGURE 4–62. Fly Bite Dermatitis. Alopecia, crusting, and serosanguineous exudate on the ear tip of a dog.

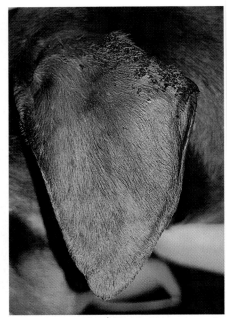

FIGURE 4–63. Fly Bite Dermatitis. Alopecia and crusting on the ear fold of a floppy-eared dog. The fly bite lesions were on the most dorsal aspect of the ear.

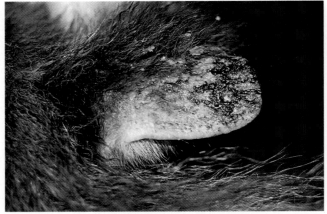

FIGURE 4–61. Fly Bite Dermatitis. Alopecia and crusting on the ear tip of a dog.

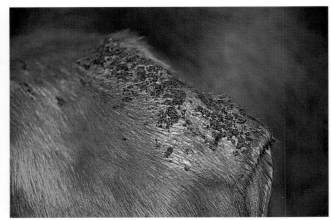

FIGURE 4–64. Fly Bite Dermatitis. Close-up of the dog in Figure 4–63. Alopecia and crusting on the dorsal ear fold.

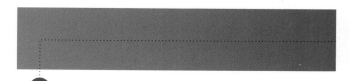

Myiasis (Figs. 4–65 and 4–66)

FEATURES

An infestation of living animals with dipteran fly larvae. Fly eggs, laid on moist skin or in wounds, hatch into larvae (maggots) that secrete proteolytic enzymes and digest cutaneous tissue. Common in cats and dogs, especially in animals that are weakened, have urine-soaked skin, and/or are paretic.

The lesions are crateriform to irregularly shaped ulcers that are most often found around the nose, eyes, anus, genitalia, or neglected wounds. Maggots are found on skin and inside lesions.

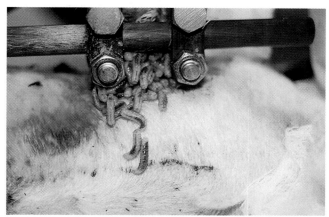

FIGURE 4–65. Myiasis. Maggots on the skin and hair of a dog with an external fixator. The limb had remained bandaged for 2 weeks on this dog living outside.

DIAGNOSIS

1. Direct visualization of maggots on skin, on hair, and in lesions.

TREATMENT AND PROGNOSIS

1. Address and correct the underlying conditions.
2. Clip and clean lesions to remove maggots.
3. Judiciously apply a pyrethrin or pyrethroid (dogs only) containing spray to lesions to kill remaining maggots. Too vigorous an application could kill a debilitated animal.
4. If animal's overall condition is stable, surgically debride wounds and follow with routine daily wound care.
5. House animal in screened, fly-free quarters.
6. Prognosis is good to guarded, depending on the predisposing factors.

FIGURE 4–66. Myiasis. Close-up of the dog in Figure 4–65. The maggots are surging out of the external fixator wound.

Hookworm Dermatitis
(ancylostomiasis and uncinariasis)
(Figs. 4–67 and 4–68)

FEATURES

A skin reaction at sites of percutaneous larval penetration in dogs previously sensitized to hookworms. The disease is caused by *Ancylostoma* in the tropics and warm temperate areas and by *Uncinaria* in temperate and subarctic areas. Uncommon to rare in dogs, with the highest incidence in dogs housed or exercised in contaminated environments such as damp kennels with cracked and porous floors or grass and dirt runs.

Lesions are characterized by mildly to intensely pruritic, papular eruptions interdigitally and on other skin areas that frequently contact the ground. Affected skin becomes uniformly erythematous, alopecic, and thickened. The feet often become swollen, hot, and painful.

TOP DIFFERENTIALS

Bacterial pododermatitis, demodicosis, dermatophytosis, hypersensitivity (food, contact, atopy), pelodera dermatitis.

DIAGNOSIS

1. Rule out other differentials.
2. Fecal flotation—Detection of hookworm ova.
3. Dermatohistopathology (rarely diagnostic)—Varying degrees of perivascular dermatitis with eosinophils and neutrophils. Larvae are rarely found but, if present, are surrounded by neutrophils, eosinophils, and mononuclear cells.
4. Response to treatment—Lesions resolve following anthelmintic therapy.

TREATMENT AND PROGNOSIS

1. Treat affected and all in-contact dogs with an anthelmintic such as fenbendazole, mebendazole, or pyrantel pamoate twice, 3–4 weeks apart.
2. Institute system of regular anthelmintic therapy for all dogs.
3. Improve environmental sanitation with frequent removal of feces and soiled bedding. Provide dry, nonporous kennel floors and runs.
4. Periodically treating dirt or graveled runs with sodium borate, 0.5 kg/m^2 (10 lb/100 ft^2), may be helpful but will kill grass.
5. Prognosis is good. A contaminated environment is a potential source of infection for other dogs and for humans.

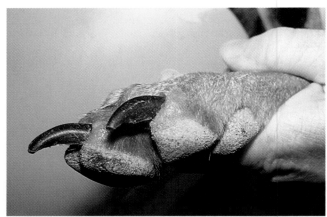

FIGURE 4–67. Hookworm Dermatitis. Alopecia and erythema with foot pad hyperkeratosis on the foot of a dog. (Courtesy of the University of Florida; case material)

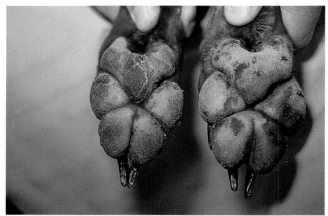

FIGURE 4–68. Hookworm Dermatitis. Close-up of the dog in Figure 4–67. Hyperkeratosis and erythema of the footpads. (Courtesy of the University of Florida; case material)

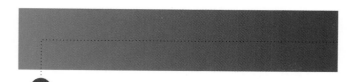

Pelodera Dermatitis (rhabditic dermatitis) (Figs. 4–69 to 4–72)

FEATURES

A cutaneous infestation with larvae of *Pelodera strongyloides*, a free-living nematode found in damp soil, decaying organic debris, straw bedding, and marsh hay. Uncommon in dogs.

There is mild to intense pruritus, with erythema, alopecia, papules, crusts, and scales on areas that contact the ground (feet, legs, ventrum, perineum, underside of the tail). Secondary pyoderma may be present.

TOP DIFFERENTIALS

Hookworm dermatitis, scabies, contact dermatitis, demodicosis, dermatophytosis, superficial pyoderma.

DIAGNOSIS

1. Microscopy (deep skin scrapings)—Detection of small, motile nematode larvae (65 μm long).
2. Dermatohistopathology—Varying degrees of perifolliculitis, folliculitis, and furunculosis with numerous eosinophils. Nematode segments are seen in hair follicles and within dermal pyogranulomas.

TREATMENT AND PROGNOSIS

1. Identify and remove the environmental source of contamination.
2. Replace all bedding, and wash down and spray kennels and cages with malathion or diazinon.
3. Bathe affected dogs to loosen crusts, and apply a scabicidal dip to entire body once weekly for 2 weeks.
4. If pruritus is severe, give prednisone, 0.5 mg/kg PO q 12–24 hours for 2–5 days.
5. For secondary pyoderma, give appropriate systemic antibiotics for 2–3 weeks.
6. Prognosis is good. Contaminated environment is a potential source of infection for other dogs and for humans.

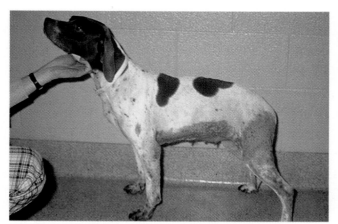

FIGURE 4–69. Pelodera Dermatitis. Alopecia and erythema on the ventrum of an adult dog. (Courtesy of J. MacDonald)

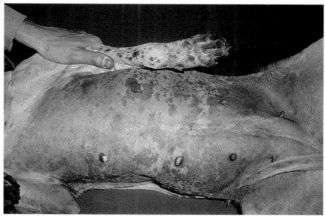

FIGURE 4–70. Pelodera Dermatitis. Close-up of the dog in Figure 4–69. Alopecia and erythema on the ventrum. (Courtesy of J. MacDonald)

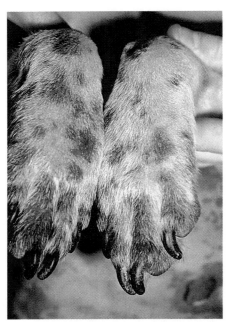

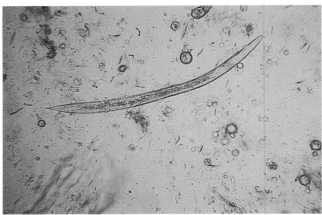

FIGURE 4–72. Pelodera Dermatitis. *P. strongyloides* from a skin scraping. (Courtesy of J. MacDonald)

FIGURE 4–71. Pelodera Dermatitis. Close-up of the dog in Figures 4–69 and 4–70. Alopecia and erythema on the distal extremities. (Courtesy of J. MacDonald)

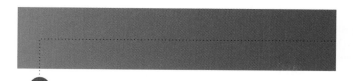

Dracunculiasis (Figs. 4–73 and 4–74)

FEATURES

A skin disease that is caused by species of *Dracunculus*, a nematode that parasitizes subcutaneous tissues. Infection occurs when the mammalian host ingests an infected microscopic crustacean (intermediate host) while drinking contaminated water. In North America, *D. insignis* primarily parasitizes raccoons, mink, and other wild mammals, with infections in dogs and cats occurring uncommonly. In North Africa and India, *D. medinensis* infects many mammals, including dogs, horses, cattle, and humans.

Lesions are painful or pruritic, chronic, single or multiple subcutaneous nodules on the legs, head, or abdomen that eventually fistulate (through which female worms are stimulated to discharge their larvae when the skin contacts water).

TOP DIFFERENTIALS

Cuterebra, bacterial or fungal infection, and neoplasia.

DIAGNOSIS

1. Cytology (fistulous exudate)—Eosinophils, neutrophils, macrophages, and 500 μm long nematode larvae that have tapered tails.
2. Dermatohistopathology—Pseudocyst containing adult and larval nematodes surrounded by eosinophilic pyogranulomatous inflammation.

TREATMENT AND PROGNOSIS

1. Surgically excise nodules.
2. Decontaminate water supplies.
3. Prognosis is good. Dracunculiasis is contagious to other animals and humans via animal-crustacean-animal transmission.

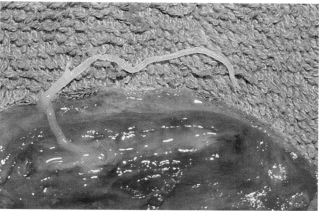

FIGURE 4–73. Dracunculiasis. The worm has been removed from the excised tissue. (Courtesy of A. Yu)

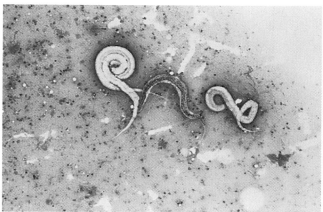

FIGURE 4–74. Dracunculiasis. *Dracunculus* sp. larvae cytology from a tissue imprint. (Courtesy of A. Yu)

Suggested Readings

Bowman DD. 1999. Georgis' Parasitology for Veterinarians. Ed. 7. W.B. Saunders, Philadelphia, PA.

Chadwick A. 1997. Use of a 0.25 Per Cent Fipronil Pump Spray Formulation to Treat Canine Cheyletiellosis. JSAP. 38: 261–262.

Chesney CJ. 1999. Short Form of *Demodex* Species Mite in the Dog: Occurrence and Measurements. J Sm Ani Pract. 40: 58–59.

Delucchi L and Castro E. 2000. Use of Doramectin for Treatment of Notoedric Mange in Five Cats. JAVMA. 216: 215–216.

Miller WH. 1995. Treatment of Generalized Demodicosis in Dogs, pp. 625–627. In Bonagura JD (ed). Kirk's Current Veterinary Therapy, XII, Small Animal Practice. W.B. Saunders, Philadelphia, PA.

Parasitic Skin Diseases, pp. 392–468. In Scott DW, Miller WH Jr, and Griffin CE. 1995. Muller & Kirk's Small Animal Dermatology. Ed. 5. W.B. Saunders, Philadelphia, PA.

Plumb DC. 1999. Veterinary Drug Handbook. Ed. 3. Iowa State University Press, Ames, IA.

5

Viral, Rickettsial, and Protozoal Skin Diseases

- **Canine Distemper**
- **Canine Papillomavirus**
- **Feline Rhinotracheitis Virus** (feline herpesvirus-1)
- **Feline Calicivirus**
- **Feline Cowpox**
- **Feline Papillomavirus**
- **Rocky Mountain Spotted Fever** (RMSF)
- **Canine Ehrlichiosis**
- **Leishmaniasis**

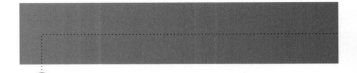

Canine Distemper (Figs. 5–1 and 5–2)

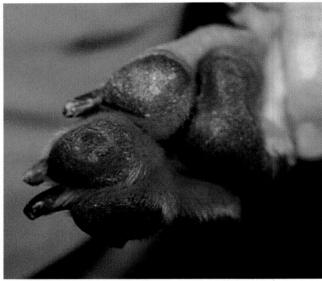

FIGURE 5–1. Canine Distemper. Hyperkeratosis and crusting of the footpads. (Courtesy of C. Greene)

FEATURES

Distemper is caused by a morbillivirus that is related to the measles and rinderpest viruses. Common in dogs, with the highest incidence in young, unvaccinated puppies.

Some affected dogs develop mild to severe nasal and digital hyperkeratosis (hard pad disease). More common symptoms include a pustular dermatitis resembling impetigo, depression, anorexia, fever, bilateral serous to mucopurulent ocular discharge, conjunctivitis, cough, dyspnea, diarrhea, and/or neurologic signs.

TOP DIFFERENTIALS

Other causes of nasodigital hyperkeratosis such as familial footpad hyperkeratosis, autoimmune skin disorders, zinc-responsive dermatosis, necrolytic migratory erythema, hypothyroidism, and idiopathic nasodigital hyperkeratosis. Other causes of pustular dermatitis such as impetigo, superficial pyoderma, and demodicosis.

DIAGNOSIS

1. Rule out other differentials.
2. Immunocytology (conjunctival scrapings, cerebrospinal fluid [CSF], blood smears)—Detection of distemper antigen.
3. Dermatohistopathology (affected footpads)—Marked orthokeratotic hyperkeratosis and mild to diffuse vacuolation of stratum spinosum with intracytoplasmic eosinophilic viral inclusion bodies.
4. Immunofluorescence or immunohistochemistry (biopsy specimens)—Detection of distemper antigen.

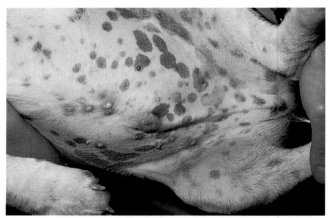

FIGURE 5–2. Canine Distemper. Multiple papules and pustules on the abdomen of a puppy. (Courtesy of C. Greene)

TREATMENT AND PROGNOSIS

1. No specific antiviral treatment is available.
2. Give supportive care and oral or parenteral broad-spectrum antibiotics to prevent secondary bacterial infections.
3. Prognosis is poor for dogs with nasodigital hyperkeratosis. Canine distemper is contagious to other dogs, but not to cats or to humans.

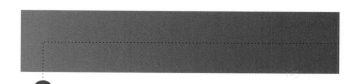

Canine Papillomavirus (Figs. 5–3 to 5–6)

FEATURES

Canine viral papillomatosis is caused by site-specific papillomaviruses that produce benign oral, ocular, or cutaneous warts. Cutaneous and ocular papillomas are rare in dogs. Oral papillomas are uncommon, with the highest incidence in dogs <1 year old. Concurrent immunosuppressive disease or use of immunosuppressive drugs may be a predisposing factor for oral papillomatosis, especially in adult-onset cases.

Oral papillomas • A few to multiple growths on oral mucosa, lips, palate, pharynx, epiglottis, and/or tongue. Lesions, which may be a few millimeters to 1 cm in diameter, begin as small, white, smooth nodules that often develop into gray, pedunculated, cauliflower-like masses. The masses eventually become pigmented and shrunken (regressing lesions). Growths typically persist for 1–5 months before regressing and are often asymptomatic. Multiple or large lesions may cause halitosis, ptyalism, dysphagia, or other signs of oral discomfort.

Ocular papillomas • Warts develop on conjunctivae, cornea, or eyelid margins.

Cutaneous papillomas • Solitary wart, plaque, or horn that can be anywhere on the body but is most common on the lower extremities, interdigitally, or on footpads.

TOP DIFFERENTIALS

Noninfectious papillomas, transmissible venereal tumor, squamous cell carcinoma, epuli.

DIAGNOSIS

1. Dermatohistopathology—Papillomatous epidermal hyperkeratosis and hyperplasia with large keratohyalin granules and koilocytes (large, pale, vacuolated keratinocytes). Basophilic intranuclear inclusion bodies within keratinocytes may be seen.
2. Immunohistochemistry (biopsy specimens)—Detection of intranuclear papillomavirus antigens in upper-layer keratinocytes.

TREATMENT AND PROGNOSIS

1. Identify and correct any underlying cause of immunosuppression.
2. Most oral papillomas do not require treatment because spontaneous regression is typical and usually begins 1–2 months after diagnosis. Occasionally, lesions persist for 6–24 months or longer before regressing.
3. For persistent oral lesions, surgically removing, freezing, or crushing 5–15 tumors may induce spontaneous regression.
4. Anecedotal reports suggest that interferon alpha, 1.0–1.5 million U/m^2 SC three times per week, continued 1 week beyond the time of clinical remission (approximately 4–8 weeks), may be effective for refractory oral papillomas.
5. Autogenous wart vaccines are usually not effective.
6. For ocular and cutaneous papillomas, surgical removal is the treatment of choice.
7. Prognosis is good, with lifelong immunity accompanying spontaneous regression. Canine viral papillomatosis is contagious to other dogs, but not to cats or to humans.

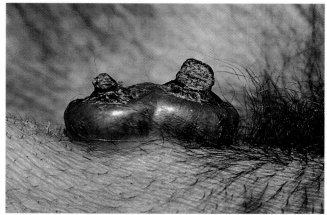

FIGURE 5–3. Canine Papillomavirus. Cutaneous horns are protruding from the papillomas on the abdomen of this 6-month-old dog.

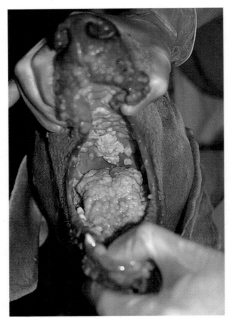

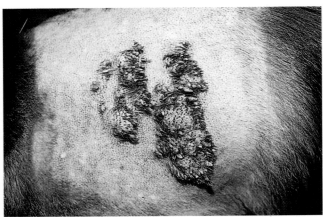

FIGURE 5–6. Canine Papillomavirus. A large papillomatous plaque on the lateral thorax of a German shepherd.

FIGURE 5–4. Canine Papillomavirus. Multiple oral papillomas have coalesced into large plaques on the tongue and hard palate of a 7-month-old weimaraer.

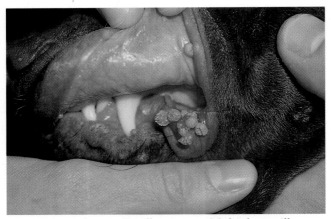

FIGURE 5–5. Canine Papillomavirus. Multiple papillomas on the lips of a young dog.

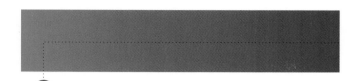

Feline Rhinotracheitis Virus

(feline herpesvirus-1) (Fig. 5–7)

FEATURES

An upper respiratory disease caused by a herpesvirus. Worldwide and common in cats, with the highest incidence in boarding facilities, catteries, and shelters. Oral and/or superficial skin ulcers on the face, trunk, and footpads can occur but are rare. Cats usually develop a severe upper respiratory disease characterized by depression, fever, anorexia, marked sneezing, conjunctivitis, and a copious serous to mucopurulent ocular and nasal discharge, with crusting of external nares and eyelids. Ulcerative or interstitial keratitis may be seen.

TOP DIFFERENTIALS

Other causes of upper respiratory disease such as feline calicivirus, *Bordetella*, *Chlamydia*, and *Mycoplasma*.

DIAGNOSIS

1. Usually based on history and clinical findings.
2. Viral isolation (oropharyngeal swabs)—Herpes virus.
3. Fluorescent antibody or polymerase chain reaction techniques (conjunctival smears)—Detection of rhinotracheitis viral antigen.
4. Dermatohistopathology—Ulcerative dermatitis with mixed inflammation. Epidermal cells may contain basophilic intranuclear inclusion bodies.

TREATMENT AND PROGNOSIS

1. No specific treatment is available.
2. Give good nursing care and broad-spectrum systemic and/or ophthalmic antibiotics to control secondary bacterial infections.
3. For refractory ulcerative keratitis, topical antiviral eye drops may be helpful.
4. Anecdotal reports suggest that antiviral medications such as interferon, 30 U PO q 24 hours on a week on–week off schedule, and/or lysine, 200–400 mg/cat PO daily, may decrease clinical signs. Continue treatment until response is seen.
5. Prognosis is usually good, with most cats recovering in 10–20 days. Some cats harbor latent infection, which may recrudesce with stress or immunosuppression. Feline rhinotracheitis virus is contagious to other cats, but not to dogs or to humans.

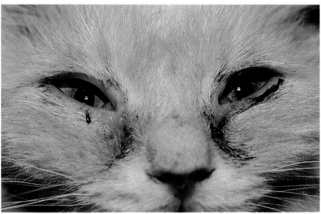

FIGURE 5–7. Rhinotracheitis Virus. Ocular discharge and superficial erosions on the eyelids of a young cat.

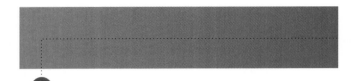

Feline Calicivirus (Fig. 5–8)

FEATURES

An upper respiratory disease caused by a small, unenveloped RNA virus. Common in cats, especially those in boarding facilities, catteries, and shelters.

Oral ulcers are common and may be the only clinical sign. Ulcers typically involve the tongue but can be anywhere in the mouth, on the lips, or on the nose. Ulcers elsewhere on the body are rare. Other symptoms include depression, fever, mild sneezing, conjunctivitis, and oculonasal discharge.

TOP DIFFERENTIALS

Other causes of upper respiratory disease such as feline rhinotracheitis virus, *Bordetella, Chlamydia,* and *Mycoplasma.*

DIAGNOSIS

1. Usually based on history and clinical findings.
2. Viral isolation (oropharyngeal swabs)—Calicivirus.
3. Fluorescent antibody testing (conjunctival smears)—Detection of caliciviral antigen.

TREATMENT AND PROGNOSIS

1. No specific treatment is available.
2. Give good nursing care and broad-spectrum systemic antibiotics to control secondary bacterial infections.
3. Prognosis is usually good. Feline calicivirus is contagious to other cats, but not to dogs or to humans.

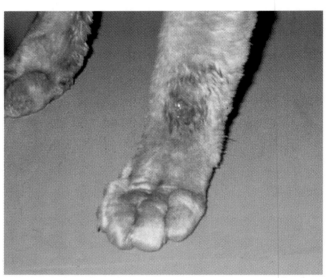

FIGURE 5–8. Feline Calicivirus. Ulcerations on the foreleg of a cat. (Courtesy of R. Malik)

Feline Cowpox (Figs. 5–9 and 5–10)

FEATURES

A poxvirus infection that is primarily seen in Europe and Asia. Uncommon in cats, with the highest incidence in rural cats that hunt rodents (reservoir host).

The initial lesion is a bite wound, usually on the head, neck, or forelimb. It is followed 1–3 weeks later by the development of widespread, randomly distributed macules and papules that enlarge into 1 cm diameter nodules. The nodules ulcerate, scab over, and gradually dry and exfoliate 4–5 weeks later. The lesions may be pruritic. Some cats have oral vesicles and ulcers. Affected cats are usually not systemically ill unless concurrent immunosuppressive disease is present.

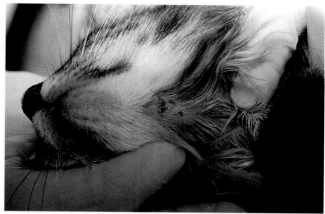

FIGURE 5–9. Feline Cowpox. Multiple crusting papular lesions on the ventral neck of a cat. (Courtesy of M. Austel)

TOP DIFFERENTIALS

Bacterial and fungal infections, eosinophilic granulomas, neoplasia.

DIAGNOSIS

1. Dermatohistopathology—Epidermal hyperplasia, ballooning and reticular degeneration, microvesicles, and necrosis with keratinocytic intracytoplasmic eosinophilic inclusion bodies.
2. Serology—Detection of antibodies against cowpox.
3. Viral isolation (from dry, scabbed material)—Feline cowpox.

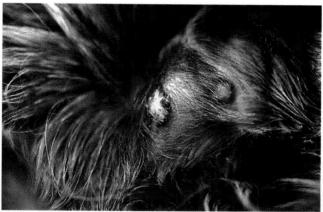

FIGURE 5–10. Feline Cowpox. Multiple papular lesions on the trunk. (Courtesy of M. Austel)

TREATMENT AND PROGNOSIS

1. No specific treatment is available.
2. Give broad-spectrum systemic antibiotics to prevent secondary bacterial infections.
3. Glucocorticosteroids are contraindicated.
4. Prognosis is good, but healed lesions may remain permanently alopecic. Infected cats are potentially contagious to other cats and to humans. However, the risk of direct transmission from cats to humans is small if basic hygienic precautions are taken.

Feline Papillomavirus (Figs. 5–11 and 5–12)

FEATURES

Feline papillomatosis is caused by a species-specific papillomavirus. Rare in cats, with the highest incidence in FIV-infected cats and cats receiving immunosuppressive therapy.

Viral papillomas are multiple, white or pigmented, slightly raised plaques several millimeters in diameter wide with rough, scaly, and/or greasy surfaces. Lesions are most common on the head, neck, and trunk.

TOP DIFFERENTIALS

Noninfectious papillomas, neoplasia.

DIAGNOSIS

1. Dermatohistopathology—Hyperkeratotic and hyperplastic epidermal plaques with koilocytes (large, pale, vacuolated keratinocytes). Intranuclear inclusion bodies within keratinocytes may be seen.
2. Immunohistochemistry (biopsy specimens)—Detection of intranuclear papillomavirus antigen in upper-layer keratinocytes.

TREATMENT AND PROGNOSIS

1. Most papillomas do not require treatment because spontaneous regression usually occurs.
2. Alternatively, anecdotal accounts report that the use of interferon alpha, 1.0–1.5 million U/m^2 SC three times per week, continued 1 week beyond clinical remission (approximately 4–8 weeks), has been successful.
3. Prognosis is usually good, although this virus has been associated with the development of multicentric squamous cell carcinoma in situ (Bowen's disease) in some cats. Feline papillomavirus is contagious to other cats, but not to dogs or to humans.

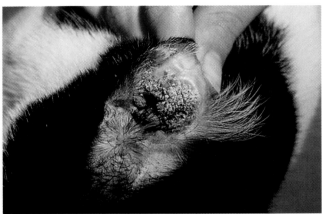

FIGURE 5–11. Feline Papillomavirus. Multiple papillomas formed a plaque on the ear of this cat. (Courtesy of A. Yu)

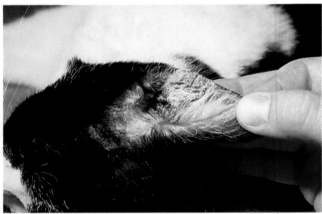

FIGURE 5–12. Feline Papillomavirus. Close-up of the cat in Figure 5–11. The raised surface of the papillomatous plaque is apparent. (Courtesy of A. Yu)

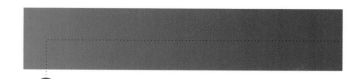

Rocky Mountain Spotted Fever (RMSF) (Figs. 5–13 and 5–14)

FEATURES

A tick-borne infection caused by *Rickettsia rickettsii*. Rickettsiae enter the circulatory system through tick bites, disseminate to various organs, and cause vascular damage by replicating in the endothelial cells of small vessels. The disease occurs in endemic areas of North America, Mexico, and Central and South America. It is most prevalent during warm months (March–October in the United States). Common in dogs living in endemic areas, with the highest incidence in young purebred dogs.

If skin lesions are present, they are characterized by edema, erythema, and sometimes ulceration and necrosis of the lips, scrotum, penile sheath, ear pinnae, extremities and, rarely, the ventral abdomen. Discrete, clear vesicles and focal, erythematous macules may appear on the buccal mucosae. Petechial and ecchymotic hemorrhages may develop on oral, genital, and ocular mucosae. Other symptoms include fever, anorexia, lethargy, peripheral lymphadenomegaly, and neurologic dysfunction (vestibular disease, seizures, coma). Occasionally there is melena, epistaxis, or hematuria.

TOP DIFFERENTIALS

Other causes of vasculitis such as other infectious agents, immune-mediated disorders, and exposure to toxins.

DIAGNOSIS

1. Hemogram—Mild to marked thrombocytopenia.
2. Dermatohistopathology—Necrotizing neutrophilic vasculitis and thrombosis.
3. Serology—Markedly elevated IgM anti-RMSF antibody titer in single serum sample or fourfold increase in IgG anti-RMSF antibody titer in paired sera taken 1–3 weeks apart.
4. Direct immunofluorescent or immunoperoxidase staining (skin biopsies of early lesions)—Detection of *Rickettsia* antigen in vascular endothelium.

TREATMENT AND PROGNOSIS

1. Remove any attached ticks.
2. The treatment of choice is either tetracycline, 22–30 mg/kg PO or IV q 8 hours, or doxycycline, 5–10 mg/kg PO or IV q 12 hours for 1–2 weeks.
3. Alternative treatments include:

Chloramphenicol (pregnant dogs or puppies <6 months old), 15–30 mg/kg PO, SC, IM, or IV q 8 hours for 1–2 weeks.

Enrofloxacin (adult dogs), 5–10 mg/kg PO or SC q 12 hours for 1–2 weeks.

4. Prognosis is good if treatment is begun early in the course of the disease. With severe necrosis, scarred and disfigured extremities may be a permanent sequela. Infected dogs are contagious to other dogs and to humans via tick vectors.

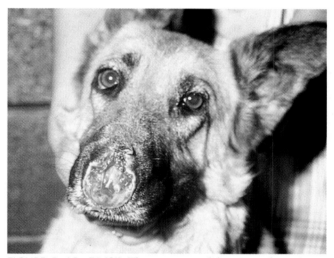

FIGURE 5–13. RMSF. The severe proliferative, ulcerating lesion has almost completely destroyed this dog's nose. (Courtesy of C. Greene)

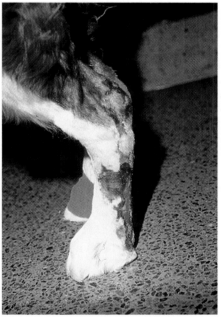

FIGURE 5–14. RMSF. Ulcerated nodular lesions on the rear leg of a dog. (Courtesy of C. Greene)

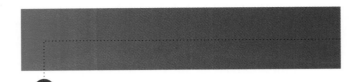

Canine Ehrlichiosis (Figs. 5–15 and 5–16)

FEATURES

A worldwide tick-borne disease caused by *Ehrlichia* spp., rickettsial organisms that infect mononuclear, granulocytic, and/or thrombocytic cells. The most common causative agent is *E. canis*, but other *Ehrlichia* species can also produce disease. Clinical and subclinical infections are common in dogs.

Infection may induce bleeding tendencies characterized by dermal petechiae and ecchymoses. Hemorrhagic diathesis, such as epistaxis, may occur. Depression, lethargy, anorexia, weight loss, and fever are common clinical signs. Other symptoms may include lymphadenomegaly, splenomegaly, hepatomegaly, and, less frequently, CNS signs, anterior and/or posterior uveitis, lameness from polyarthritis, and limb edema.

TOP DIFFERENTIALS

RMSF and other causes of thrombocytopenia.

DIAGNOSIS

1. Hemogram—Normochromic, normocytic nonregenerative anemia, thrombocytopenia, and/or leukopenia is common.
2. Serology—Positive IgG anti-*Ehrlichia* antibody titer.

TREATMENT AND PROGNOSIS

1. Give supportive care (fluids, blood transfusions, etc.) if needed.
2. The treatment of choice is either doxycycline, 5–10 mg/kg PO or IV q 12 hours, or minocycline, 10 mg/kg PO or IV q 12 hours for 10–21 days.
3. Alternative treatments include:

   Tetracycline, 22 mg/kg PO q 8 hours for 14–21 days.

   Chloramphenicol (i.e., puppies <6 months old), 15–25 mg/kg PO, SC, or IV q 8 hours for 14–21 days.

   Imidocarb diprorionate, 5 mg/kg IM twice, 2–3 weeks apart.

4. Clinical improvement should be seen 48–72 hours after initiating treatment.
5. Institute a strict tick control program for dogs and premises.
6. In endemic areas, long-term tetracycline, 6.6 mg/kg PO q 24 hours, has been used prophylactically to prevent reinfection.
7. Prognosis is good if treatment is initiated early in the course of the disease. Prognosis is poor for dogs with chronic and/or severe disease. Infected dogs are contagious to other dogs via tick vectors and if their blood is used for transfusions.

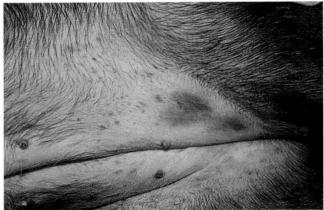

FIGURE 5–15. Canine Ehrlichiosis. Petechia and ecchymotic hemorrhages caused by thrombocytopenia resulting from the infection.

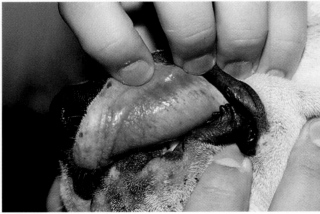

FIGURE 5–16. Canine Ehrlichiosis. Close-up of the dog in Figure 5–15. Bruising on the oral mucosa.

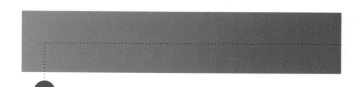

Leishmaniasis (Figs. 5–17 to 5–20)

FEATURES

A protozoal infection transmitted by certain species of blood-sucking sandflies. The disease occurs worldwide but is most prevalent in endemic areas where vector sandflies are found—in countries around the Mediterranean basin, in Portugal, and in regions of Central and South America. In endemic areas, infection is common in dogs but rare in cats. Infections also occur sporadically in nonendemic regions (United States, Canada, many European countries), usually in dogs that have been imported or have visited endemic areas.

Dogs. A visceral and cutaneous disease that develops a few months to several years after the initial infection. A progressive, symmetric alopecia and exfoliative dermatitis with dry, silvery-white scaling is common. Lesions usually begin on the head, then develop on the ear pinnae and extremities and may become generalized. Some dogs develop periocular alopecia, nasal or pinnal ulcers, and/or nasodigital hyperkeratosis. Less common cutaneous symptoms include mucocutaneous ulcers, cutaneous or mucosal nodules, pustules, and abnormally long or brittle nails. Noncutaneous signs are variable but often include insidious, progressive mental dullness, exercise intolerance, weight loss, anorexia, muscle wasting, abnormal locomotion, conjunctivitis, signs of renal failure, and lymphadenomegaly.

Cats. Nodules or crusted ulcers develop on the ear pinnae, eyelids, lips and/or nose.

TOP DIFFERENTIALS

Dogs. Leishmaniasis may mimic many other causes of seborrheic, nodular, and erosive/ulcerative skin diseases. Specific differentials depend on the clinical presentation.

Cats. Bacterial or deep fungal infections, neoplasia.

DIAGNOSIS

1. Cytology (lymph node and bone marrow aspirates)—*Leishmania* organisms (amastigotes) free or in macrophages.
2. Dermatohistopathology—Variable findings with orthokeratotic and parakeratotic hyperkeratosis, granulomatous perifolliculitis, superficial and deep granulomatous perivasculitis, and/or granulomatous interstitial dermatitis. Extracellular and intracellular (in macrophages) leishmaniae (small round to oval organisms with a round, basophilic nucleus and a rod-like kinetoplast) may be difficult to find and are more easily seen with Giemsa stains.
3. Serology—High antibody titer against *Leishmania* is usually seen, but false-positive and false-negative results can occur.
4. Immunohistochemistry (skin biopsies)—Detection of *Leishmania* antigen.
5. Polymerase chain reaction technique (skin biopsy or bone marrow specimens)—Detection of leishmanial DNA.
6. Tissue culture—*Leishmania* spp.

TREATMENT AND PROGNOSIS

1. There are no reported treatments for cats.
2. Dogs are traditionally treated with either meglumine antimonate, 100 mg/kg IV or SC q 24 hours for 3–4 weeks, or sodium stibogluconate, 30–50 mg/kg IV or SC q 24 hours for 3–4 weeks.
3. An alternative treatment for dogs is to give long-term allopurinol, PO 6–8 mg/kg q 8 hours or 15 mg/kg q 12 hours for 6–9 months.
4. Combination therapy with allopurinol and an antimony compound may result in a better response than when either is used alone.
5. Antifungal agents (amphotericin B, ketoconazole, itraconazole) have been used with variable success. In humans, liposome-encapsulated amphotericin B has been effective in cases unresponsive to antimonials, but only a partial response to this drug has been noted in infected dogs.
6. Regardless of the treatment used, the disease is not curable. All long-term survivors require periodic retreatments when they relapse.
7. Prevention—Leave dogs at home when traveling to endemic areas. In endemic areas, keep dogs indoors from 1 hour before sunset to 1 hour after dawn, use fine-mesh screens on kennels and home, and use topical repellants and insecticides on dogs.
8. Prognosis is good for dogs without renal insufficiency. Following their initial treatment, they have a 75% chance of surviving for more than 4 years with a good quality of life if they are periodically retreated as needed. Prognosis is poor for dogs with renal insufficiency. Infected dogs are contagious to other dogs and to humans via sandfly vectors. Direct transmission from dogs to humans or between dogs is rare.

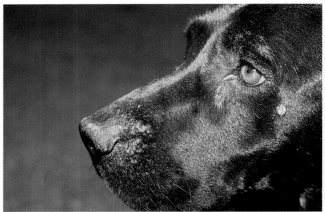

FIGURE 5-17. Leishmaniasis. Alopecia and crusting on the nose and periocular skin of a Labrador. Note the mild nature of the lesions.

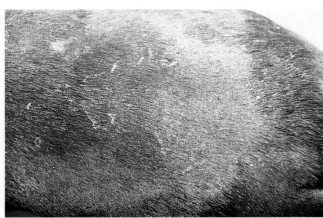

FIGURE 5-19. Leishmaniasis. Superficial flakes and scale (mild seborrhea) caused by the infection.

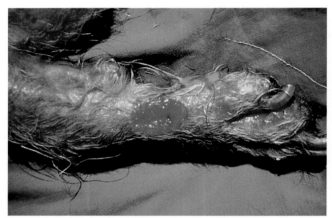

FIGURE 5-18. Leishmaniasis. Severe ulceration with tissue proliferation on the distal limb of a dog. (Courtesy of A. Wolf)

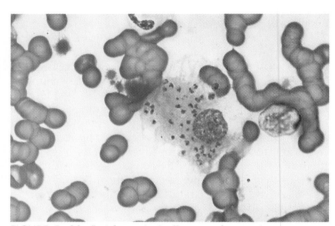

FIGURE 5-20. Leishmaniasis. Protozoal amastigotes viewed with a 100× objective (Diff Quick stain).

Suggested Readings

Ciaramella P, Oliva G, De Luna RR, Gradonni L, Ambrosio R, Cortese L, Scalone A, and Persechino A. 1997. A Retrospective Clinical Study of Canine Leishmaniasis in 150 Dogs Naturally Infected by *Leishmania infantum*. Vet Rec. 141: 539–543.

Font A, Roura X, Fondevila D, Closa J, Mascort J, and Ferrer L. 1996. Canine Mucosal Leishmaniasis. J Am Anim Hosp Assoc. 32: 131–137.

Ginel P, Lucena R, Lopez R, and Molleda J. 1998. Use of Allopurinol for Maintenance of Remission in Dogs with Leishmaniasis. J Small Anim Pract. 39: 271–274.

Harrus S, Bark H, and Waner T. 1997. Canine Monocytic Ehrlichiosis: An Update. Compend Cont Edu Pract Vet. 19: 431–444.

Miller WH. 1995. Epidermal Dysplastic Disorders of Dogs and Cats, pp. 597–599. In Bonagura JD (ed). Kirk's Current Veterinary Therapy, XII, Small Animal Practice. W.B. Saunders, Philadelphia, PA.

Plumb DC. 1999. Veterinary Drug Handbook. Ed. 3. Iowa State University Press, Ames, IA.

Sainz A, Tesouro MA, Amusategui I, Rodriguez F, Mazzucchelli F, and Rodriguez M. 2000. Prospective Comparative Study of 3 Treatment Protocols Using Doxycycline or Imidocard Dipropionate in Dogs with Naturally Occurring Ehrlichiosis. J Vet Intern Med. 14:134–139.

Viral, Rickettsial, Chlamydial, and Mycoplasmal Diseases, Section I, pp. 1–177. In Green CE (ed). 1998. Infectious Diseases of the Dog and Cat. Ed. 2. W.B. Saunders, Philadelphia, PA.

Viral, Rickettsial, and Protozoal Skin Diseases, pp. 469–483. In Scott DW, Miller WH Jr, and Griffin CE. 1995. Muller & Kirk's Small Animal Dermatology. Ed. 5. W.B. Saunders, Philadelphia, PA.

6

Hypersensitivity Disorders

- **Urticaria and Angioedema** (hives)
- **Canine Atopy** (allergic inhalant dermatitis)
- **Canine Food Hypersensitivity**
- **Flea Allergy Dermatitis**
- **Feline Atopy**
- **Feline Food Hypersensitivity**
- **Mosquito Bite Hypersensitivity**
- **Canine Eosinophilic Furunculosis of the Face**
- **Contact Dermatitis** (allergic contact dermatitis)

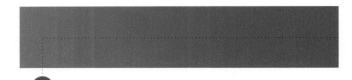

Urticaria and Angioedema (hives)
(Figs. 6–1 to 6–4)

FEATURES

A cutaneous hypersensitivity reaction to immunologic and nonimmunologic stimuli such as drugs, vaccines, bacterins, food or food additives, stinging or biting insects, plants, excessive heat or cold, sunlight, and psychologic stresses. Uncommon in dogs and rare in cats.

Usually there is an acute onset of variably pruritic wheals (urticaria) or large, edematous swellings (angioedema). Urticarial lesions may resolve and appear elsewhere on the body. Angioedema is usually localized, especially to the head, whereas urticaria may be localized or generalized. Affected skin is often erythematous, but hair loss does not occur. Dyspnea from pharyngeal, nasal, or laryngeal angioedema may be present. Rarely, anaphylactic shock with hypotension, collapse, gastrointestinal signs, and/or death may develop.

TOP DIFFERENTIALS

Urticaria—Folliculitis (bacterial, dermatophyte, *Demodex*), vasculitis, erythema multiforme, neoplasia (lymphoreticular, mast cell).

Angioedema—Juvenile cellulitis, bacterial or fungal cellulitis, neoplasia, snake bite.

DIAGNOSIS

1. Usually based on history and clinical findings.
2. Dermatohistopathology (usually nondiagnostic)—Vascular dilatation and edema in superficial and middle dermis or superficial perivascular to interstitial dermatitis with varying numbers of mononuclear cells, neutrophils, mast cells, and, rarely, eosinophils.

TREATMENT AND PROGNOSIS

1. Give prednisone or prednisolone, 2 mg/kg PO or IM once.
2. Concurrently giving diphenhydramine, 2 mg/kg PO or IM q 8 hours for 2–3 days, may be helpful.
3. If animal is dyspneic, give epinephrine (1:1000), 0.1–0.5 ml SC, IM, or IV once. If necessary, treat for anaphylactic shock.
4. Identify and avoid future exposure to the suspected cause.
5. Long-term antihistamine therapy may help prevent or control chronic urticaria of unknown cause.
6. Prognosis is good for animals that do not develop anaphylactic shock.

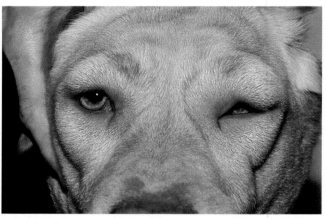

FIGURE 6–1. Angioedema. The severe swelling of the face and periocular tissue developed after a venomous insect sting.

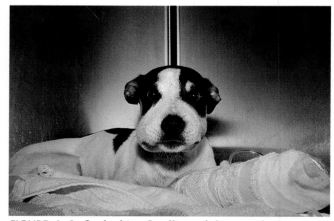

FIGURE 6–2. Snake bite. Swelling of the muzzle resembling angioedema.

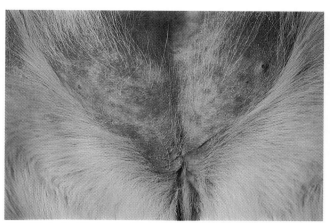

FIGURE 6–3. Urticaria. These intensely erythematous macules were caused by an acute urticarial reaction.

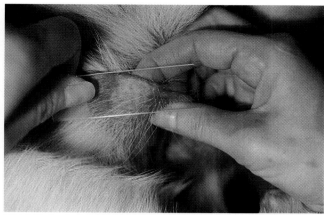

FIGURE 6–4. Urticaria. Diascopy being performed on the dog in Figure 6–3. The blanching indicates vasodilatation rather than ecchymotic hemorrhage.

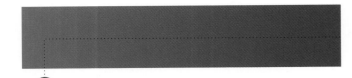

Canine Atopy (allergic inhalant dermatitis) (Figs. 6-5 to 6-18)

FEATURES

A type 1 hypersensitivity reaction to inhaled or cutaneously absorbed environmental antigens (allergens) in genetically predisposed individuals. Common in dogs, with age of onset ranging from 3 months to 7 years. However, in most atopic dogs, symptoms first appear between 1 and 3 years of age.

Symptoms begin as skin erythema and pruritus (licking, chewing, scratching, rubbing) which may be seasonal or nonseasonal, depending on the offending allergen. The distribution of the pruritus usually involves the feet, flanks, groin, axillae, face, and/or ears. Self-trauma often results in secondary skin lesions including salivary staining, alopecia, excoriations, scales, crusts, hyperpigmentation, and lichenification. Secondary pyoderma, *Malassezia* dermatitis, and otitis externa are common. Chronic acral lick dermatitis, recurrent pyotraumatic dermatitis, conjunctivitis, hyperhidrosis (sweating), and, rarely, allergic bronchitis or rhinitis may be seen.

TOP DIFFERENTIALS

Other hypersensitivities (food, flea bite, contact), parasites (scabies, cheyletiellosis, pediculosis), folliculitis (bacteria, dermatophyte, *Demodex*), *Malassezia* dermatitis.

DIAGNOSIS

1. Usually based on history and clinical findings, but other differentials should be ruled out.
2. Allergy testing (intradermal, serologic)—Positive reactions to grass, weed, tree, mold, insect, dander, and/or indoor environmental allergens. False-negative and false-positive reactions can occur.
3. Dermatohistopathology (nondiagnostic)—Superficial perivascular dermatitis that may be spongiotic or hyperplastic. Inflammatory cells are predominantly lymphocytes and histiocytes. Eosinophils are uncommon. Neutrophils or plasma cells suggest secondary infection.

TREATMENT AND PROGNOSIS

1. Reduce exposure to offending allergens by removing them from environment, if possible. Use high-efficiency particulate (HEPA) air and charcoal filters to reduce pollens, molds, and dust in the home.
2. Treat any secondary pyoderma, otitis externa, and *Malassezia* dermatitis with appropriate therapies. Controlling secondary infection is an essential component of managing atopic dogs.
3. Institute a flea control program to prevent flea bites from aggravating the pruritus.
4. Control pruritus with topical therapy, antihistamines, essential fatty acid supplements, glucocorticoids, and/or immunotherapy.
5. Topical therapy with shampoos, conditioners, and sprays (containing oatmeal, pramoxine, aloe vera, antihistamines, and/or glucocorticoids) q 2-7 days or as needed may help reduce clinical symptoms.
6. Systemic antihistamine therapy reduces clinical symptoms in 20-35% of cases (Table 6-1). Antihistamines can be used alone or in combination with glucocorticoids and/or essential fatty acids for a synergistic effect. One- to 2-week-long therapeutic trials with different antihistamines may be required in order to find the one that is most effective.
7. Oral essential fatty acid supplements help control pruritus in 20-50% of cases, with beneficial effect usually occurring within 3-4 weeks of initiating therapy. A synergistic effect may be seen when essential fatty acid supplements are given in combination with glucocorticoids or antihistamines.
8. Systemic glucocorticoid therapy is often effective in controlling pruritus. It is a therapeutic option if the allergy season is short (<4 months), but may result in unacceptable side effects, especially if used long-term. Give prednisone, 0.25-0.5 mg/kg (or methylprednisolone, 0.2-0.4 mg/

TABLE 6-1 Oral Antihistamine Therapy in Dogs

Antihistamine	Dose
Amitriptyline (Elavil)	1-2 mg/kg q 12 hours
Brompheniramine (Dimetane-DX)	0.5-2 mg/kg q 12 hours
Cetirizine (Zyrtec)	0.5-1 mg/kg q 24 hours
Chlorpheniramine (Chlor-Trimeton)	4-8 mg/dog q 12 hours
Clemastine (Tavist)	0.05 mg/kg q 12 hours
Cyproheptadine (Periactin)	1.0 mg/kg q 8-12 hours
Diphenhydramine (Benadryl)	2-4 mg/kg q 8 hours
Doxepin (Sinequan)	0.5-1 mg/kg q 8-12 hours
Hydroxyzine (Atarax)	2 mg/kg q 8 hours
Loratadine (Claritin)	0.5 mg/kg q 24 hours
Trimeprazine (Temaril-P)	Up to 20 kg: 0.5 mg/kg q 12 hours Over 20 kg: 15 mg/dog q 12 hours Reduce dose by one half after 4 days

kg) PO q 12 hours, until pruritus ceases (approximately 3–10 days). Then give prednisone, 0.5–1.0 mg/kg (methylprednisolone, 0.4–0.8 mg/kg) PO q 48 hours for 3–7 days. Continue tapering dosage until <0.5 mg/kg prednisone (<0.4 mg/kg methylprednisolone) is being given q 48 hours if long-term maintenance therapy is needed.

9. With immunotherapy (allergy shots), 50–75% of atopic dogs show a good (some medical therapy still needed) to excellent (no other therapy needed) response. Clinical improvement is usually noted within 6–8 months of initiating immunotherapy, but it can take up to 1 year in some dogs.

10. Alternative therapies that may be helpful in controlling pruritus include:

Cyclosporin A (Neoral), 5 mg/kg PO q 24 hours for 6 weeks, then slowly tapered to the lowest dose/frequency that controls clinical signs.

Misoprostol, 6 μg/kg PO q 8 hours.

11. Prognosis is good, although lifelong therapy for control is needed in most dogs. Relapses (pruritic flare-ups with/without secondary infections) are common, so individualized treatment adjustments to meet patient's needs may be required periodically. In dogs that become poorly controlled, rule out secondary infections (bacteria, *Malassezia*, dermatophyte), sarcoptic mange, demodicosis, concurrent food, flea bite, and/or contact hypersensitivies, and recently acquired hypersensitivity to additional environmental allergens.

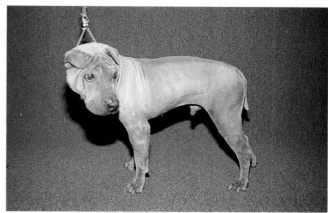

FIGURE 6–6. Canine Atopy. Alopecia, erythema, and excoriations on the face, extremities, and flank of an adult shar pei.

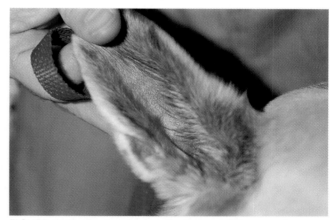

FIGURE 6–7. Canine Atopy. Erythema of the ear pinnae (with or without otitis externa) is a common clinical finding.

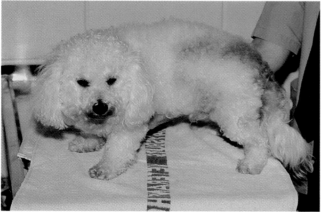

FIGURE 6–5. Canine Atopy. Salivary staining of the fur coat caused by chronic licking. The pattern of discoloration (feet and lumbar region) is typical of atopy, food allergy, and flea allergy dermatitis.

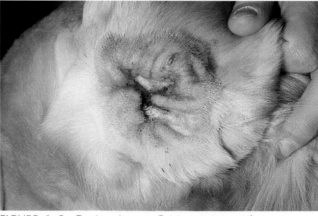

FIGURE 6–8. Canine Atopy. Otitis externa with a waxy exudate caused by a secondary *Malassezia* infection associated with the allergic disease. (Courtesy of D. Angarano.)

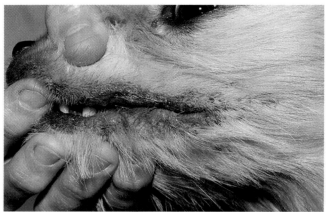

FIGURE 6–9. Canine Atopy. Perioral dermatitis with erythema and alopecia caused by pruritic secondary bacterial and yeast infections.

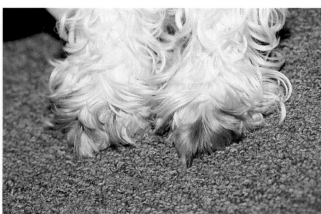

FIGURE 6–12. Canine Atopy. Salivary staining of the fur coat caused by chronic licking and chewing.

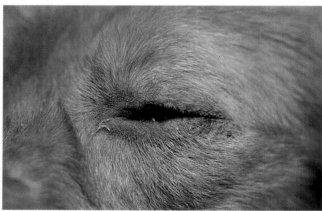

FIGURE 6–10. Canine Atopy. Periocular alopecia, erythema, hyperpigmentation, and lichenification caused by pruritus.

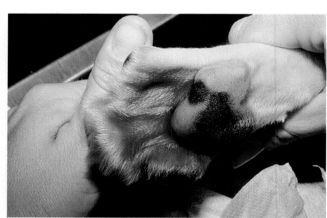

FIGURE 6–13. Canine Atopy. Erythema, alopecia, and salivary staining of the interdigital spaces associated with pododermatitis. Secondary bacterial and yeast overgrowth leads to increased pruritus.

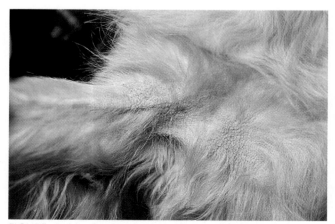

FIGURE 6–11. Canine Atopy. Alopecia and erythema in the axillary area are common dermatologic findings in atopic dogs.

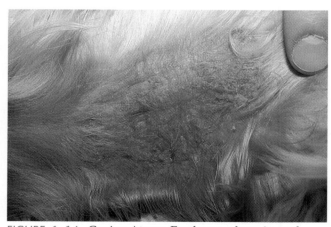

FIGURE 6–14. Canine Atopy. Erythema, alopecia, and lichenification on the ventral neck of an atopic cocker spaniel. This lesion is typical of secondary yeast dermatitis caused by *Malassezia* organisms.

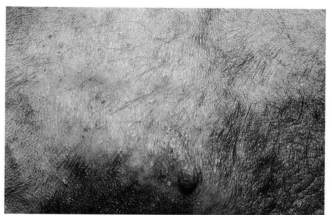

FIGURE 6–15. Canine Atopy. Alopecia with a crusting papular rash typical of folliculitis. This superficial pyoderma was secondary to the allergic dermatitis.

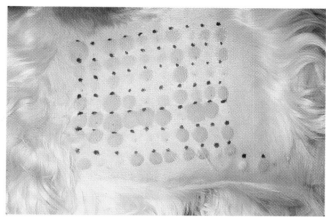

FIGURE 6–17. Canine Atopy. An intradermal allergy test showing the classic positive reactions. (Courtesy of D. Angarano.)

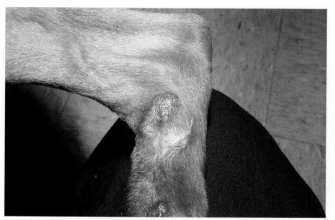

FIGURE 6–16. Canine Atopy. An acral lick granuloma (dermatitis) on the lateral hock. The lesion resolved with medical management of the dog's atopy.

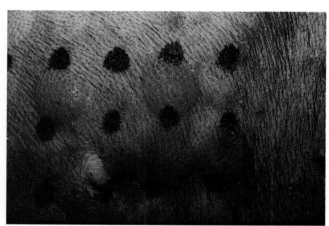

FIGURE 6–18. Canine Atopy. A close-up of an intradermal allergy test demonstrating the positive (bee sting-like) reactions.

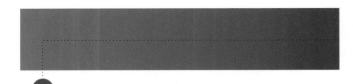

Canine Food Hypersensitivity
(Figs. 6–19 to 6–32)

FEATURES

An immunologically mediated adverse reaction to a food or food additive. It can occur at any age. Common in dogs.

It is characterized by nonseasonal pruritus that may or may not respond to steroid therapy. The pruritus may be regional or generalized and usually involves the ears, feet, inguinal or axillary areas, face, neck, and/or perineum. Affected skin is often erythematous, and a papular rash may be present. Self-trauma-induced lesions include alopecia, excoriations, scales, crusts, hyperpigmentation, and/or lichenification. Secondary superficial pyoderma, *Malassezia* dermatitis, and/or otitis externa are common. Other symptoms that may be seen are acral lick dermatitis, chronic seborrhea, and recurring pyotraumatic dermatitis. Some dogs are minimally pruritic and have symptoms only of recurrent pyoderma and/or otitis externa. Occasionally, urticaria or angioedema may occur. Concurrent gastrointestinal signs (vomiting, diarrhea, flatulence) are occasionally present.

TOP DIFFERENTIALS

Other hypersensitivities (atopy, flea bite, contact), parasites (scabies, cheyletiellosis, pediculosis), folliculitis (bacteria, dermatophyte, *Demodex*), *Malassezia* dermatitis.

DIAGNOSIS

1. Rule out other differentials.
2. Dermatohistopathology (nondiagnostic)—Varying degrees of superficial perivascular dermatitis. Mononuclear cells or neutrophils may predominate.
3. Food allergy testing (intradermal, serologic)—Not recommended because test results are unreliable.

4. Response to hypoallergenic diet trial—Symptoms improve within 10–12 weeks of initiating a strict home-cooked or commercially prepared restricted diet (one protein and one carbohydrate source). The diet should not contain food ingredients previously fed in dog food, treats, or table scraps (Table 6–2).
5. Provocative challenge—Recurrence of symptoms within 7–10 days of reintroducing suspect allergen into diet.

TREATMENT AND PROGNOSIS

1. Treat any secondary pyoderma, otitis externa, and *Malassezia* dermatitis with appropriate therapies. Controlling secondary infection is an essential component of managing food-allergic dogs.
2. Institute a flea control program to prevent flea bites from aggravating the pruritus.
3. Avoid offending dietary allergen(s). Feed a balanced, home-cooked diet or a commercial hypoallergenic diet. To identify offending substances to be avoided, add one new food item to the hypoallergenic diet every 2–4 weeks. If the item is allergenic, clinical symptoms will recur within 7–10 days. Note: some dogs (approximately 20%) must be fed home-cooked diets in order to remain symptom-free. For these dogs, commercial hypoallergenic diets are ineffective, presumably because of food additive hypersensitivity.
4. Alternatively, medical therapy alone with systemic glucocorticoids, antihistamines, fatty acids, or topical therapies as described for canine atopy can be attempted. However, response is often poor.
5. For some dogs whose only symptom is recurring superficial pyoderma, control may be achieved with long-term, low-dose antibiotic therapy alone. Cephalexin is given PO, 20 mg/kg q 8 hours or 30 mg/kg q 12 hours (minimum 4 weeks), and continued at least 1 week beyond complete clinical resolution. It is then continued as maintenance therapy at 20 mg/kg PO q 24 hours.
6. Prognosis is good. In dogs that become poorly controlled, rule out owner noncompliance, development of hypersensitivity to ingredient in hypoallergenic diet, secondary infections (bacteria, Malassezia, dermatophyte), scabies, demodicosis, atopy, flea-allergic dermatitis, and contact hypersensitivity.

TABLE 6–2 Commercial Hypoallergenic Diets for Dogs

Manufacturer	Product	How Supplied	Main Ingredients
Hills	Prescription Diet Canine d/d Lamb & Rice	canned	rice, lamb, lamb liver, rice flour, powdered cellulose, vegetable oil
	Prescription Diet Canine d/d Whitefish & Rice	canned	whitefish, rice, rice flour, animal fat, powdered cellulose, vegetable oil
	Prescription Diet Canine d/d Rice & Salmon	dry	brewer's rice, salmon, rice protein concentrate, animal fat, vegetable oil, sucrose
	Prescription Diet Canine d/d Rice & Duck	dry	brewer's rice, duck by-products, rice protein concentrate, animal fat, vegetable oil, sucrose
	Prescription Diet Canine d/d Rice & Egg	dry	brewer's rice, dried egg product, animal fat, vegetable oil, sucrose
	Prescription Diet Canine z/d	dry	dried potato products, hydrolyzed chicken liver, potato starch, vegetable oil, hydrolyzed chicken
	Prescription Diet Canine z/d Ultra	dry	starch, hydrolyzed chicken liver, vegetable oil, hydrolyzed chicken
Iams	Eukanuba Veterinary Diets Response FP Formula	canned	catfish, herring meal, modified potato starch, dried beet pulp, corn oil
		dry	potato, herring meal, catfish, animal fat, dried beet pulp, fish digest
	Eukanuba Response KO Kangaroo & Oatmeal	dry	oat flour, kangaroo, canola meal, animal fat, dried beet pulp, fish oil
Innovative Pet Foods	Nature's Recipe Easy-to-Digest Lamb, Lamb meal, Rice & Barley Formula	canned	lamb stock, lamb, soybean meal, ground rice, potatoes, carrots, lamb by-products, canola oil, lamb liver, ground barley
		dry	lamb meal, ground rice, cracked pearl barley, animal fat, natural flavor, tomato puree
	Nature's Recipe Allergy Vegetarian Formula	canned	soybean meal, ground rice, carrots, potatoes, ground barley, canola oil
		dry	ground rice, soy flour, cracked pearl barley, canola oil
	Nature's Recipe Allergy Venison Meal & Rice Formula	canned	venison stock, venison meal, venison by-products, potatoes, carrots, ground rice, canola oil, peas, ground barley
Innovative Veterinary Diets	Limited Ingredient Lamb and Potato	canned	potato, lamb stock, lamb, lamb by-products, canola oil, salmon oil
		dry	dehydrated potatoes, lamb, lamb meal, potato protein, canola oil, potato fiber, salmon oil
	Limited Ingredient Venison & Potato	canned	potato, venison stock, venison, venison by-products, canola oil, salmon oil
		dry	dehydrated potatoes, venison, potato protein, canola oil, potato fiber, salmon oil
	Limited Ingredient Rabbit & Potato	canned	potato, rabbit, rabbit stock, rabbit by-products, canola oil, salmon oil
		dry	dehydrated potatoes, rabbit, potato protein, canola oil, potato fiber, salmon oil
	Limited Ingredient Duck & Potato	canned	potatoes, duck, duck stock, duck by-products, canola oil, salmon oil
		dry	dehydrated potatoes, duck, duck meal, potato fiber, canola oil, salmon oil
	Limited Ingredient Whitefish & Potato	canned	potatoes, whitefish, fish stock, canola oil, salmon stock
Pet Products Plus, Inc	Sensible Choice with Lamb & Rice	canned	lamb, brewers rice
		dry	lamb meal, brewer's rice, rice flour, rice gluten, poultry fat
	Sensible Choice Lamb Meal and Rice Puppy	dry	lamb meal, brewer's rice, rice gluten, rice flour, poultry fat
Purina	CNM HA-Formula	dry	corn starch, modified isolated soy protein, coconut oil, canola oil
	CNM LA-Formula	dry	brewers rice, salmon meal, trout, canola meal, tallow, brewer's dried yeast, canola oil, fish oil
Waltham	Waltham Veterinary Diet Selected Protein with Lamb & Rice	canned	lamb by-products, lamb, rice
	Waltham Veterinary Diet Selected Protein with Rice and Catfish	dry	rice, catfish meal, rice gluten, cellulose powder, catfish, vegetable oil
Nutro Products, Inc	Natural Choice Lamb & Rice Formula	canned	lamb broth, lamb, lamb liver, rice gluten, ground rice, dried egg product
		dry	lamb meal, ground rice, rice bran, rice flour, sunflower oil, rice gluten, dried egg product
	Natural Choice Lite Lamb & Rice Formula	canned	lamb broth, lamb, barley, defatted rice bran, rice gluten, ground rice, peas, lamb liver
		dry	rice flour, lamb meal, rice bran, ground rice, sunflower oil, dried egg product, rice gluten
	Natural Choice Puppy, Lamb & Rice Formula	canned	lamb broth, lamb liver, lamb, lamb kidney, dried egg product, ground rice, rice gluten

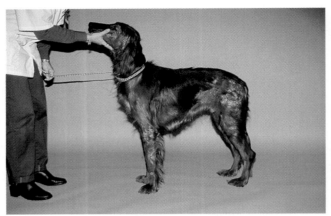

FIGURE 6–19. Canine Food Hypersensitivity. Alopecia, erythema, and excoriations on the face, extremities, and flank of an Irish setter. Note the similarity to atopy and scabies.

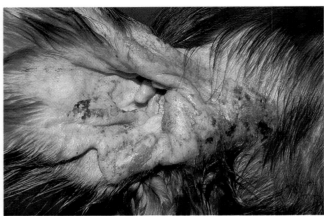

FIGURE 6–22. Canine Food Hypersensitivity. Close-up of the dog in Figures 6–19 to 6–21. Erythema, alopecia, and papular rash involving the ear pinnae. There is no infectious otitis, only external lesions associated with the underlying allergy.

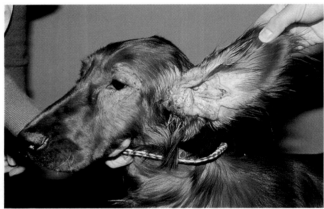

FIGURE 6–20. Canine Food Hypersensitivity. Close-up of the dog in Figure 6–19. Alopecia, erythema, and excoriations around the eye and ear. The crusting papular rash is due to a secondary superficial pyoderma associated with the allergic disease.

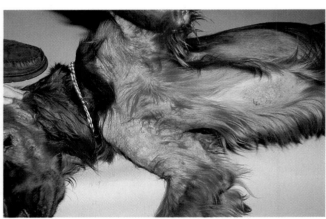

FIGURE 6–23. Canine Food Hypersensitivity. Alopecia and erythema in the axillary area. The mild hyperpigmentation and lichenification are caused by a secondary yeast dermatitis. Note the similarity to lesions seen with atopy.

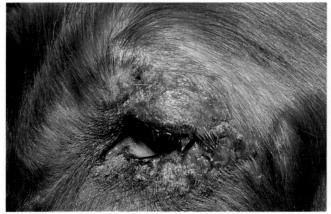

FIGURE 6–21. Canine Food Hypersensitivity. Close-up of the dog in Figures 6–19 and 6–20. Erythema, alopecia, and papular rash around the eye.

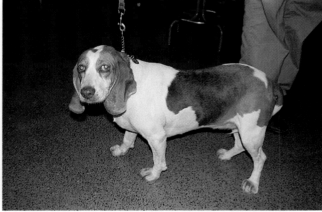

FIGURE 6–24. Canine Food Hypersensitivity. This food-allergic dog demonstrates few gross lesions when observed from a distance. There is mild pododermatitis (see Figure 6–25).

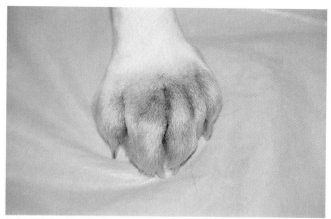

FIGURE 6–25. Canine Food Hypersensitivity. Close-up of the dog in Figure 6–24. Erythema, alopecia, and salivary staining of the foot.

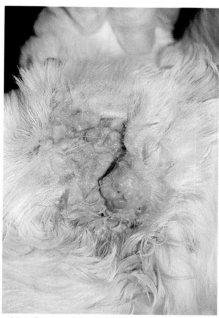

FIGURE 6–27. Canine Food Hypersensitivity. Severe allergic otitis with a secondary bacterial infection in a cocker spaniel. The previous lateral ear canal resection without dietary therapy failed to resolve the otitis.

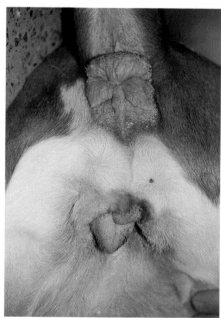

FIGURE 6–26. Canine Food Hypersensitivity. Close-up of the dog in Figures 6–24 and 6–25. Perianal alopecia and lichenification are common in food-allergic dogs.

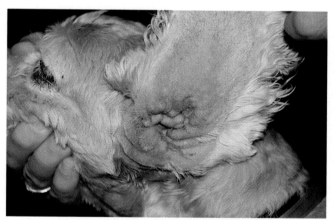

FIGURE 6–28. Canine Food Hypersensitivity. Lichenification and hypertrophy of the ear canal caused its occlusion. The moist exudate is due to a secondary bacterial infection.

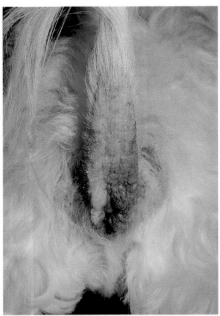

FIGURE 6–29. Canine Food Hypersensitivity. Perianal dermatitis with alopecia and lichenification.

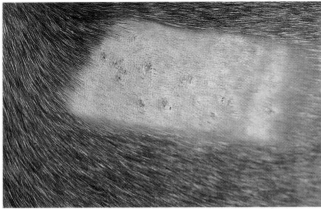

FIGURE 6–31. Canine Food Hypersensitivity. Crusting papular rash caused by a secondary superficial pyoderma. The lesions were not visible until the haircoat was clipped.

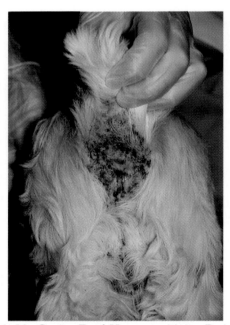

FIGURE 6–30. Canine Food Hypersensitivity. Perianal dermatitis in a food-allergic cocker spaniel.

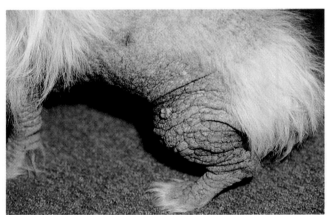

FIGURE 6–32. Canine Food Hypersensitivity. Severe alopecia, lichenification, and hyperpigmentation caused by a secondary yeast infection.

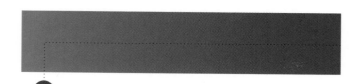

Flea Allergy Dermatitis

(Figs. 6–33 to 6–44)

FEATURES

A common skin disease in dogs and cats sensitized to flea bites. Symptoms are usually seasonal (warm weather months) in temperate zones and often non-seasonal in subtropical and tropical areas.

Dogs. Lesions include pruritic, papular, crusting eruptions with secondary erythema, seborrhea, alopecia, excoriations, pyoderma, hyperpigmentation, and/or lichenification. The distribution typically involves the caudodorsal lumbosacral area, dorsal tail-head, caudomedial thighs, abdomen, and flanks.

Cats. Commonly present with pruritic miliary dermatitis with secondary excoriations, crusting, and alopecia of the neck, dorsal lumbosacral area, caudomedial thighs, and/or ventral abdomen. Other symptoms include symmetrical alopecia secondary to excessive grooming and eosinophilic granuloma complex lesions.

TOP DIFFERENTIALS

Atopy, food hypersensitivity, other ectoparasites (scabies, cheyletiellosis, pediculosis, demodicosis), superficial pyoderma, dermatophytosis, *Malassezia* dermatitis.

DIAGNOSIS

1. Usually based on history and clinical findings, but rule out other differentials.
2. Visualization of fleas or flea excreta on body—May be difficult to find on flea-allergic animals.
3. Allergy testing (intradermal, serologic)—Positive skin test reaction to flea antigen or positive serum IgE anti-flea antibody titer is highly suggestive, but false-negative results are possible.
4. Dermatohistopathology (nondiagnostic)—Varying degrees of superficial or deep perivascular to interstitial dermatitis, with eosinophils often predominating.
5. Response to flea therapy—Symptoms resolve.

TREATMENT AND PROGNOSIS

1. Treat affected and all in-contact dogs and cats with adulticidal flea sprays, solutions, or dips q 7–30 days as instructed on label. Products containing fipronil or imidocloprid are especially efficacious when used every 3–4 weeks.
2. Insect growth regulators (lufenuron, pyriproxifen, methoprene) may be effective alone or in combination with adulticidal therapy.
3. Continue flea control therapy from spring until first snowfall or year-round in warm climates.
4. In heavily flea-infested environments, treat areas where pets spend the most time. Treat indoor premises with an adulticidal insecticide and insect growth regulator (methoprene, pyriproxifen). Treat outdoor environment with insecticidal or biologic products designed for such use.
5. To help resolve pruritus, consider glucocorticoid therapy. Give prednisone, 0.5 mg/kg (dogs) or 1.0 mg/kg (cats) PO q 12 hours for 3–7 days, then q 24 hours for 3–7 days, then q 48 hours for 3–7 days. Alternatively, give cats repositol methylprednisolone acetate, 20 mg/cat or 4 mg/kg SC once or twice at a 2- to 3-week interval.
6. For secondary pyoderma, give appropriate systemic antibiotics for at least 3–4 weeks.
7. Prognosis is good if strict flea control is practiced. Fleas can infest other in-contact animals and humans.

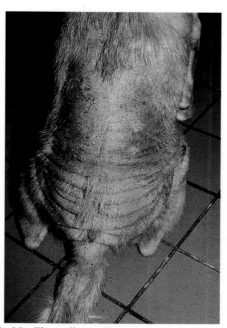

FIGURE 6–33. Flea Allergy Dermatitis. Alopecia with hyperpigmentation and lichenification on the lumbar region. Most lesions associated with flea allergy dermatitis are caudal to the rib cage.

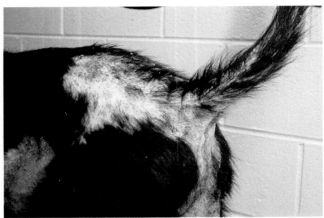

FIGURE 6–34. Flea Allergy Dermatitis. Alopecia, papules, and crusts on the lumbar region and tail head. (Courtesy of N. White-Weithers)

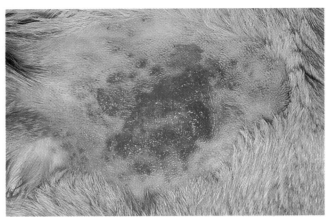

FIGURE 6–37. Flea Allergy Dermatitis. Pyotraumatic dermatitis (hot spot) caused by flea allergy dermatitis.

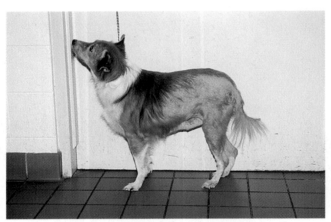

FIGURE 6–35. Flea Allergy Dermatitis. Alopecia affecting the lumbar region.

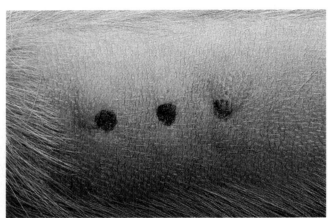

FIGURE 6–38. Flea Allergy Dermatitis. An intradermal allergy test using flea antigen (right) was positive in this flea-allergic dog. Histamine (left) and saline (middle) were used as positive and negative controls.

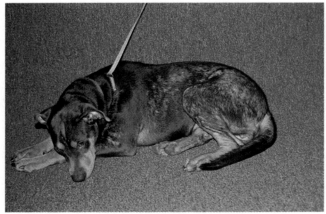

FIGURE 6–36. Flea Allergy Dermatitis. Moth-eaten alopecia on the lumbar region.

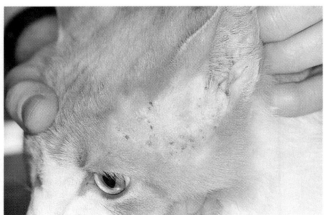

FIGURE 6–39. Flea Allergy Dermatitis. The papular rash, alopecia, and crusting on the head of this cat are typical of miliary dermatitis.

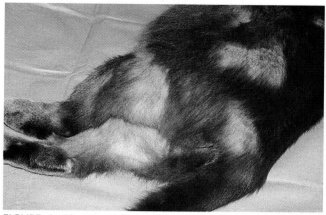

FIGURE 6-40. Flea Allergy Dermatitis. Alopecia on the lumbar region of a cat.

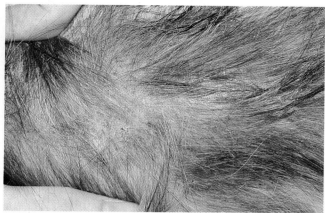

FIGURE 6-43. Flea Allergy Dermatitis. Small focal crusts associated with miliary dermatitis and a small erosion on the dorsum of a flea-allergic cat.

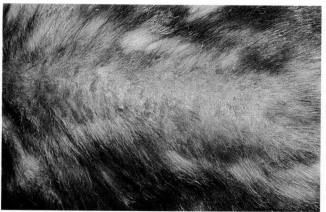

FIGURE 6-41. Flea Allergy Dermatitis. Severe alopecia and crusting dermatitis on the dorsal lumbar region of a flea-allergic cat.

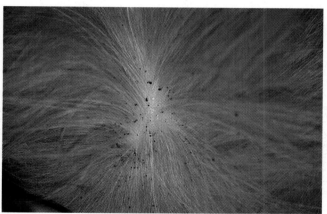

FIGURE 6-44. Flea Allergy Dermatitis. Digested blood passed as feces forms a dark coagulate typical of "flea dirt."

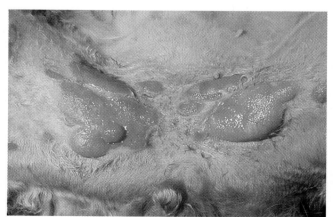

FIGURE 6-42. Flea Allergy Dermatitis. Multiple eosinophilic plaques on the ventral abdomen of a flea-allergic cat.

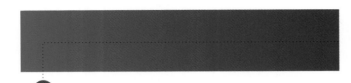

Feline Atopy (Figs. 6–45 to 6–52)

FEATURES

A type 1 hypersensitivity reaction to environmental antigens (allergens). Uncommon in cats.

The primary symptom is pruritus (chewing, scratching, excessive grooming), which may be seasonal or nonseasonal, depending on the offending allergens. The pruritus may concentrate around the head, neck, and ears or it may involve other areas such as the ventral abdomen, caudal thighs, forelegs, and/or lateral thorax. Self-trauma usually results in alopecia that can be bilaterally symmetric. Remaining hairs are broken off and do not epilate easily. The alopecic skin may appear otherwise normal or may be secondarily excoriated. Miliary dermatitis, ceruminous otitis externa, and/or eosinophilic granuloma complex lesions are common. With chronicity, secondary pyoderma and/or peripheral lymphadenomegaly may develop. Atopy may be linked with chronic bronchitis or asthma in some cats.

TOP DIFFERENTIALS

Other hypersensitivities (food, flea bite, mosquito bite), dermatophytosis, ectoparasites (cheyletiellosis, ear mites, feline scabies, demodicosis), and psychogenic alopecia.

DIAGNOSIS

1. Rule out other differentials.
2. Allergy testing (intradermal)—Positive reactions to grass, tree, mold, weed, insect, dander, feathers, or indoor environmental allergens. False-negative reactions are common. False-positive reactions can occur.
3. Dermatohistopathology (nondiagnostic)—Variably mild to marked perivascular or diffuse inflammation with lymphocytes, mast cell hyperplasia, and/or eosinophils. Epidermal hyperplasia, spongiosis, erosions, ulcers, and/or serocellular crusts may be present.

TREATMENT AND PROGNOSIS

1. Reduce exposure to offending allergens by removing them from the environment if possible. Use HEPA air and charcoal filters to reduce pollens, molds, and dust in the home.

TABLE 6–3 Oral Antihistamine Therapy for Cats

Antihistamine	Dose
Amitriptyline (Elavil)	5–10 mg/cat q 12–24 hours
Chlorpheniramine (Chlor-Trimeton)	2–4 mg/cat q 12–24 hours
Clemastine (Tavist)	0.68 mg/cat q 12 hours
Cyproheptadine (Periactin)	2 mg/cat q 12 hours
Diphenhydramine (Benadryl)	2–4 mg/cat q 12 hours
Hydroxyzine (Atarax)	5–10 mg/cat q 8–12 hours

2. Treat any secondary pyoderma or otitis with appropriate therapies for 2–4 weeks.
3. Institute a flea control program to prevent flea bites from aggravating the pruritus.
4. Control pruritus with systemic glucocorticoids, antihistamines, essential fatty acid supplements, and/or immunotherapy.
5. Systemic glucocorticoids control pruritus in most cases. Effective therapies include:

   Repositol methylprednisolone acetate, 20 mg/cat or 4 mg/kg SC or IM q 2–3 months as needed.

   Triamcinolone acetonide, 5 mg/cat SC or IM q 2–3 months as needed.

   Prednisone, 2 mg/kg PO q 24 hours until pruritus and lesions resolve (approximately 2–8 weeks), then 2 mg/kg PO q 48 hours for 2–4 weeks, then taper down to lowest possible alternate-day dosage if long-term maintenance therapy is needed.

6. Systemic antihistamines may reduce clinical symptoms in 40–70% of cases. They can be used alone or in combination with glucocorticoids and essential fatty acids. A beneficial effect should occur within 1–2 weeks of instituting therapy (Table 6–3).
7. Oral essential fatty acid supplements may help control pruritus in 20–50% of cases. A beneficial effect should occur within 3–4 weeks of initiating therapy. A synergistic effect may be seen when essential fatty acid supplements are given in combination with glucocorticoids or antihistamines.
8. Immunotherapy (allergy shots) is indicated if medical therapy is ineffective, unacceptable to the owner, or results in undesirable side effects. Fifty to 70% of atopic cats show favorable responses to immunotherapy. Clinical improvement is usually noted within 6–8 months but can take up to 1 year in some cats.
9. Prognosis is good for most cats, but successful management usually requires lifelong therapy.

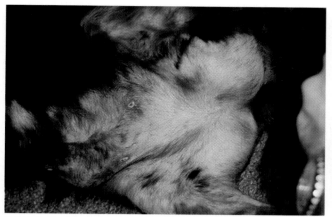

FIGURE 6–45. Feline Atopy. Alopecia on the abdomen of an atopic cat. Cutaneous inflammation can be mild and easily overlooked.

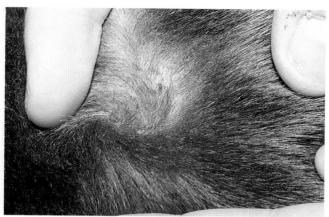

FIGURE 6–48. Feline Atopy. Small focal crusts typical of miliary dermatitis in an atopic cat.

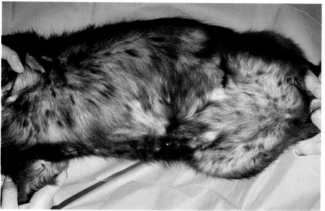

FIGURE 6–46. Feline Atopy. Generalized moth-eaten alopecia on the trunk of an atopic cat.

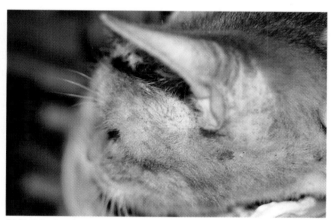

FIGURE 6–49. Feline Atopy. Diffuse alopecia with miliary crusts on the head of an allergic cat.

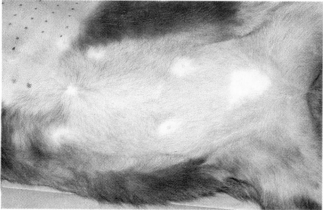

FIGURE 6–47. Feline Atopy. Complete alopecia on the abdomen of a cat. Similar alopecic lesions with excessive grooming can be caused by flea allergy, food allergy, mite infestations, and psychogenic alopecia.

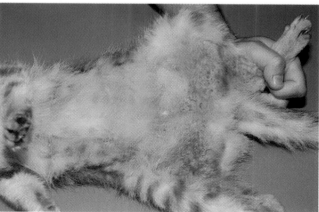

FIGURE 6–50. Feline Atopy. Alopecia and early eosinophilic plaques on the abdomen of an allergic cat.

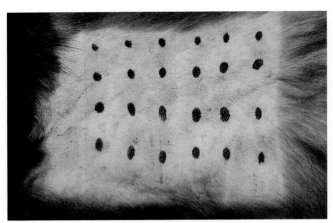

FIGURE 6–51. Feline Atopy. This intradermal allergy skin test demonstrates several positive reactions. Note the subtlety of the reactions, which is typical in cats.

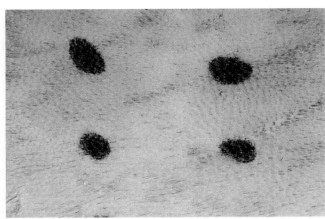

FIGURE 6–52. Feline Atopy. Close-up of the allergy skin test in Figure 6–51. The positive reactions appear as erythematous macules.

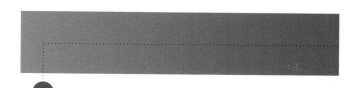

Feline Food Hypersensitivity
(Figs. 6–53 to 6–60)

FEATURES

An immunologically mediated adverse reaction to a food or food additive. It can occur at any age. Uncommon in cats.

It is characterized by nonseasonal pruritus that may or may not respond to glucocorticoid therapy. The distribution of the pruritus may be localized to the head and neck, or it may be generalized and involve the trunk, ventrum, and limbs. Skin lesions are variable and may include alopecia, erythema, miliary dermatitis, eosinophilic granuloma complex lesions, excoriations, crusts, and scales. *Malassezia* or ceruminous otitis externa may be seen. Concurrent gastrointestinal symptoms (diarrhea, vomiting) may be present.

TOP DIFFERENTIALS

Flea allergy dermatitis, atopy, mosquito bite hypersensitivity, dermatophytosis, ectoparasites (cheyletiellosis, ear mites, feline scabies, demodicosis), and psychogenic alopecia.

DIAGNOSIS

1. Rule out other differentials.
2. Dermatohistopathology (nondiagnostic)—Varying degrees of superficial or deep perivascular dermatitis in which eosinophils or mast cells often predominate.
3. Food allergy testing (intradermal or serologic)—Not recommended because test results are unreliable.
4. Response to hypoallergenic diet trial—Symptoms improve within 10–12 weeks of initiating a strict home-cooked or commercially prepared restricted diet (one protein and one carbohydrate source). The diet should not contain food ingredients previously fed in cat food, treats, or table scraps (Table 6–4).
5. Provocative challenge—Symptoms recur within 7–10 days of reintroducing suspected allergen into diet.

TREATMENT AND PROGNOSIS

1. Treat any secondary skin or ear infections with appropriate therapies.

TABLE 6–4 Commercial Hypoallergenic Diets for Cats

Manufacturer	Product	How Supplied	Main Ingredients
Hill's	Prescription Diet Feline d/d	canned	lamb by-products, lamb liver, rice
	Prescription Diet Feline z/d	dry	brewers rice, rice gluten, rice protein concentrate, hydrolyzed chicken liver, vegetable oil, hydrolyzed chicken
Iams	Eukanuba Veterinary Diets Response Formula LB	canned	lamb liver, lamb tripe, lamb, ground pearled barley, lamb meal, dried beet pulp, corn oil
Innovative Veterinary Diets	Limited Ingredient Diets Green Peas and Lamb	canned	lamb by-products, lamb stock, lamb, whole dried peas, canola oil, salmon oil, evening primrose oil
		dry	whole dried peas, lamb meal, natural flavor, lamb, canola oil, salmon oil, evening primrose oil
	Limited Ingredient Diets Green Peas and Venison	canned	venison by-products, venison stock, venison, whole dried peas, canola oil, salmon oil, evening primrose oil
		dry	whole dried peas, venison meal, natural flavor, venison, canola oil, salmon oil, evening primrose oil
	Limited Ingredient Diets Green Peas and Rabbit	canned	rabbit liver, rabbit stock, rabbit, whole dried peas, canola oil, salmon oil, evening primrose oil
		dry	whole dried peas, rabbit meal, rabbit, canola oil, natural flavor, salmon oil, evening primrose oil
	Limited Ingredient Diets Green Peas and Duck	canned	duck stock, duck, duck by-products, whole dried peas, canola oil, salmon oil, evening primrose oil
		dry	whole dried peas, duck meal, duck, natural flavor, canola oil, salmon oil, evening primrose oil
Waltham	Waltham Veterinary Diet Selected Protein Diet with Rice & Duck	dry	rice, duck by-product meal, rice gluten, digest of duck by-products, vegetable oil
	Waltham Veterinary Diet Selected Protein with Venison & Rice	canned	venison, venison by-products, rice, sunflower oil

2. Institute a flea control program to prevent flea bites from aggravating the pruritus.
3. Avoid offending dietary allergen(s). Feed balanced, home-cooked or commercially prepared hypoallergenic foods.
4. If cat refuses to eat hypoallergenic foods, long-term therapy with systemic glucocorticoids, antihistamines, and fatty acid supplements, as described for feline atopy, can be tried. However, medical therapy alone is often ineffective.
5. Prognosis is good if the cat accepts the hypoallergenic diet. If the cat relapses, rule out owner noncompliance, development of food hypersensitivity to the new diet, dermatophytosis, ectoparasites, concurrent atopy, and flea allergy dermatitis.

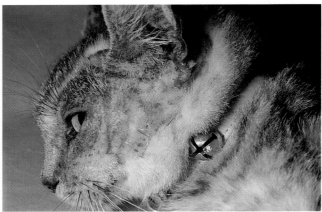

FIGURE 6–55. Feline Food Hypersensitivity. Alopecia and crusting on the head of a food-allergic cat. (Courtesy of J. MacDonald)

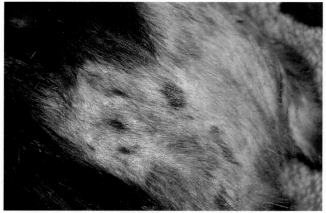

FIGURE 6–53. Feline Food Hypersensitivity. Alopecia on the lumbar and caudal thigh regions of a food-allergic cat.

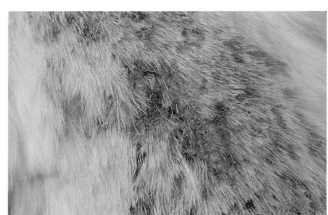

FIGURE 6–56. Feline Food Hypersensitivity. Severe miliary dermatitis and alopecia on the dorsum of a food-allergic cat. (Courtesy of D. Angarano)

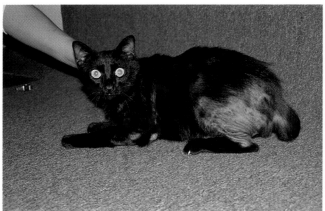

FIGURE 6–54. Feline Food Hypersensitivity. Close-up of the cat in Figure 6–53. The alopecia is often the predominant lesion. Note that the skin is in good condition, with little inflammation.

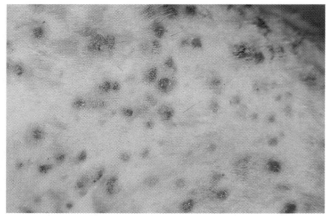

FIGURE 6–57. Feline Food Hypersensitivity. Severe eosinophilic papular dermatitis on the trunk of a cat. The rash covered the majority of the cat's body.

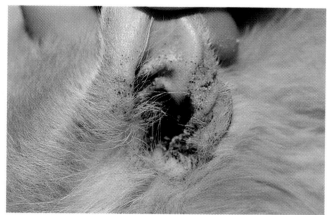

FIGURE 6-58. Feline Food Hypersensitivity. Otitis externa caused by a secondary bacterial and yeast infection associated with allergy. The otitis resolved after a dietary food trial.

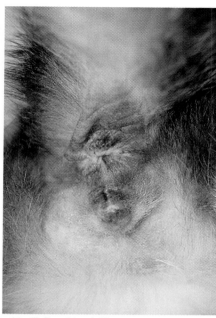

FIGURE 6-60. Feline Food Hypersensitivity. The perianal dermatitis in this cat was intensely pruritic. Perianal dermatitis is a common finding in food-allergic animals.

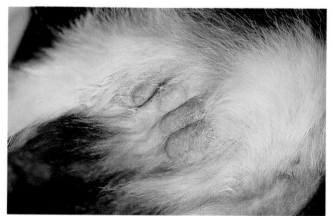

FIGURE 6-59. Feline Food Hypersensitivity. An eosinophilic plaque on the abdomen of a food-allergic cat.

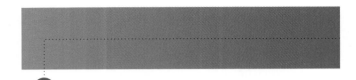

Mosquito Bite Hypersensitivity (Figs. 6–61 to 6–64)

FEATURES

An uncommon seasonal disease in cats sensitized to mosquito bites.

Mildly to severely pruritic papules, pustules, erosions, and crusts appear on the bridge of the nose and on the outer ear pinnae. Lesions may be hypo- or hyperpigmented and symmetric. The bridge of the nose is often swollen. The footpads, especially the outer margins, may be hyperkeratotic, hyper- or hypopigmented, fissured, painful, swollen, and/or ulcerated. Fever and peripheral lymphadenomegaly may be present.

TOP DIFFERENTIALS

Atopy, food hypersensitivity, flea allergy dermatitis, dermatophytosis, ear mites, demodicosis, plasma cell pododermatitis, and autoimmune skin disorders.

DIAGNOSIS

1. Usually based on seasonal history, clinical findings, and response to confinement of cat to a mosquito-free environment. Lesions improve within 4–7 days.
2. Dermatohistopathology—Hyperplastic, superficial perivascular to diffuse eosinophilic dermatitis.

TREATMENT AND PROGNOSIS

1. Keep cat confined indoors, especially at dawn and dusk, when mosquitoes are most active.
2. Keep cat away from known mosquito breeding grounds such as marshes and ponds.
3. If cat cannot be confined, treat symptomatically with prednisone, 3–5 mg/kg PO q 24 hours, until lesions heal (approximately 1–3 weeks), then maintain therapy with the lowest possible alternate-day dosage for the duration of the mosquito season.
4. Alternatively, repositol methylprednisolone acetate, 20 mg/cat or 4 mg/kg SC or IM, can be administered q 2–3 months as needed during the mosquito season.
5. To repel mosquitoes, apply a water-based pyrethrin spray topically, to affected areas q 24 hours. Topical mosquito repellants marketed for human use (i.e. DEET) are generally ineffective and can be toxic to cats.
6. Prognosis is good, but permanent scarring is a potential sequela in severely affected cats.

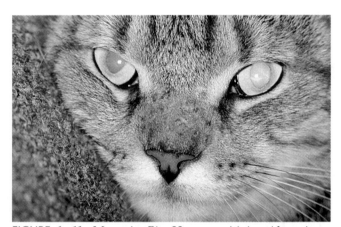

FIGURE 6–61. Mosquito Bite Hypersensitivity. Alopecia and crusts on the bridge of the nose caused by biting mosquitoes.

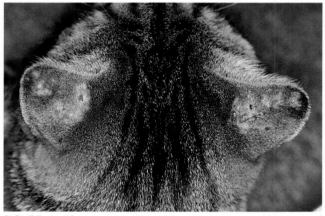

FIGURE 6–62. Mosquito Bite Hypersensitivity. Close-up of the cat in Figure 6–61. Alopecia and crusts on the ear pinnae. Note the similarity to autoimmune skin diseases.

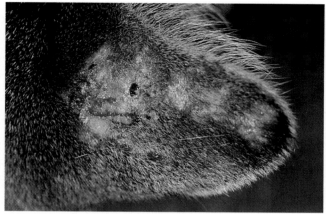

FIGURE 6–63. Mosquito Bite Hypersensitivity. Close-up of the cat in Figures 6–61 and 6–62. Alopecia and crusts on the ear pinnae.

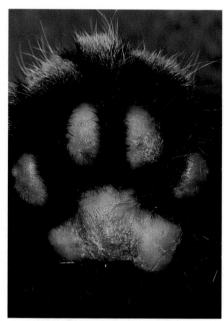

FIGURE 6–64. Feline Mosquito Bite Hypersensitivity. Close-up of the cat in Figures 6–61 to 6–63. Hyperkeratosis and crusting of the footpads. Note the similarity to plasma cell pododermatitis.

Canine Eosinophilic Furunculosis of the Face (Figs. 6–65 to 6–68)

FEATURES

An acute, usually self-limiting disease of the face. Although its exact pathogenesis is not known, a hypersensitivity reaction to insect stings or spider bites is suspected. Uncommon to rare in dogs, with the highest incidence in medium-sized and large-breed dogs.

Blisters, erythematous papules and nodules, ulceration, crusts, and hemorrhage develop acutely and usually peak in severity within 24 hours. Lesions are minimally pruritic to nonpruritic but may be painful and typically involve the muzzle, bridge of the nose, and periocular areas. Occasionally, the ventral abdomen, chest, and/or ear pinnae may be involved.

TOP DIFFERENTIALS

Nasal pyoderma, dermatophytosis, demodicosis, autoimmune skin diseases.

DIAGNOSIS

1. Usually based on history, clinical findings, and ruling out other differentials.
2. Cytology (blister, pustule, exudates)—Numerous eosinophils are seen. Neutrophils and bacteria may also be seen if lesions are secondarily infected.
3. Dermatohistopathology—Eosinophilic perifolliculitis, folliculitis, and furunculosis. Infiltration with neutrophils, lymphocytes, and macrophages, and areas of dermal hemorrhage and collagen degeneration are also common.

TREATMENT AND PROGNOSIS

1. Treat any secondary pyoderma with appropriate systemic antibiotics for 3–4 weeks.
2. Give prednisone, 1–2 mg/kg PO q 24 hours, until lesions are markedly improved (approximately 7–10 days), then give 1–2 mg/kg PO q 48 hours for 10 more days.
3. Prognosis is good. Without glucocorticoid treatment, spontaneous recovery usually occurs within 3 weeks, but giving systemic prednisone hastens resolution of the lesions.

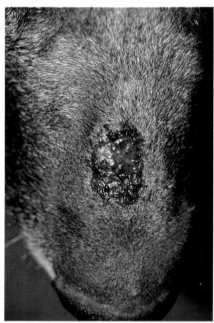

FIGURE 6-65. Canine Eosinophilic Furunculosis of the Face. This focal ulcerative lesion on the nose developed acutely.

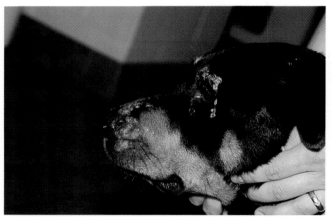

FIGURE 6-67. Canine Eosinophilic Furunculosis of the Face. Same dog as in Figure 6-66. Alopecia, erythema, and papules on the muzzle and around the eye.

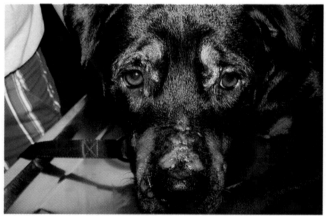

FIGURE 6-66. Canine Eosinophilic Furunculosis of the Face. Alopecia, erythema, and swelling of the nose and periocular tissue caused by venomous insect stings.

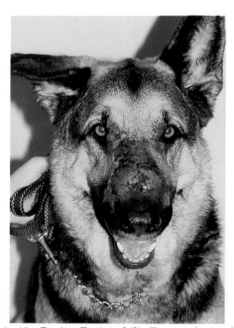

FIGURE 6-68. Canine Eosinophilic Furunculosis of the Face. Severe swelling, erythema, and alopecia on the nose. (Courtesy of D. Angarano)

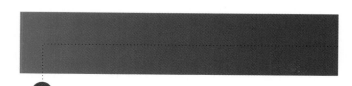

Contact Dermatitis (allergic

contact dermatitis) (Figs. 6–69 to 6–73)

FEATURES

A reaction that usually requires prolonged contact with the offending allergen. Contact hypersensitivity can develop to plants, carpet deodorizers, detergents, floor waxes, fabric cleaners, fertilizers, mulch, concrete, plastic dishes, rubber chew toys, leather/rawhide, and wool or synthetic carpets and rugs. Uncommon to rare in dogs and cats.

Mildly to intensely pruritic skin lesions may include erythema, macules, papules, alopecia, plaques, vesicles, excoriations, hyperpigmentation, lichenification, and crusts. Secondary pyoderma and *Malassezia* dermatitis may be present. Thin-haired skin that frequently contacts the ground (interdigital areas, axillae, groin, scrotum, pressure points, perineum, chin, ear flaps) is usually affected, but haired skin can be involved if the offending allergen is a liquid. The lips and muzzle are typically affected if the offending allergen is rawhide, a rubber chew toy, or a plastic dish.

TOP DIFFERENTIALS

Parasites (canine scabies, demodicosis, pelodera, hookworm dermatitis), atopy, food hypersensitivity, pyoderma, dermatophytosis, *Malassezia* dermatitis.

DIAGNOSIS

1. Rule out other differentials.
2. Dermatohistopathology (nondiagnostic)—Varying degrees of superficial perivascular dermatitis. Mononuclear cells or neutrophils may predominate. Evidence of pyoderma or seborrhea may also be present.
3. Patch testing—A skin reaction (erythema, swelling, macules, and/or papules) develops 48–72 hours after suspected allergen is applied to shaved skin site. False-negative and false-positive reactions can occur.
4. Avoidance/provocative exposure—Removing animal from its environment and hospitalizing it in a stainless steel cage for 3–5 days results in significant clinical improvement. Symptoms recur shortly after reintroduction into regular environment.

TREATMENT AND PROGNOSIS

1. Bathe animal with a hypoallergenic shampoo to remove surface contact allergens.
2. Treat any secondary pyoderma or *Malassezia* dermatitis with appropriate therapies.
3. Identify and remove or avoid contact with the offending allergen.
4. If the allergen cannot be identified or avoided, using mechanical barriers such as socks and a T-shirt may be effective.
5. For short-term control of pruritus, apply glucocorticoid-containing topical preparation to affected areas q 12 hours or give prednisone, 1 mg/kg (dogs) or 2 mg/kg (cats) PO q 24 hours for 5–10 days.
6. For long-term control (if allergen cannot be identified or avoided), systemic glucocorticoid therapy, as described for canine and feline atopy, can be attempted. However, steroids may lose their effectiveness over time.
7. Alternatively, long-term treatment with pentoxyfylline (dogs), 10 mg/kg PO q 12 hours, may be effective in controlling pruritus.
8. Prognosis is good if offending allergen is identified and avoided. Prognosis is poor if allergen cannot be identified or avoided.

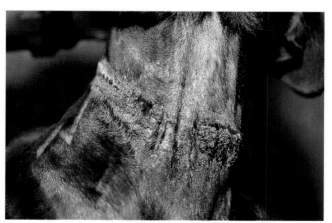

FIGURE 6–69. Contact Dermatitis. The deep erosions, crusts, and alopecia around the neck of this dog were caused by a flea collar that was fastened too tightly. The combination of the pressure and an insecticide acting as an irritant created the severe dermatitis.

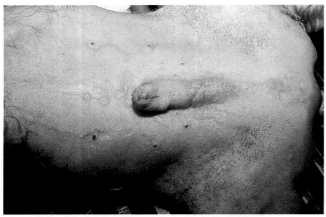

FIGURE 6–70. Contact Dermatitis. Acute urticarial reaction on the abdomen of a dachshund following the application of an iodine surgical scrub.

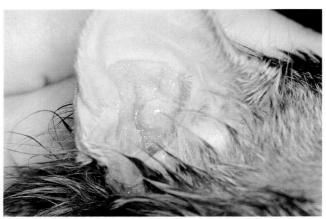

FIGURE 6–72. Contact Dermatitis. Focal erythema and edema caused by a topical otic medication.

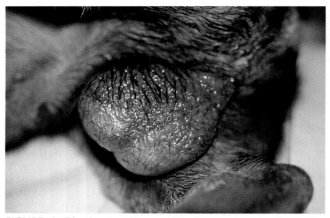

FIGURE 6–71. Contact Dermatitis. Severe erosive dermatitis on the scrotum of a dog.

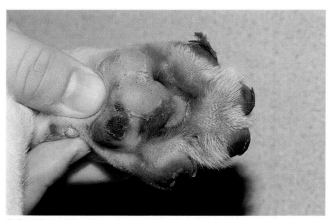

FIGURE 6–73. Contact Dermatitis. Erythema, alopecia, and crusting of the feet caused by chronic exposure to wet concrete cleaned with bleach. The stratum corneum of the footpads is peeling off.

Suggested Readings

Bond R and Llyod DH. 1994. Combined Treatment with Concentrated Essential Fatty Acids and Prednisolone in the Management of Canine Atopy. Vet Rec. 134: 30–32.

Buerger RG. 1995. Insect and Arachnid Hypersensitivity Disorders of Dogs and Cats, pp. 631–634. In Bonagura JD (ed). Kirk's Current Veterinary Therapy, XII, Small Animal Practice. W.B. Saunders, Philadelphia, PA.

Friberg CA and Lewis DT. 1998. Insect Hypersensitivity in Small Animals. Compend Cont Edu Pract Vet. 20: 1121–1132.

Genchi C, Traldi G, and Bianciardi P. 2000. Control of Flea Allergy Dermatitis. Compend Cont Edu Pract Vet. 22: 12–14.

Glivry T, Olivry T, Guaguère E, and Héripret D. 1996. Treatment of Canine Atopic Dermatitis with Misoprostol, a Prostaglandin E Analogue: An Open Study. Proc AAVD & ACVD Ann. Mtg. Las Vegas, NV, pp. 9–10.

Immunologic Skin Diseases, pp. 497-556. In Scott DW, Miller WH Jr, and Griffin CE. 1995. Muller & Kirk's Small Animal Dermatology. Ed. 5. W.B. Saunders, Philadelphia, PA.

Marsella R. 1999. Pentoxyfylline: Drug of the Nineties? TNAVC 1999 Proceedings, pp. 151–152.

Marsella R, Kunkle G, and Lewis D. 1997. Use of Pentoxifylline in the Treatment of Allergic Contact Reactions to Plants of the Commelinceae Family in Dogs. Vet Derm. 8: 121–126.

Nutall T, Thoday K, van den Broek AA, Jackson H, Sture G, and Halliwell R. Retrospective Survey of Allergen Immunotherapy in Canine Atopy. Vet Rec. 143: 139–142.

Plumb DC. 1999. Veterinary Drug Handbook. Ed. 3. Iowa State University Press, Ames, IA.

Scott DW and Miller WH Jr. 1999. Antihistamines in the Management of Allergic Pruritis in Dogs and Cats. J Small Anim Pract. 40: 359–364.

White PD. 1993. Essential Fatty Acids: Use in Management of Canine Atopy. Compend Cont Edu Pract Vet. 15: 451–457.

7

Autoimmune Skin Diseases

- **Pemphigus Foliaceus**

- **Pemphigus Erythematosus**

- **Pemphigus Vulgaris**

- **Bullous Pemphigoid**

- **Discoid Lupus Erythematosus** (DLE)

- **Systemic Lupus Erythematosus** (SLE)

- **Canine Uveodermatologic Syndrome** (Vogt-Koyanagi-Harada-like syndrome, VKH)

- **Alopecia Areata**

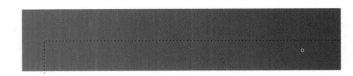

Pemphigus Foliaceus (Figs. 7–1 to 7–20)

FEATURES

An autoimmune skin disease that is characterized by the production of autoantibodies against antigen(s) in or near the epidermal cell membranes. The deposition of antibody in intercellular spaces causes the cells to detach from each other within the uppermost epidermal layers (acantholysis).

Pemphigus foliaceus is probably the most common autoimmune skin disease in dogs and cats.

The primary lesions are superficial pustules. However, intact pustules are often difficult to find because they are obscured by the haircoat, are fragile, and rupture easily. Secondary lesions include superficial erosions, crusts, scales, epidermal collarettes, and alopecia. The disease often begins on the bridge of the nose, around the eyes, and on the ear pinnae before becoming generalized. Nasal depigmentation frequently accompanies facial lesions. Skin lesions are variably pruritic and may wax and wane. Footpad hyperkeratosis is common and may be the only symptom in some dogs. Oral lesions are rare. Mucocutaneous involvement is usually minimal in dogs. In cats, lesions around the nail beds and nipples may be seen. Concurrent lymphadenomegaly, fever, anorexia, and/or depression may be present.

TOP DIFFERENTIALS

Demodicosis, superficial pyoderma, dermatophytosis, systemic lupus erythematosus, subcorneal pustular dermatosis, drug eruption, dermatomyositis, zinc-responsive dermatosis, cutaneous epitheliotropic lymphoma, superficial necrolytic migratory erythema, mosquito bite hypersensitivity (cats).

DIAGNOSIS

1. Rule out other differentials.
2. Cytology (pustule)—Neutrophils and acantholytic cells are seen. Eosinophils may also be present.
3. Dermatohistopathology—Subcorneal pustules containing neutrophils and acantholytic cells, with variable numbers of eosinophils.
4. Immunofluorescence or immunohistochemistry (skin biopsy specimens)—Detection of intercellular antibody deposition is suggestive, but false-positive and false-negative results are common. Positive results should be confirmed histologically.
5. Bacterial culture (pustule)—Usually sterile, but occasionally contaminant bacteria are isolated.

TREATMENT AND PROGNOSIS

1. Symptomatic shampoo therapy to remove crusts may be helpful.
2. To treat or prevent secondary pyoderma, give appropriate long-term systemic antibiotics (minimum 4 weeks). Continue giving antibiotics until concurrent immunosuppressive therapy has the pemphigus under control.
3. To treat the pemphigus, give immunosuppressive doses of oral prednisone or methylprednisolone daily (Table 7–1). After lesions resolve (approximately 2–8 weeks), gradually taper dosage over a period of several (8–10) weeks until the lowest possible alternate-day dosage that maintains remission is being given. If no significant improvement is seen within 2–4 weeks of initiating therapy, rule out a concurrent skin infection and then consider alternative and/or additional immunosuppressive medications.
4. Alternative steroids for refractory cases include triamcinolone and dexamethasone (Table 7–1).
5. Although glucocorticoid therapy alone may be effective in maintaining remission, the dosages needed may result in undesirable side effects. For this reason, the use of nonsteroidal immunosuppressive drugs, either alone or in combination with glucocorticoids, is usually recommended for long-term maintenance.

TABLE 7–1 Glucocorticosteroid Therapies for Autoimmune Skin Diseases

Drug	Species	Induction Dosage	Maintenance Dosage
Prednisone	Dogs and cats	1–3 mg/kg PO q 12 hours	0.5–2 mg/kg PO q 48 hours
Methylprednisolone	Dogs and cats	0.8–2.4 mg/kg PO q 12 hours	0.4–1.6 mg/kg PO q 48 hours
Triamcinolone	Dogs and cats	0.2–0.3 mg/kg PO q 12 hours	0.1–0.2 mg/kg PO q 48–72 hours
Dexamethasone	Dogs and cats	0.1–0.2 mg/kg PO q 12 hours	0.05–0.1 mg/kg PO q 48–72 hours
Methylprednisolone sodium succinate (pulse therapy)	Dogs and cats	1 mg/kg IV over a 3–4 hour period q 24 hours for 2–3 consecutive days	Alternate-day oral glucocorticosteroid

TABLE 7–2 Nonsteroidal Immunosuppressive Drugs for the Treatment of Autoimmune Skin Diseases

Drug	Species	Induction Dosage	Maintenance Dosage
Azathioprine (Imuran)	Dogs	2 mg/kg PO q 24 hours	2 mg/kg PO q 48–72 hours
Chlorambucil (Leukeran)	Dogs and cats	0.1–0.2 mg/kg PO q 24 hours	0.1–0.2 mg/kg PO q 48 hours
Cyclophosphamide (Cytoxan)	Dogs and cats	50 mg/m² PO q 48 hours	25–50 mg/m² PO q 48 hours
Aurothioglucose (Solganal)	Dogs and cats	1 mg/kg IM q 7 days	1 mg/kg IM q 2–4 weeks
Cyclosporin (Neoral)	Dogs	2.5–5 mg/kg PO q 12 hours	Unknown
Tetracycline and niacinamide	Dogs >10 kg	500 mg of each drug PO q 8 hours	500 mg of each drug PO q 12–24 hours
	Dogs <10 kg	250 mg of each drug PO q 8 hours	250 mg of each drug PO q 12–24 hours

6. Nonsteroidal immunosuppressive drugs that may be effective include azathioprine (dogs only), chlorambucil, aurothioglucose, cyclophosphamide, and cyclosporin (Table 7–2). A beneficial response should be noted within 8–12 weeks of initiating therapy. Once remission is achieved, gradually attempt to taper the dosage and frequency of the nonsteroidal immunosuppressive drug for long-term maintenance (Table 7–2).

7. Prognosis is fair to good, but lifelong therapy is usually required to maintain remission. Regular monitoring of clinical signs, hemograms, and serum biochemistry panels with treatment adjustments as needed are essential. Potential complications of immunosuppressive therapy include unacceptable drug side effects and immunosuppression-induced bacterial infections, dermatophytosis, or demodicosis.

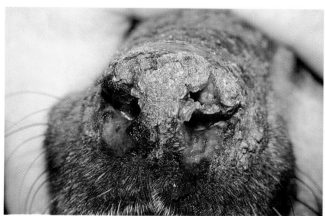

FIGURE 7–2. Pemphigus Foliaceus. Close-up of the dog in Figure 7–1. Severe ulcerations with crust formation on the nasal planum. (Courtesy of A. Yu)

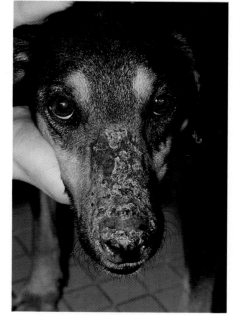

FIGURE 7–1. Pemphigus Foliaceus. Extensive alopecia, erosions, and crusting on the face and nasal planum are typical of many autoimmune skin diseases. (Courtesy of A. Yu)

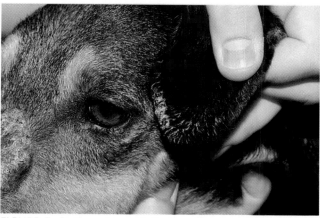

FIGURE 7–3. Pemphigus Foliaceus. Close-up of the dog in Figures 7–1 and 7–2. Alopecia and crusting on the ear pinnae. (Courtesy of A. Yu)

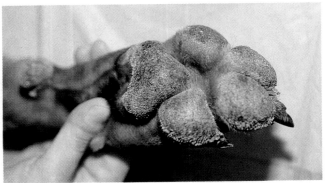

FIGURE 7–4. Pemphigus Foliaceus. Close-up of the dog in Figures 7–1 to 7–3. Hyperkeratosis and crusting of the footpads. Footpad lesions are common in autoimmune skin diseases. (Courtesy of A. Yu)

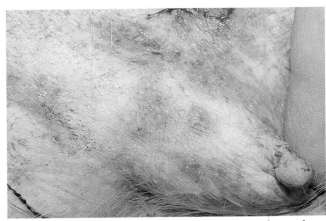

FIGURE 7–7. Pemphigus Foliaceus. Pustules and papules on the abdomen of a dog. Note the similarity to lesions caused by folliculitis. (Courtesy of A. Yu)

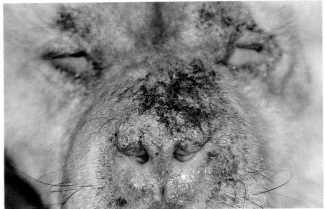

FIGURE 7–5. Pemphigus Foliaceus. Alopecic, erosive lesions on the nasal planum and face of an adult chow chow.

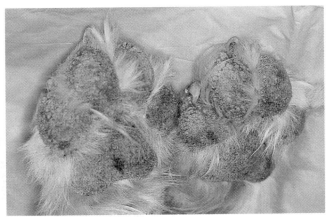

FIGURE 7–8. Pemphigus Foliaceus. Hyperkeratosis and crusting of the footpads.

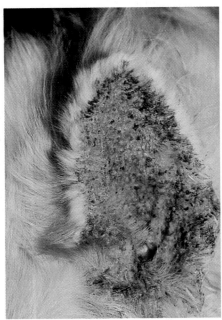

FIGURE 7–6. Pemphigus Foliaceus. Severe papular lesions with crusting on the ear pinnae. (Courtesy of D. Angarano)

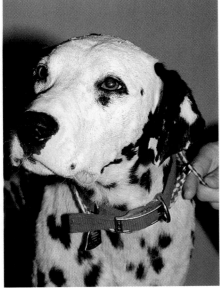

FIGURE 7–9. Pemphigus Foliaceus. This 2-year-old dalmatian developed generalized papules and crusts over a period of a several weeks. The papules are causing the rippled appearance of the hair coat.

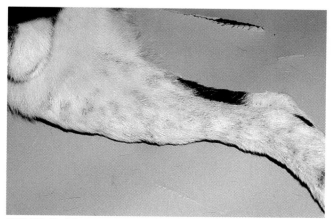

FIGURE 7–10. Pemphigus Foliaceus. Close-up of the dog in Figure 7–9. Papular crusting lesions on the medial thigh.

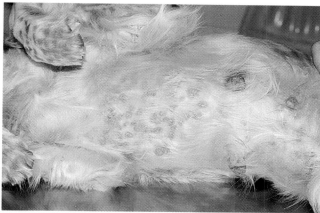

FIGURE 7–13. Pemphigus Foliaceus. Large pustules on the ventrum of a dog. (Courtesy of A. Yu)

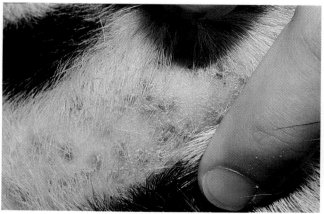

FIGURE 7–11. Pemphigus Foliaceus. Close-up of the dog in Figures 7–9 and 7–10. Papular crusting lesions.

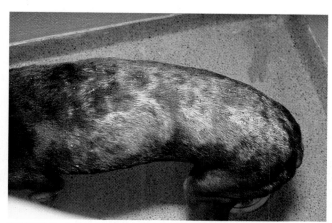

FIGURE 7–14. Pemphigus Foliaceus. Alopecia and cutaneous depigmentation on the dorsum of a dog.

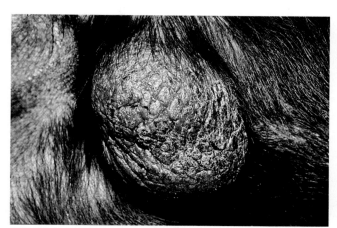

FIGURE 7–12. Pemphigus Foliaceus. Hyperkeratosis and lichenification of the scrotum.

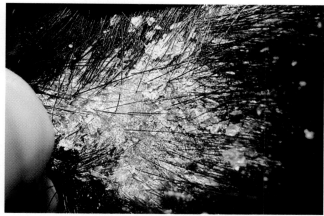

FIGURE 7–15. Pemphigus Foliaceus. Alopecia with crusts and scale are typical lesions caused by pemphigus foliaceus.

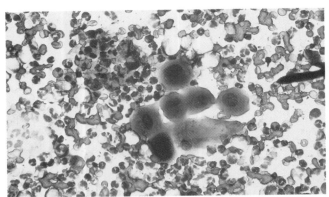

FIGURE 7–16. Pemphigus Foliaceus. Cytology from an impression smear demonstrating large basophilic, nucleated keratinocytes (acantholytic cells).

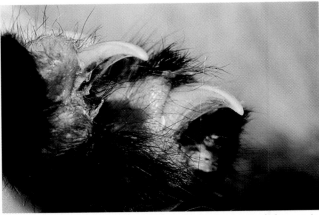

FIGURE 7–19. Pemphigus Foliaceus. Close-up of the cat in Figures 7–17 and 7–18. Paronychia is a common feature of pemphigus foliaceus in cats.

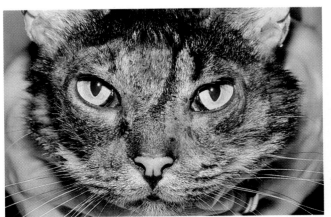

FIGURE 7–17. Pemphigus Foliaceus. Diffuse alopecia and crusting on the face of an adult cat.

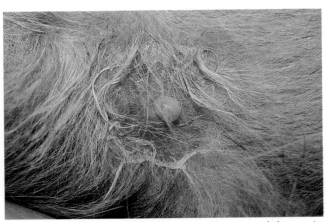

FIGURE 7–20. Pemphigus Foliaceus. Close-up of the cat in Figures 7–17 to 7–19. Alopecia, erythema, and scaling around the nipple.

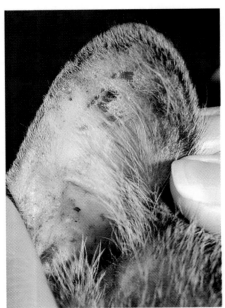

FIGURE 7–18. Pemphigus Foliaceus. Close-up of the cat in Figure 7–17. Papules and crusts on the ear pinnae are typical lesions.

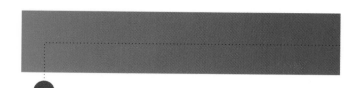

Pemphigus Erythematosus
(Figs. 7–21 to 7–24)

FEATURES

This disease may be a benign form of pemphigus foliaceus or a crossover between pemphigus and lupus erythematosus. Uncommon in cats. Common in dogs, with an increased incidence in German shepherds, collies, and Shetland sheepdogs.

The disease is usually limited to the face (bridge of the nose and around the eyes) and ear pinnae. Superficial erosions, scales, and/or crusts are typical. Pustules may be present but are usually difficult to find. The skin lesions may be minimally to mildly pruritic. Concurrent nasal depigmentation is common. Occasionally, the footpads are hyperkeratotic. The oral cavity is not involved.

TOP DIFFERENTIALS

Demodicosis, nasal pyoderma, dermatophytosis, discoid lupus erythematosus, pemphigus foliaceus, dermatomyositis, nasal solar dermatitis, mosquito bite hypersensitivity (cats), uveodermatologic syndrome, and zinc-responsive dermatosis.

DIAGNOSIS

1. Rule out other differentials.
2. Cytology (pustule)—Neutrophils and acantholytic cells are seen. Eosinophils may also be present.
3. Antinuclear antibody (ANA) test—May be positive; however, a positive result is only supportive, and not pathognomonic for pemphigus erythematosus because positive titers can be associated with many other chronic diseases.
4. Dermatohistopathology—Subcorneal pustules containing neutrophils and acantholytic cells with/without eosinophils. Lichenoid infiltration with mononuclear cells, plasma cells, neutrophils, and/or eosinophils may also be present.
5. Immunofluorescence or immunohistochemistry (skin biopsy specimens)—Detection of intercellular antibody deposition. Antibody deposition along the dermal-epidermal junction may also be present. False-positive and false-negative results are common. Positive results should be confirmed histologically.
6. Bacterial culture (pustule)—Usually sterile, but occasionally contaminant bacteria are isolated.

TREATMENT AND PROGNOSIS

1. Avoid sunlight exposure and use topical sunscreens to prevent ultraviolet light from exacerbating nasal lesions.
2. For mild cases, topically applied glucocorticoids may be effective. Initially, use a potent glucocorticoid (i.e., betamethasone or fluocinolone) q 12 hours until lesions resolve (approximately 4–6 weeks), then gradually decrease the frequency of applications and the potency of the glucocorticoid as much as possible for maintenance therapy. Permanent alopecia and cutaneous atrophy at the site of application are possible side effects of high-potency, frequently applied topical glucocorticoids.
3. For mild to moderate cases, systemic therapy with fatty acid supplements, vitamin E, or combination niacinamide and tetracycline may be effective (Table 7–2). Significant improvement should be seen within 8–12 weeks of initiating therapy.
4. For severe or refractory cases, give immunosuppressive doses of oral prednisone or methylprednisolone daily (Table 7–1). After lesions resolve (approximately 2–8 weeks), gradually taper dosage over a period of several (8–10) weeks until the lowest possible alternate-day dosage that maintains remission is being given. If no significant improvement is seen within 2–4 weeks of initiating therapy, rule out a concurrent skin infection and then consider alternative and/or additional immunosuppressive medications.
5. Although systemic glucocorticoid therapy alone may be effective in maintaining remission, the dosages needed may result in undesirable side effects. For this reason, the use of nonsteroidal immunosuppressive drugs, either alone or in combination with glucocorticoids, is usually recommended for long-term maintenance.
6. Nonsteroidal immunosuppressive drugs that may be effective include azathioprine (dogs only), chlorambucil, aurothioglucose, cyclophosphamide, and cyclosporin (Table 7–2). A beneficial response should be noted within 8–12 weeks of initiating therapy. Once remission is achieved, gradually attempt to taper the dosage and frequency of the nonsteroidal immunosuppressive drug for long-term maintenance (Table 7–2).
7. Prognosis is good because even without treatment, this disease usually remains benign and localized. If systemic immunosuppressive drugs are used, regular monitoring of clinical signs, hemograms, and serum biochemistry panels with treatment adjustments as needed are essential. Potential complications of systemic immunosuppressive therapy include unacceptable drug side effects and immunosuppression-induced secondary bacterial infections, dermatophytosis, or demodicosis.

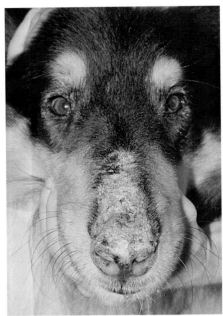

FIGURE 7–21. Pemphigus Erythematosus. Alopecia, erosions, crusting, and depigmentation on the nasal planum, bridge of the nose, and around the eyes. (Courtesy of D. Angarano)

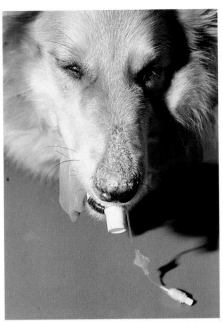

FIGURE 7–23. Pemphigus Erythematosus. Alopecia, erythema, and depigmentation affecting the nasal planum and bridge of the nose.

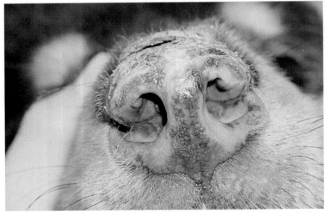

FIGURE 7–22. Pemphigus Erythematosus. Close-up of the dog in Figure 7–21. Nasal depigmentation and erosions. (Courtesy of D. Angarano)

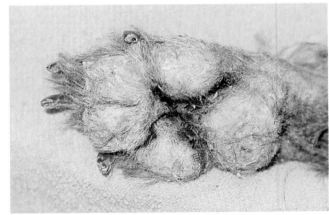

FIGURE 7–24. Pemphigus Erythematosus. Severe crusting and hyperkeratosis of the footpads. (Courtesy of D. Angarano)

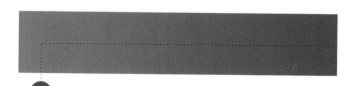

Pemphigus Vulgaris (Figs. 7–25 to 7–31)

FEATURES

An autoimmune skin disease that is characterized by the production of autoantibodies against antigen(s) in or near the epidermal cell membranes. The deposition of antibody in intercellular spaces causes cell detachment within the deeper epidermal layers (acantholysis). The most severe form of pemphigus. Rare in dogs and cats.

Erosions, ulcers, and, rarely, vesicles and bullae occur on the skin (especially the axillae and groin), mucocutaneous junctions (nailbeds, lips, nares, eyelids), and mucous membranes (oral cavity, anus, vulva, prepuce, conjunctiva). Concurrent fever, depression, and anorexia are common.

TOP DIFFERENTIALS

Bullous pemphigoid, systemic lupus erythematosus, erythema multiforme/toxic epidermal necrolysis, drug reaction, infection (bacterial, fungal), cutaneous epitheliotrophic lymphoma.

DIAGNOSIS

1. Rule out other differentials.
2. Dermatohistopathology—Suprabasilar clefts and vesicles with varying degrees of perivascular, interstitial, or lichenoid inflammation.
3. Immunofluorescence or immunohistochemistry (skin biopsy specimens)—Detection of intercellular antibody deposition. False-positive and false-negative results are common. Positive results should be confirmed histologically.
4. Bacterial culture (vesicle, bulla)—Usually sterile, but occasionally contaminant bacteria are isolated.

TREATMENT AND PROGNOSIS

1. Symptomatic shampoo therapy to remove crusts may be helpful.
2. To treat or prevent secondary pyoderma, give appropriate long-term systemic antibiotics (minimum 4 weeks). Continue giving antibiotics until concurrent immunosuppressive therapy has the pemphigus under control.
3. To treat the pemphigus, give immunosuppressive doses of oral prednisone or methylprednisolone daily (Table 7–1). After lesions resolve (approximately 4–10 weeks), gradually taper dosage over a period of several (8–10) weeks until the lowest possible alternate-day dosage that maintains re-

mission is being given. If no significant improvement is seen within 2–4 weeks of initiating therapy, rule out a concurrent skin infection and then consider alternative and/or additional immunosuppressive medications.
4. Alternative glucocorticoids for refractory cases include triamcinolone and dexamethasone (Table 7–1).
5. Although glucocorticoid therapy alone may be effective in maintaining remission, the dosages needed may result in undesirable side effects. For this reason, the use of nonsteroidal immunosuppressive drugs in combination with glucocorticoids is usually recommended for long-term maintenance.
6. Nonsteroidal immunosuppressive drugs that may be effective include azathioprine (dogs only), chlorambucil, cyclophosphamide, and cyclosporin (Table 7–2). A beneficial response should be noted within 8–12 weeks of initiating therapy. Once remission is achieved, gradually attempt to taper the dosage and frequency of the nonsteroidal immunosuppressive drug for long-term maintenance (Table 7–2).
7. Prognosis is fair to poor, and lifelong therapy is usually required to maintain remission. Regular monitoring of clinical signs, hemograms, serum biochemistry panels, and treatment adjustments as needed are essential. Potential complications of immunosuppressive therapy include unacceptable drug side effects and immunosuppression-induced bacterial infections, dermatophytosis, or demodicosis.

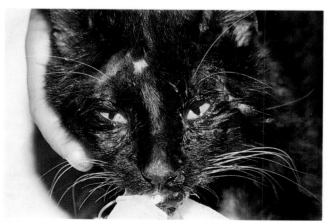

FIGURE 7–25. Pemphigus Vulgaris. These deep ulcerations on the face of an adult cat are typical of this deeper form of pemphigus. (Courtesy of A. Yu)

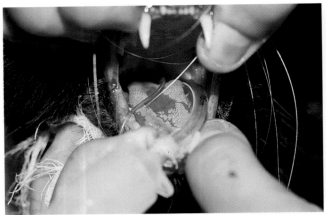

FIGURE 7–26. Pemphigus Vulgaris. Close-up of the cat in Figure 7–25. Erosions and ulcerations on the tongue. Mucosal erosions and ulcerations are common in patients with pemphigus vulgaris. (Courtesy of A. Yu)

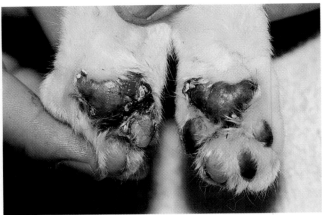

FIGURE 7–29. Pemphigus Vulgaris. Close-up of the cat in Figures 7–25 to 7–28. Crusting, erosive footpad lesions. (Courtesy of A. Yu)

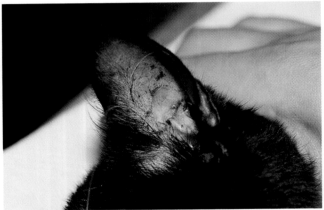

FIGURE 7–27. Pemphigus Vulgaris. Close-up of the cat in Figures 7–25 and 7–26. Erosions and ulcerations on the ear pinnae. (Courtesy of A. Yu)

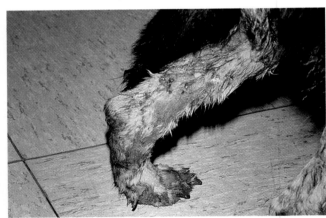

FIGURE 7–30. Pemphigus Vulgaris. Alopecia and erosions on the rear leg of a young mixed-breed German shepherd.

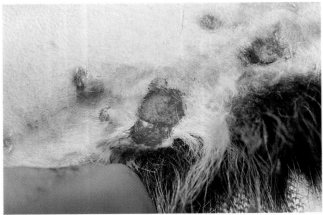

FIGURE 7–28. Pemphigus Vulgaris. Close-up of the cat in Figures 7–25 to 7–27. The deep ulcerations are characteristic of pemphigus vulgaris. (Courtesy of A. Yu)

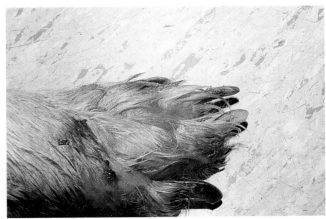

FIGURE 7–31. Pemphigus Vulgaris. Close-up of the dog in Figure 7–30. Alopecic erosions on the dorsal foot.

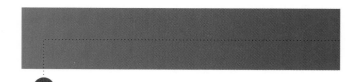

Bullous Pemphigoid (Figs. 7–32 to 7–36)

FEATURES

An autoimmune skin disease characterized by the production of autoantibodies against basement membrane zone (lamina lucida) antigens that cause the epidermis to separate from the underlying dermis. Fragile vesicles and bullae form and rupture, leaving ulcerated lesions. Rare in dogs.

An ulcerative disease of skin (especially on the head, neck, axillae, ventral abdomen), mucocutaneous junctions (nares, eyelids, lips), mucous membranes (oral cavity, anus, vulva, prepuce, conjunctiva), and footpads. Vesicles and bullae are rare. Severely affected dogs may be anorectic, depressed, and febrile.

TOP DIFFERENTIALS

Pemphigus vulgaris, systemic lupus erythematosus, erythema multiforme/toxic epidermal necrolysis, drug eruption, cutaneous epitheliotropic lymphoma, infection (bacterial, fungal).

DIAGNOSIS

1. Rule out other differentials.
2. Dermatohistopathology—Subepidermal clefts and vesicles with a mild perivascular to marked lichenoid mononuclear and neutrophilic inflammation. Eosinophils may also be present.
3. Immunofluorescence or immunohistochemistry (skin biopsy specimens)—Deposition of immunoglobulin along the dermoepidermal junction. False-positive and false-negative results are common. Positive results should be confirmed histologically.
4. Bacterial culture (vesicle, bulla)—Usually sterile, but occasionally contaminant bacteria are isolated.

TREATMENT AND PROGNOSIS

1. Symptomatic shampoo therapy to remove crusts may be helpful.
2. To treat or prevent secondary pyoderma, give appropriate long-term systemic antibiotics (minimum 4 weeks). Continue giving antibiotics until concurrent immunosuppressive therapy has the pemphigoid under control.
3. To treat the bullous pemphigoid, give immunosuppressive doses of oral prednisone or methylprednisolone daily (Table 7–1). After lesions resolve (approximately 4–8 weeks), gradually taper dosage over a period of several (8–10) weeks until the lowest possible alternate-day dosage that maintains remission is being given. If no significant improvement is seen within 2–4 weeks of initiating therapy, rule out a concurrent skin infection and then consider alternative and/ or additional immunosuppressive medications.
4. Alternative glucocorticoids for refractory cases include triamcinolone and dexamethasone (Table 7–1).
5. Although glucocorticoid therapy alone may be effective in maintaining remission, the dosages needed may result in undesirable side effects. For this reason, the use of nonsteroidal immunosuppressive drugs, either alone or in combination with glucocorticoids, is usually recommended for long-term maintenance.
6. Nonsteroidal immunosuppressive drugs that may be effective include azathioprine, chlorambucil, aurothioglucose, cyclophosphamide, and cyclosporin (Table 7–2). A beneficial response should be noted within 8–12 weeks of initiating therapy. Once remission is achieved, gradually attempt to taper the dosage and frequency of the nonsteroidal immunosuppressive drug for long-term maintenance (Table 7–2).
7. Prognosis is fair to good, but lifelong therapy is usually required to maintain remission. Regular monitoring of clinical signs, hemograms, and serum biochemistry panels with treatment adjustments as needed are essential. Potential complications of immunosuppressive therapy include unacceptable drug side effects and immunosuppression-induced bacterial infections, dermatophytosis, or demodicosis.

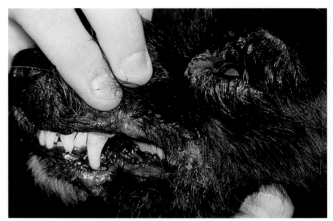

FIGURE 7–32. Bullous Pemphigoid. Alopecia, ulcers, and crusts around the mouth and eye of an adult Scottie.

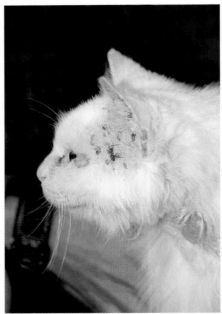

FIGURE 7–33. Bullous Pemphigoid. Alopecia and ulcers on the face of an adult cat.

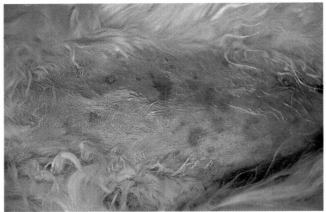

FIGURE 7–35. Bullous Pemphigoid. Close-up of the cat in Figures 7–33 and 7–34. Numerous ulcers were present on the trunk.

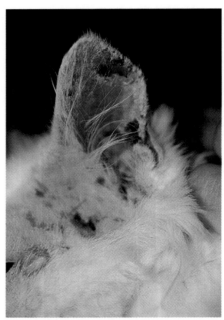

FIGURE 7–34. Bullous Pemphigoid. Close-up of the cat in Figure 7–33. Alopecia, erythremia, and ulcers on the ear pinnae.

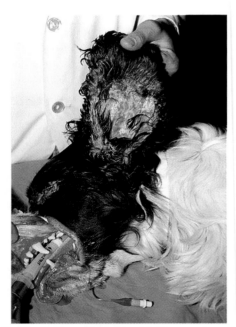

FIGURE 7–36. Bullous Pemphigoid. Severe ulceration on the oral mucosa, mucocutaneous junction, face, and ear pinnae. (Courtesy of D. Angarano)

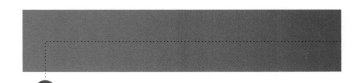

Discoid Lupus Erythematosus

(DLE) (Figs. 7–37 to 7–42)

FEATURES

This disease is considered by many to be a benign variant of systemic lupus erythematosus. Common in dogs and rare in cats.

Dogs. Nasal depigmentation, erythema, scaling, erosions, ulcerations and/or crusting are characteristic. Similar lesions may involve the lips, the bridge of the nose, periocular skin, ear pinnae, and, less commonly, the distal limbs or genitalia. Hyperkeratotic footpads and oral ulcers are rarely present.

Cats. Erythema, alopecia, and crusting on the face and ear pinnae. Nasal lesions are uncommon.

TOP DIFFERENTIALS

Nasal pyoderma, demodicosis, dermatophytosis, pemphigus erythematosus or foliaceus, dermatomyositis, uveodermatologic syndrome, nasal solar dermatitis, nasal depigmentation, mosquito bite hypersensitivity (cats).

DIAGNOSIS

1. Rule out other differentials.
2. Dermatohistopathology—Findings may include hydropic and/or lichenoid interface dermatitis, focal thickening of basement membrane zone, pigmentary incontinence, apoptotic keratinocytes, and perivascular and periadnexal accumulations of mononuclear and plasma cells.
3. Immunofluorescence or immunohistochemistry (skin biopsy specimens)—Patchy deposition of immunoglobulin or complement at the basement membrane zone. Not diagnostic in itself because false-positive results are possible and false-negative results are common.

TREATMENT AND PROGNOSIS

1. Avoid sunlight exposure and use topical sunscreens to prevent ultraviolet light from exacerbating nasal lesions.
2. For mild cases, topically applied glucocorticoids may be effective. Initially, use a potent glucocorticoid (i.e., betamethasone or fluocinolone) q 12 hours until lesions resolve (approximately 4–6 weeks), then gradually decrease the frequency of applications and the potency of the glucocorticoid as much as possible for maintenance therapy. Permanent alopecia and cutaneous atrophy at the site of application are possible side effects of high-potency, frequently applied topical glucocorticoids.
3. As an alternative to topical glucocorticoids, topically applied 1–2% cyclosporin solution q 8–12 hours may be effective in some cases. Beneficial response should be seen within 1–2 months. Then use as infrequently as needed to retain remission.
4. For mild to moderate cases, systemic therapy with fatty acid supplements, vitamin E, or combination of niacinamide and tetracycline may be effective (Table 7–2). Significant improvement should be seen within 8–12 weeks of initiating therapy.
5. For moderate to severe cases, give prednisone PO, 2 mg/kg q 24 hours or 1 mg/kg q 12 hours, until lesions resolve (approximately 4 weeks). Then give 2 mg/kg PO q 48 hours for approximately 2–4 weeks, and then gradually taper down to the lowest possible alternate-day dosage needed for maintenance therapy.
6. Treatment with combined systemic glucocorticoid and nonsteroidal immunosuppressive drugs is rarely necessary.
7. Prognosis is good, but lifelong treatment is usually necessary. Permanent scarring or leukoderma (depigmentation) and, rarely, squamous cell carcinoma are possible sequelae.

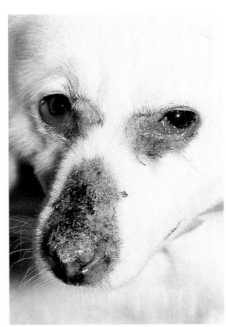

FIGURE 7–37. Discoid Lupus Erythematosus. Severe erosive crusting lesions affecting the nasal planum, bridge of the nose, and periocular tissue. (Courtesy of D. Angarano)

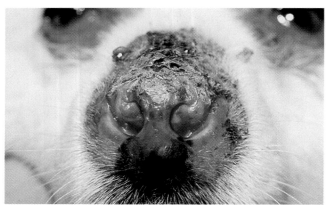

FIGURE 7–38. Discoid Lupus Erythematosus. Close-up of the dog in Figure 7–37. Severe ulcerative lesions on the nose. (Courtesy of D. Angarano)

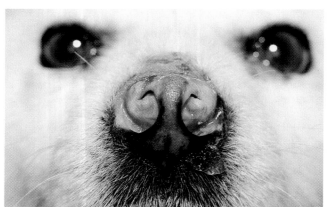

FIGURE 7–39. Discoid Lupus Erythematosus. Close-up of the dog in Figures 7–37 and 7–38. Residual depigmentation and scarring following treatment. (Courtesy of D. Angarano)

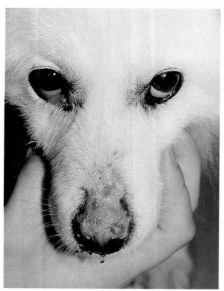

FIGURE 7–40. Discoid Lupus Erythematosus. Close-up of the dog in Figures 7–37 to 7–39. Residual alopecia, depigmentation, and scarring can be a sequelae of the disease. (Courtesy of D. Angarano)

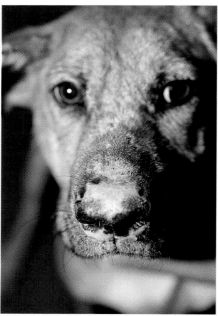

FIGURE 7–41. Discoid Lupus Erythematosus. Focal alopecia and depigmentation.

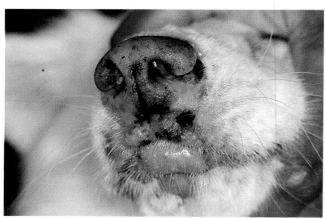

FIGURE 7–42. Discoid Lupus Erythematosus. Early lesions consisting of focal depigmentation and inflammation without erosions or crusts.

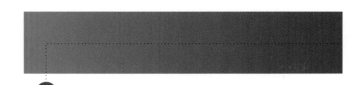

Systemic Lupus Erythematosus (SLE) (Figs. 7–43 to 7–52)

FEATURES

A multisystemic immune-mediated disease characterized by the production of a variety of autoantibodies (i.e., ANA, rheumatoid factor, antiRBC antibodies) that form circulating immune-complexes. Rare in cats. Uncommon in dogs, with collies, Shetland sheepdogs, and German shepherds possibly predisposed.

Dogs. Symptoms are often nonspecific and may wax and wane. Cutaneous signs are common, variable, and often mimic those seen in many other skin disorders. Mucocutaneous and/or mucosal erosions and ulcers may be present. Skin lesions may include erosions, ulcers, scales, erythema, alopecia, crusting, and scarring. Lesions may be multifocal or diffuse. They can occur anywhere on the body, but the face, ears, and distal extremities are most commonly affected. Peripheral lymphadomegaly is often present.

Other symptoms include fluctuating fever, polyarthritis, polymyositis, renal failure, blood dyscrasias, pleuritis, pneumonitis, pericarditis or myocarditis, central or peripheral neuropathy, and lymphedema.

Cats. Cutaneous lesions are variable and may include an erythematous, alopecic, scaling, crusting, and scarring dermatosis, an exfoliative erythroderma, or excessive scaling (seborrhea). Lesions can be anywhere on the body, but the face, ear pinnae, and paws are most often affected. Oral ulcers may be present. Other symptoms may include fever, polyarthritis, renal failure, neurologic or behavioral abnormalities, hematologic abnormalities, and myopathy.

TOP DIFFERENTIALS

Other causes of polysystemic disease such as drug reaction, infections (viral, bacterial, rickettsial, fungal), neoplasia, and other autoimmune and immune-mediated disorders.

DIAGNOSIS

1. A definitive diagnosis is often difficult to make. All other differentials must be ruled out. The following findings are supportive and, when several are present, highly suggestive of systemic lupus erythematosus:
   Hemogram—Anemia (that may or may not be Coombs' positive), thrombocytopenia, leukopenia, or leukocytosis.
   Urinalysis—Proteinuria.
   Arthrocentesis (polyarthritis)—Sterile purulent inflammation (may or may not be rheumatoid factor positive).
   ANA test—A good screening test because most patients with systemic lupus erythematosus have positive ANA titers. However, a positive result is only supportive, not pathognomonic for systemic lupus erythematosus, because positive titers can be associated with many other chronic diseases.
   Lupus erythematosus (LE) cell test—A positive result is highly suggestive, but this is not a good screening test because false-negative results are common.
2. Dermatohistopathology—Focal thickening of basement membrane zone, subepidermal vacuolation, hydropic or lichenoid interface dermatitis, and/or leukocytoclastic vasculitis are characteristic. However, these changes are not always seen, and findings may be nonspecific.
3. Immunofluorescence or immunohistochemistry (skin biopsy specimens)—Patchy deposition of immunoglobulin or complement at the basement membrane zone. Not diagnostic in itself because false-positive results are possible and false-negative results are common.

TREATMENT AND PROGNOSIS

1. Symptomatic shampoo therapy to remove crusts may be helpful.
2. To treat or prevent secondary pyoderma, give appropriate long-term systemic antibiotics (minimum 4 weeks). Continue giving antibiotics until concurrent immunosuppressive therapy has the lupus under control.
3. To treat the lupus, give immunosuppressive doses of oral prednisone or methylprednisolone daily (Table 7–1). Continue daily induction dosage until lesions resolve (approximately 4–8 weeks). Then gradually taper dosage over a period of several (8–10) weeks until the lowest possible alternate-day dosage that maintains remission is being given. If no significant improvement is seen within 2–4 weeks of initiating therapy, rule out a concurrent skin infection and then consider alternative and/or additional immunosuppressive medications.
4. Alternative glucocorticoids for refractory cases include triamcinolone and dexamethasone (Table 7–1).
5. Although glucocorticoid therapy alone may be effective in maintaining remission, the dosages needed may result in undesirable side effects. For this reason, the use of nonsteroidal immunosuppressive drugs in combination with glucocorticoids is usually recommended for long-term maintenance.
6. Nonsteroidal immunosuppressive drugs that may be effective include azathioprine (dogs only), chlorambucil, cyclophosphamide, and cyclosporin (Table 7–2). A beneficial response should be

noted within 8–12 weeks of initiating therapy. Once remission is achieved, gradually attempt to taper the dosage and frequency of the nonsteroidal immunosuppressive drug for long-term maintenance (Table 7–2).

7. Prognosis is guarded if hemolytic anemia, thrombocytopenia, or glomerulonephritis is present. In up to 40% of these cases, death occurs during the first year of treatment from renal failure, a poor response to therapy, drug complications, or secondary systemic infections (pneumonia, sepsis). Prognosis is more favorable for animals that respond to glucocorticoid therapy alone, with approximately 50% of them having long-term survival times. Regular monitoring of clinical signs, hemograms, and serum biochemistry panels with treatment adjustments as needed are essential.

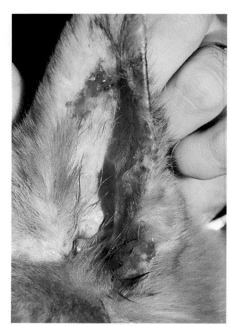

FIGURE 7–45. Systemic Lupus Erythematosus. Close-up of the dog in Figures 7–43 and 7–44. Erosive lesions on the ear pinnae.

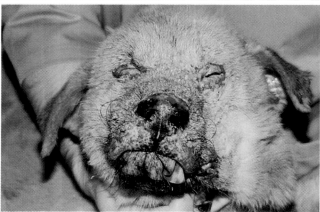

FIGURE 7–43. Systemic Lupus Erythematosus. Deep erosions and ulcerations on the nasal planum and face of a young mixed-breed female chow.

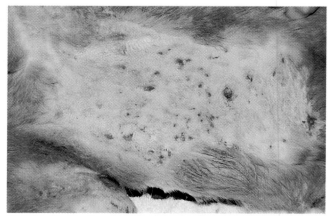

FIGURE 7–46. Systemic Lupus Erythematosus. Close-up of the dog in Figures 7–43 to 7–45. Multiple punctate erosions were present over the entire cutaneous surface.

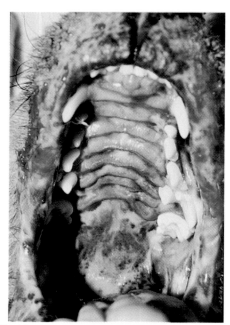

FIGURE 7–44. Systemic Lupus Erythematosus. Close-up of the dog in Figure 7–43. Erosions on the hard palate and mucocutaneous junction.

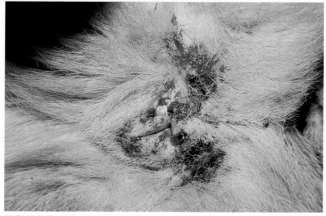

FIGURE 7–47. Systemic Lupus Erythematosus. Close-up of the dog in Figures 7–43 to 7–46. Erosive lesions on the mucocutaneous junction of the vulva.

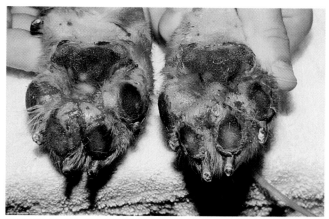

FIGURE 7–48. Systemic Lupus Erythematosus. Close-up of the dog in Figures 7–43 to 7–47. Deep erosive lesions on the feet, with crusting and sloughing of the footpad.

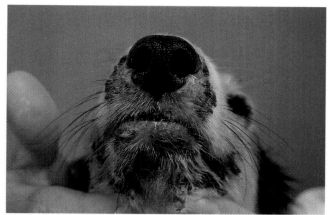

FIGURE 7–51. Systemic Lupus Erythematosus. Alopecia and erythema with depigmentation on the muzzle of a dog. (Courtesy of D. Angarano)

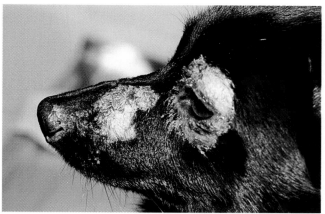

FIGURE 7–49. Systemic Lupus Erythematosus. Alopecia, erythema, and crusting, erosive lesions on the nose and face of a dog.

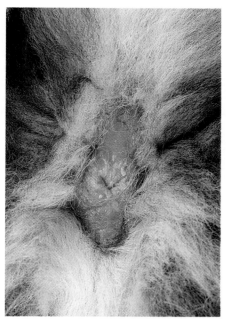

FIGURE 7–52. Systemic Lupus Erythematosus. Erosive dermatitis affecting the perianal tissue and mucocutaneous junction of a dog. (Courtesy of D. Angarano)

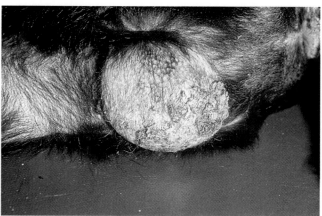

FIGURE 7–50. Systemic Lupus Erythematosus. Crusting erosions on the scrotum of a dog. (Courtesy of D. Angarano)

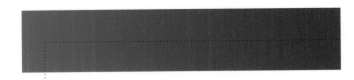

Canine Uveodermatologic Syndrome (Vogt-Koyanagi-Harada-like syndrome, VKH) (Figs. 7–53 to 7–56)

FEATURES

An autoimmune disorder characterized by the production of autoantibodies against melanocytes that result in granulomatous panuveitis, leukoderma (skin depigmentation), and leukotrichia (hair depigmentation). Rare in dogs, with the highest incidence in young adult and middle-aged Akitas, Samoyeds, Siberian huskies, Irish setters, and Chow chows.

Acute onset of uveitis (blepharospasm, conjunctivitis, corneal edema, miosis, serous ocular discharge) which can develop shortly before, concurrent with, or subsequent to well-demarcated symmetrical depigmentation of the nose, lips, and eyelids. Occasionally the scrotum or vulva, anus, footpads, and/or hard palate also are depigmented. Rarely, lesions become eroded, ulcerated, and crusted. In some dogs, generalized skin and haircoat depigmentation may develop.

TOP DIFFERENTIALS

Vitiligo, other autoimmune skin diseases, and other causes of uveitis.

DIAGNOSIS

1. Usually based on history, clinical findings, and ruling out other differentials.
2. Ophthalmic findings—Sterile uveitis and chorioretinitis.
3. Dermatohistopathology—Pigmentary incontinence and lichenoid interface dermatitis composed of large histiocytes, small mononuclear cells, and multinucleated giant cells. Occasionally, plasma cells and lymphocytes may predominate.

TREATMENT AND PROGNOSIS

1. To prevent blindness, early and aggressive treatment is essential.
2. Treat eyes with topical or subconjunctival glucocorticoids until the uveitis has resolved. Effective therapies include:

    0.1% Dexamethasone ophthalmic solution OU q 4 hours.

    1% Prednisone ophthalmic solution OU q 4 hours.

    Dexamethasone, 1–2 mg subconjunctivally OU q 24 hours.

    Triamcinolone, 10–20 mg subconjunctivally OU once.

    Depot betamethasone, 6 mg subconjunctivally OU once.

3. Also instill a topical cycloplegic (1% atropine ophthalmic solution) OU q 6–24 hours or to effect.
4. Give immunosuppressive doses of oral prednisone or methylprednisolone (Table 7–1). After ocular lesions resolve (approximately 4–8 weeks), gradually taper dosage over a period of several (8–10) weeks until the lowest possible alternate-day dosage that maintains remission is being given. If no significant improvement is seen within 2 weeks of initiating therapy, consider alternative and/or additional immunosuppressive medications.
5. Alternative glucocorticoids for refractory cases include triamcinolone and dexamethasone (Table 7–1).
6. If systemic glucocorticoid therapy alone is ineffective or if undesirable side effects develop, treatment with oral azathioprine or cyclophosphamide may be effective (Table 7–2). A beneficial response should be noted within 8–12 weeks of initiating treatment. Once remission is achieved, taper the azathiaprine or cyclophosphamide dosage and frequency of administration for long-term maintenance therapy (Table 7–2).
7. Prognosis is guarded to fair. Lifelong therapy is usually needed. If the uveitis is not treated early and aggressively or is poorly controlled, glaucoma, cataracts, and blindness are likely sequelae. The cutaneous depigmentation is usually a cosmetic problem only, and may be permanent or incompletely improved in some cases.

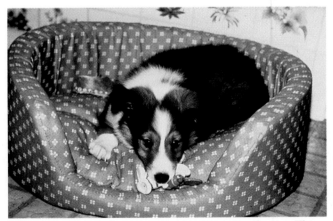

FIGURE 7–53. Canine Uveodermatologic Syndrome. This young sheltie was diagnosed early. As the disease progressed, the cutaneous pigmentation was lost (see Figure 7–54). (Courtesy of K. Campbell; Campbell K and McLaughlin S: Generalized Leukoderma and Poliosis Following Uveitis in a Dog. J Am Anim Hosp Assoc. 22: 121, 1986)

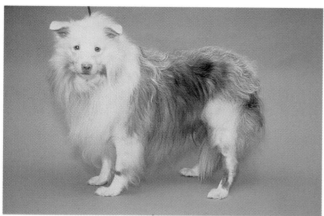

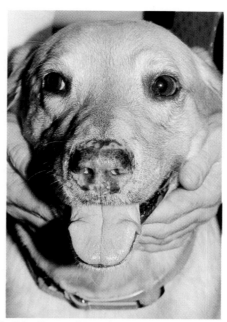

FIGURE 7–54. Canine Uveodermatologic Syndrome. The same dog as in Figure 7–53. The depigmentation has progressed over several years. (Courtesy of K. Campbell; Campbell K and McLaughlin S: Generalized Leukoderma and Poliosis Following Uveitis in a Dog. J Am Anim Hosp Assoc. 22: 121, 1986)

FIGURE 7–56. Canine Uveodermatologic Syndrome. Moderate depigmentation affecting the nose and lips. Note the ocular lesions (uveitis), which can progress rapidly, causing blindness.

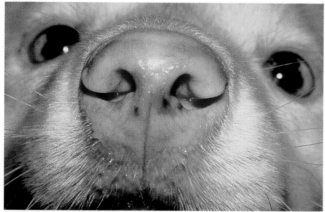

FIGURE 7–55. Canine Uveodermatologic Syndrome. Close-up of the dog in Figures 7–53 and 7–54. The nasal depigmentation has progressed and is almost complete. (Courtesy of K. Campbell; Campbell K and McLaughlin S: Generalized Leukoderma and Poliosis Following Uveitis in a Dog. J Am Anim Hosp Assoc. 22: 121, 1986)

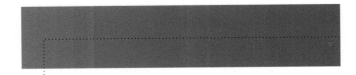

Alopecia Areata (Figs. 7–57 to 7–60)

FEATURES

An autoimmune skin disease characterized by the production of autoantibodies against hair follicle antigens that result in hair loss. Rare in dogs and cats.

Focal to multifocal, well-circumscribed patches of alopecia that may gradually enlarge. Lesions may occur anywhere on the body but are most common on the head and neck. The alopecic skin may gradually become hyperpigmented but otherwise appears normal.

TOP DIFFERENTIALS

Dermatophytosis, demodicosis, superficial pyoderma, injection reaction, topical steroid reaction, traction alopecia.

DIAGNOSIS

1. Rule out other differentials.
2. Dermatohistopathology—Findings depend on the stage of the lesion. Early lesions have peri- and intrafollicular accumulations of lymphocytes, histiocytes, and plasma cells. Older lesions show a predominance of catagen, telogen, and atrophic hair follicles. In chronic lesions there is an absence of hair follicles, with residual fibrous tracts.

TREATMENT AND PROGNOSIS

1. No specific treatment is known.
2. Topical, intralesional, and/or systemic therapy with immunosuppressive doses of glucocorticoids is usually ineffective.
3. Spontaneous hair regrowth may be seen in some cases, but this can take months to years to occur.
4. Prognosis for hair regrowth is guarded. This is a cosmetic disease that does not affect the animal's quality of life.

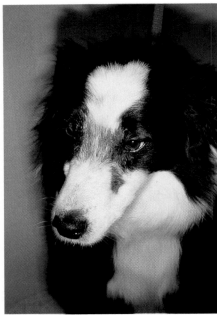

FIGURE 7–57. Alopecia Areata. Focal alopecia on the face of an adult dog. (Courtesy of A. Yu)

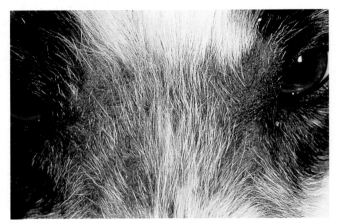

FIGURE 7–58. Alopecia Areata. Close-up of the dog in Figure 7–57. Alopecia with no evidence of concurrent infections. (Courtesy of A. Yu)

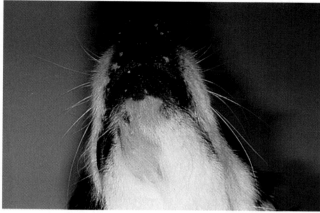

FIGURE 7–59. Alopecia Areata. Close-up of the dog in Figures 7–57 and 7–58. Focal alopecia and erythema on the chin. (Courtesy of A. Yu)

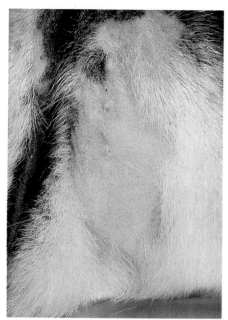

FIGURE 7–60. Alopecia Areata. Close-up of the dog in Figures 7–57 to 7–59. Alopecia and erythema. (Courtesy of A. Yu)

Suggested Readings

Chabanne L, Fournel C, Monier J-C, Rigal D, and Monestier M. 1999. Canine Systemic Lupus Erythematosus. Part I. Clinical and Biologic Aspects. Compend Cont Edu Pract Vet. 21: 135–144.

Immunologic Skin Diseases, pp. 558–588, 607–609, 611–613. In Scott DW, Miller WH Jr, and Griffin CE. 1995. Muller & Kirk's Small Animal Dermatology. Ed. 5. W.B. Saunders, Philadelphia, PA.

Kummel BA. 1995. Medical Treatment of Canine Pemphigus-Pemphigoid, pp. 636–638. In Bonagura JD (ed). Kirk's Current Veterinary Therapy, XII, Small Animal Practice. W.B. Saunders, Philadelphia, PA.

Masella R. 2000. Canine Pemphigus Complex: Diagnosis and Therapy. Compend Cont Edu Pract Vet. 22: 680–689.

Morgan R. 1989. Vogt-Koyannagi-Harada Syndrome in Human and Dog. Compend Cont Edu Pract Vet. 11(10): 1211–1218.

Plumb DC. 1999. Veterinary Drug Handbook. Ed. 3. Iowa State University Press, Ames, IA.

Vitale C, Ihrke P, Gross T, and Werner L. 1997. Systemic Lupus Erythematosus in a Cat: Fulfillment of the American Rheumatism Association Criteria with Supportive Skin Histopathology. Vet Dermatol. 8: 133–138.

Werner AH. 1999. Recognizing and Treating Discoid Lupus Erythematosus and Pemphigus Foliaceus in Dogs. Vet Med. November:995–966.

8

Immune-Mediated Skin Diseases

- **Canine Juvenile Cellulitis** (juvenile pyoderma, puppy strangles)

- **Sterile Nodular Panniculitis**

- **Idiopathic Sterile Granuloma and Pyogranuloma**

- **Vasculitis**

- **Erythema Multiforme and Toxic Epidermal Necrolysis** (TEN)

- **Cutaneous Drug Reaction** (drug eruption)

Canine Juvenile Cellulitis

(juvenile pyoderma, puppy strangles)
(Figs. 8–1 to 8–6)

FEATURES

An idiopathic skin disease that primarily occurs in puppies between 3 weeks and 6 months of age. Uncommon in dogs, with the highest incidence in dachshunds, golden retrievers, Labrador retrievers, beagles, and pointers. More than one puppy in the litter may be affected.

Vesicles, pustules, serous to purulent exudation, crusts, cellulitis, and alopecia develop on the lips, muzzle, and eyelid margins. The ear pinnae may be swollen and exudative. In some dogs, lesions may also involve the anus and prepuce. Lesions may be mild to severe, and are often painful but not pruritic. Marked regional to diffuse lymphadenomegaly is common, and lymph node abscessation can occur. Severely affected puppies are usually depressed and often anorectic and febrile.

TOP DIFFERENTIALS

Canine acne, demodicosis, deep pyoderma, angioedema.

DIAGNOSIS

1. Usually based on signalment, history, clinical findings, and ruling out other differentials.
2. Cytology (skin or ear exudate)—Purulent to pyogranulomatous inflammation. Bacterial cocci may be seen but are secondary contaminants.
3. Cytology (lymph node aspirate)—Suppurative, pyogranulomatous, or granulomatous inflammation. No infectious agents are seen.
4. Dermatohistopathology—Diffuse (pyo)granulomatous dermatitis and panniculitis. Infectious agents are not seen.
5. Bacterial culture (exudate)—Bacteria may be isolated, but a poor response is seen to antibiotic therapy alone.

TREATMENT AND PROGNOSIS

1. Use daily, gentle, topical warm water soaks to remove crusts and exudate.
2. Give prednisone, 2 mg/kg PO q 24 hours, until lesions resolve (approximately 1–4 weeks), then give 2 mg/kg PO q 48 hours for 2–3 weeks, then taper off completely over the next few weeks. If the prednisone therapy is tapered or discontinued too soon, a relapse may occur.
3. Prophylactically give cephalexin, 20 mg/kg PO q 8 hours or 30 mg/kg PO q 12 hours, for the duration of the prednisone therapy.
4. Prognosis is good if response to therapy is seen within 4–5 days. In severe cases, even with treatment, permanent scarring may be a sequela. Death may occur if the disease is not treated.

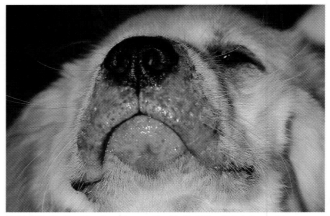

FIGURE 8–1. Canine Juvenile Cellulitis. Moist, erythematous papular lesions with alopecia on the muzzle. (Courtesy of D. Angarano)

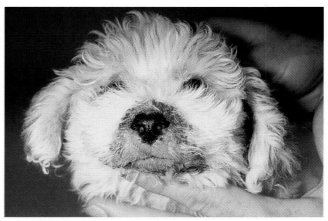

FIGURE 8–2. Canine Juvenile Cellulitis. Moist, alopecic papular dermatitis on the muzzle.

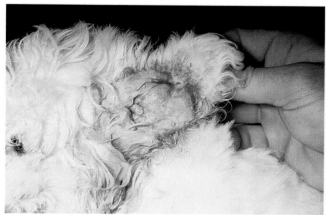

FIGURE 8–3. Canine Juvenile Cellulitis. Close-up of the dog in Figure 8–2. Moist papular lesions in the ear canal.

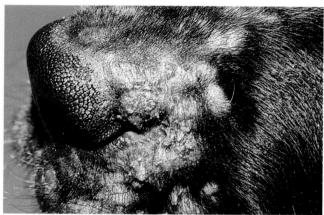

FIGURE 8–5. Canine Juvenile Cellulitis. Close-up of the dog in Figure 8–4. Papular crusting lesions on the nose.

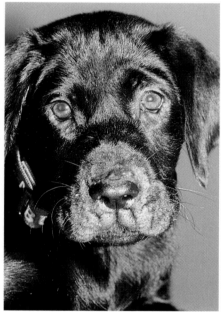

FIGURE 8–4. Canine Juvenile Cellulitis. Alopecic papular lesions on the nose and face.

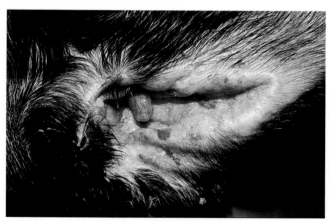

FIGURE 8–6. Canine Juvenile Cellulitis. Close-up of the dog in Figures 8–4 and 8–5. Papular crusting lesions on the ear pinnae.

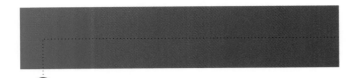

Sterile Nodular Panniculitis
(Figs. 8–7 to 8–12)

FEATURES

An idiopathic inflammatory disease of subcutaneous fat. Rare in dogs and cats.

Lesions are characterized by one or more deep-seated subcutaneous nodules that may be a few millimeters to a few centimeters in diameter. The nodules may be painful, fluctuant to firm, and may ulcerate and drain a yellowish, oily exudate. Lesions can occur anywhere on the body and in some dogs may wax and wane. Concurrent fever, anorexia, and depression may be present.

TOP DIFFERENTIALS

Infection (bacterial, fungal), foreign body reaction, drug reaction, postinjection reaction, systemic lupus erythematosus, neoplasia, and vitamin E deficiency (steatitis in cats).

DIAGNOSIS

1. Rule out other differentials.
2. Cytology (aspirate)—Neutrophils and foamy (lipid-containing) macrophages. No microorganisms are seen.
3. Dermatohistopathology (excisional biopsy)—Suppurative, pyogranulomatous, granulomatous, eosinophilic, necrotizing, or fibrosing septal and/or diffuse panniculitis. Special stains do not reveal infectious agents.
4. Microbial cultures (tissue)—Negative for anaerobic and aerobic bacteria, mycobacteria, and fungi.

TREATMENT AND PROGNOSIS

1. If lesion is solitary, complete surgical excision is usually curative.
2. Treatment with combination tetracycline and niacinamide may be effective in some cases. A beneficial response should be seen within 2–3 months of initiating treatment. Give 500 mg of each drug (dogs >10 kg) or 250 mg of each drug (dogs <10 kg) PO q 8 hours until lesions resolve (approximately 2–3 months). Then give each drug q 12 hours for 4–6 weeks, then attempt to decrease frequency to q 24 hours for maintenance.
3. For severe or refractory cases, give prednisone, 2 mg/kg (dogs) or 4 mg/kg (cats) PO q 24 hours, or give methylprednisolone, 1.6 mg/kg (dogs) PO q 24 hours. After lesions resolve (approximately 2–8 weeks), gradually taper dosage over a period of several (8–10) weeks until the lowest possible alternate-day dosage that maintains remission is being given. In many cases, the steroid therapy can eventually be discontinued.
4. Prognosis following treatment is good, although healed lesions may leave scars.

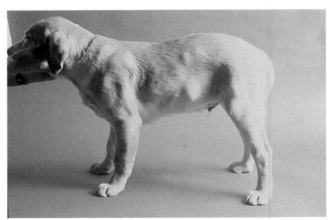

FIGURE 8–7. Sterile Nodular Panniculitis. The multiple nodules on the trunk of this young Labrador slowly enlarged and eventually drained. (Courtesy of J. MacDonald)

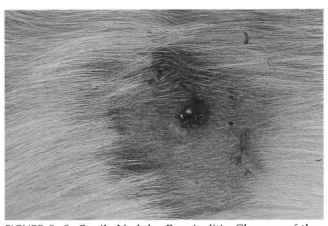

FIGURE 8–8. Sterile Nodular Panniculitis. Close-up of the dog in Figure 8–7. The nodular lesions drained a clear, oily fluid. (Courtesy of J. MacDonald)

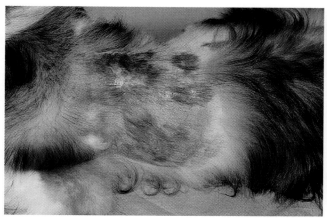

FIGURE 8–9. Sterile Nodular Panniculitis. Multiple nodules on the trunk of a young adult Shetland sheepdog. (Courtesy of A. Yu)

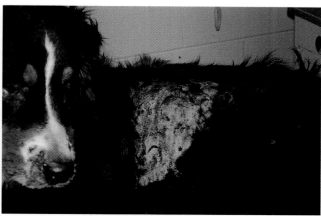

FIGURE 8–11. Sterile Nodular Panniculitis. An adult Bernese mountain dog with multiple nodules, draining tracts, and crust formation.

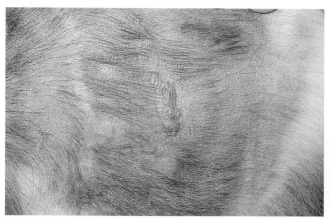

FIGURE 8–10. Sterile Nodular Panniculitis. Close-up of the dog in Figure 8–9. Alopecic nodules on the trunk. (Courtesy of A. Yu)

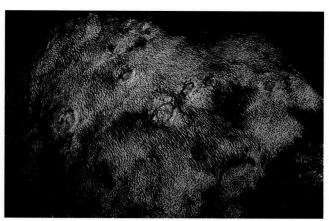

FIGURE 8–12. Sterile Nodular Panniculitis. Close-up of the dog in Figure 8–11. Multiple nodules and draining tracts.

Idiopathic Sterile Granuloma and Pyogranuloma (Figs. 8–13 and 8–14)

FEATURES

A skin disease that is thought to be immune-mediated, although its exact pathogenesis is unknown. Uncommon in dogs, with the highest incidence in collies, golden retrievers, boxers, and large, short-coated breeds.

Nonpainful and nonpruritic, firm dermal papules and nodules that may become alopecic or ulcerated. Lesions can be anywhere on the body but are most commonly found on the bridge of the nose, muzzle, around the eyes, ear pinnae, and/or the feet.

TOP DIFFERENTIALS

Infection (bacteria, fungus), parasite (leishmaniasis, tick bites), foreign body reaction, neoplasia.

DIAGNOSIS

1. Rule out other differentials.
2. Cytology (aspirate)—(Pyo)granulomatous inflammation with no microorganisms.
3. Dermatohistopathology—Nodular to diffuse (pyo)granulomatous dermatitis. Special stains do not reveal infectious agents.
4. Microbial cultures (tissue)—Negative for anaerobic and aerobic bacteria, mycobacteria, and fungi.

TREATMENT AND PROGNOSIS

1. Surgically excise solitary lesions if possible.
2. For nonsurgical or multiple lesions, give prednisone, 1–2 mg/kg PO q 12 hours. Significant improvement should be seen within 1–2 weeks. After lesions resolve (approximately 2–6 weeks), gradually taper the steroid dosage over a period of several (8–10) weeks until the lowest alternate-day dosage possible is being given that maintains remission. In some dogs, steroid therapy can eventually be discontinued.
3. Alternatively, treatment with combination tetracycline and niacinamide may be effective. A beneficial response should be seen within 2–3 months of initiating therapy. Give 500 mg of each drug (dogs >10 kg) or 250 mg of each drug (dogs <10 kg) PO q 8 hours until lesions completely resolve. Then gradually taper the frequency of administration by giving each drug q 12 hours for 4–6 weeks, followed by q 24 hours for 4–6 weeks,

and then stop therapy if lesions have not recurred.
4. Other treatments that may be effective include:

Azathioprine, 2 mg/kg PO q 24 hours, until lesions resolve (approximately 4–8 weeks) and then 2 mg/kg PO q 48 hours for maintenance.

L-Asparginase, 10,000 IU IM q 7 days, until lesions resolve (usually 1–2 weeks) and then as needed.

5. Prognosis is good for most dogs, although lifelong therapy may be needed in some dogs.

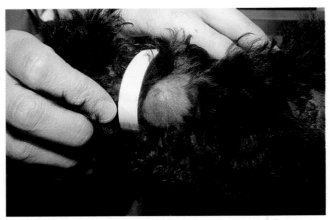

FIGURE 8–13. Idiopathic Sterile Granuloma and Pyogranuloma. This granuloma developed over several weeks.

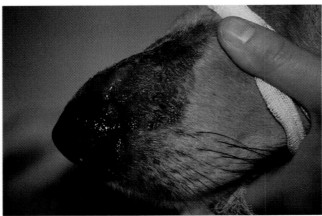

FIGURE 8–14. Idiopathic Sterile Granuloma and Pyogranuloma. An alopecic, eroded granuloma on the nose of a dog.

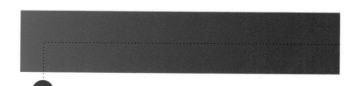

Vasculitis (Figs. 8–15 to 8–20)

FEATURES

An inflammatory disease of blood vessels that is usually secondary to immune complex deposition within the vessel walls. Vasculitis may be associated with underlying infection (bacterial, rickettsial, viral, fungal), malignancy, drug reaction, rabies vaccination (dogs), metabolic disease (diabetes mellitus, uremia), systemic lupus erythematosus, or exposure to cold (cold agglutinin disease), or it may be idiopathic. Uncommon in dogs and rare in cats.

Clinical signs include purpura, necrosis, and punctate ulcers, especially on the ear pinnae, lips, oral mucosa, paws, tail, and scrotum. In vasculitis associated with rabies vaccination, a focal area of alopecia and hyperpigmentation at the site of vaccination may be followed weeks to months later by the development of multifocal lesions. Occasionally acrocyanosis is seen. Anorexia, depression, fever, arthropathy, myopathy, and/or pitting edema of the extremities may be present.

TOP DIFFERENTIALS

Systemic lupus erythematosus, erythema multiforme/toxic epidermal necrolysis, bullous pemphigoid, pemphigus vulgaris, frostbite, urticaria, and cutaneous drug reactions.

DIAGNOSIS

1. Rule out other differentials.
2. Dermatohistopathology—Neutrophilic or lymphocytic vasculitis.

TREATMENT AND PROGNOSIS

1. Identify and correct any underlying cause.
2. Give prednisone, 1–2 mg/kg (dogs) or 2–4 mg/kg (cats) PO q 12 hours, until lesions resolve (approximately 2–4 weeks). Then gradually taper the steroid dosage over a period of several (8–10) weeks until the lowest alternate-day dosage possible is being given that maintains remission.
3. Alternative therapies that may be effective in prednisone-nonresponsive cases include:

   Dapsone (dogs only), 1 mg/kg PO q 8 hours, until lesions resolve (approximately 2–3 weeks). Once remission is achieved, slowly taper dosage by giving 1 mg/kg PO q 12 hours for 2 weeks, then give 1 mg/kg PO q 24 hours for 2 weeks, followed by 1 mg/kg PO q 48 hours.

   Sulfasalazine, 10–20 mg/kg (maximum 3 g/day) PO q 8 hours, until lesions resolve (approximately 2–4 weeks). Once remission is achieved, taper dosage by giving 10 mg/kg PO q 12 hours for 3 weeks, followed by 10 mg/kg PO q 24 hours.

   Tetracycline and niacinamide, 500 mg of each (dogs >10 kg) or 250 mg of each (dogs <10 kg) PO q 8 hours, until lesions resolve (approximately 2–3 months). Once remission is achieved, decrease frequency of administration of both drugs to q 12 hours for 4–6 weeks and then to q 24 hours if possible.

4. Pentoxifylline 200–400 mg/day PO q 8–12 hours or 10 mg/kg PO q 8–12 hours may be effective.
5. Treatment with azathioprine (dogs only), cyclophosphamide, or chlorambucil, alone or in combination with steroid therapy, may be indicated when other therapeutic measures have failed (see Table 7–2).
6. Regardless of the drug used, in some patients the therapy can be eventually discontinued after 4–6 months. In others, long-term maintenance therapy is needed.
7. Prognosis is variable, depending on the underlying cause, the extent of the cutaneous lesions, and the degree of involvement of other organs.

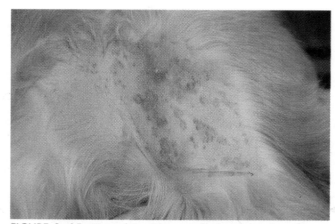

FIGURE 8–15. Vasculitis. These well-demarcated, erythematous lesions developed acutely on the lateral thigh of this adult golden retriever.

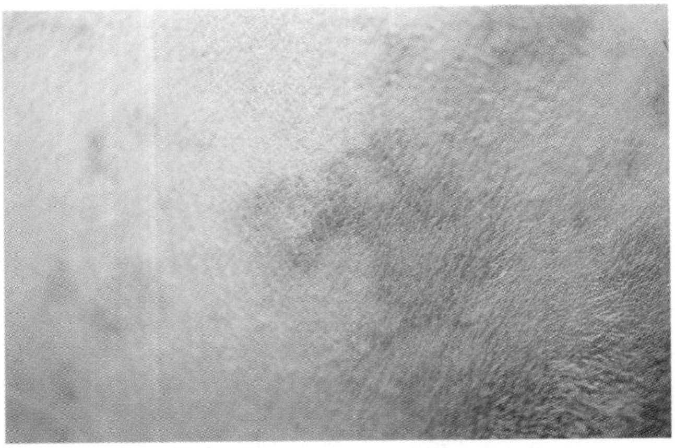

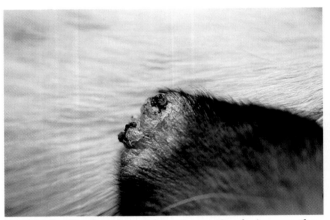

FIGURE 8–16. Vasculitis. Close-up of the dog in Figure 8–15. The well-demarcated serpentine margin of the lesion is typical of vasculitis or drug reactions.

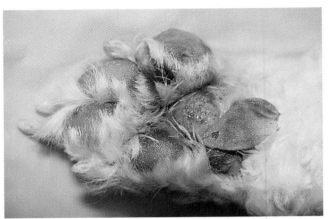

FIGURE 8–19. Vasculitis. Sloughing of the footpad caused by vascular injury.

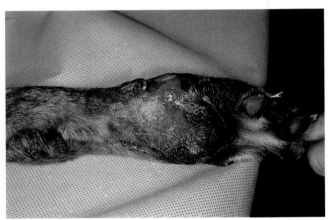

FIGURE 8–17. Vasculitis. Alopecic crusting lesions on the ear tip of a Jack Russell terrier. The distal margin has necrosed, leaving a notched ear pinna.

FIGURE 8–20. Vasculitis. Ulcerative lesions on the distal limb of a greyhound with idiopathic vasculitis (Shorter-Rott syndrome).

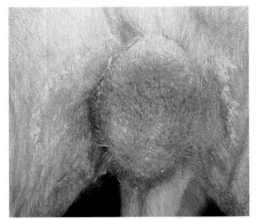

FIGURE 8–18. Vasculitis. Scrotal dermatitis caused by cold agglutinin disease. (Courtesy of G. Kunkle)

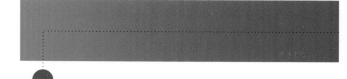

Erythema Multiforme and Toxic Epidermal Necrolysis

(TEN) (Figs. 8–21 to 8–30)

FEATURES

The exact pathogenesis of these two diseases is unknown, but an immune-mediated reaction to or a direct toxic effect of chemicals, drug therapy, infection, or malignancy has been suggested. Many investigators believe that toxic epidermal necrolysis is a more severe form of erythema multiforme. Uncommon in dogs and rare in cats.

Lesions usually occur acutely and are multifocal to diffuse. The skin, mucocutaneous junctions, and/or oral cavity may be involved. Erythema multiforme is characterized by erythematous macules to slightly raised papules that spread peripherally and clear centrally to produce annular or serpiginous "target" or "bulls-eye" lesions. There is usually no associated scaling, crusting, or alopecia. Toxic epidermal necrolysis is characterized by painful vesicles, bullae, ulcers, and/or epidermal necrosis. Concurrent depression, anorexia, and fever may be present, especially with toxic epidermal necrolysis.

TOP DIFFERENTIALS

Urticaria, deep infection (bacterial, fungal), thermal burn, bullous pemphigoid, pemphigus vulgaris, systemic lupus erythematosus, vasculitis, epitheliotrophic lymphoma, cutaneous drug reaction.

DIAGNOSIS

1. Rule out other differentials.
2. Dermatohistopathology—Single-cell to full-thickness necrosis of epidermis. The epithelial cells of outer root sheaths of hair follicles may be similarly affected.

TREATMENT AND PROGNOSIS

1. Identify and correct any underlying cause.
2. Give appropriate symptomatic and supportive care (i.e., whirlpool baths, antibiotics, fluids, electrolytes, parenteral nutrition) as needed.
3. Mild cases of erythema multiforme may resolve spontaneously within 3–4 weeks.
4. In more severe cases, treatment with prednisone, 2 mg/kg (dogs) or 4 mg/kg (cats) PO q 24 hours, may be helpful. Significant improvement should be seen within 1–2 weeks. After lesions resolve (approximately 2–8 weeks), gradually taper dosage over a period of 4–6 weeks. In most cases, the steroid therapy can be discontinued.
5. In rare animals that require long-term maintenance therapy to remain in remission, alternate-day steroid therapy, alone or in combination with azathioprine (dogs only) or cyclosporin, may be effective (see Table 7–2).
6. Prognosis is good to guarded, depending on extent and severity of lesions and whether or not an underlying cause can be found.

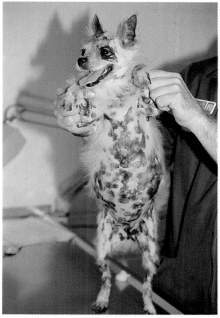

FIGURE 8–21. Erythema Multiforme. Generalized alopecia with well-demarcated areas of erosion and hyperpigmentation.

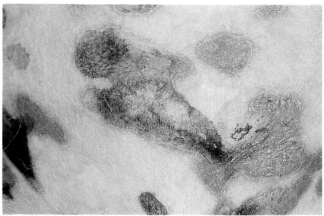

FIGURE 8–22. Erythema Multiforme. Close-up of the dog in Figure 8–19. Well-demarcated areas of erythema, erosion, and hyperpigmentation.

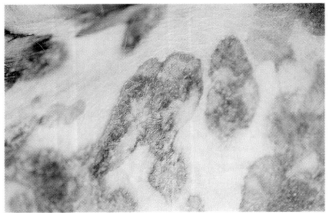

FIGURE 8–23. Erythema Multiforme. Close-up of the dog in Figures 8–21 and 8–22. The serpentine margins of these lesions are suggestive of a drug reaction.

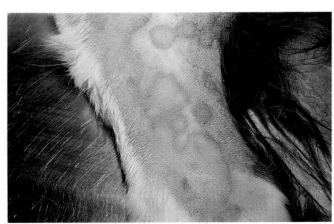

FIGURE 8–26. Erythema Multiforme. Well-demarcated, erythematous lesions on the distal limb of an adult dog.

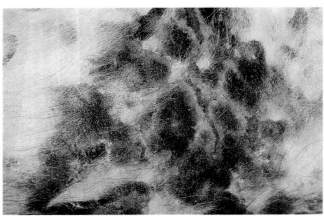

FIGURE 8–24. Erythema Multiforme. Close-up of the dog in Figures 8–21 to 8–23. The resolving lesions became hyperpigmented.

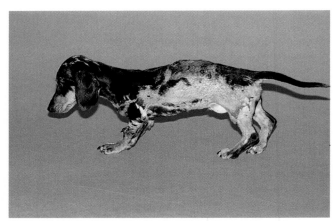

FIGURE 8–27. Toxic Epidermal Necrolysis. Alopecia, crusting, ulceration, and granulation tissue on the dorsum of a 6-month-old dachshund. The epidermal necrosis developed over several weeks following routine vaccination.

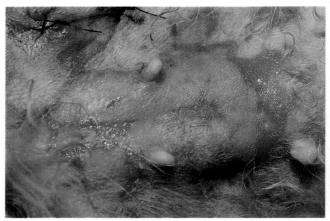

FIGURE 8–25. Erythema Multiforme. These erosive, erythematous lesions on the abdomen developed acutely. Note the well-demarcated margins typical of cutaneous drug reactions.

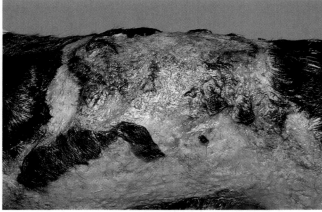

FIGURE 8–28. Toxic Epidermal Necrolysis. Close-up of the dog in Figure 8–27. The lesion is beginning to form granulation tissue. The remaining skin is necrotic and will eventually slough.

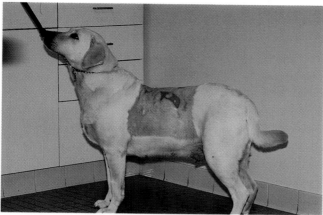

FIGURE 8–29. Toxic Epidermal Necrolysis. The alopecia, crusting, and ulcerations developed on the dorsum of this Labrador after it was anesthetized for a cesarean section. (Courtesy of D. Angarano)

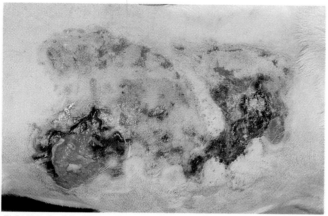

FIGURE 8–30. Toxic Epidermal Necrolysis. Close-up of the dog in Figure 8–29. Alopecia, crusting, ulceration, and granulation tissue. (Courtesy of D. Angarano)

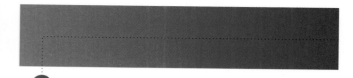

Cutaneous Drug Reaction
(drug eruption) (Figs. 8–31 to 8–37)

FEATURES

A cutaneous/mucocutaneous reaction to a topical, oral, or injectable drug. An adverse drug reaction can occur after one treatment, after several treatments, or after years of treatment. Uncommon in dogs and cats.

Clinical signs are extremely variable and may include papules, plaques, pustules, vesicles, bullae, purpura, erythema, urticaria, angioedema, alopecia, erythema multiforme or toxic epidermal necrolysis lesions, scaling/exfoliation, erosions, ulcerations, and/or otitis externa. Lesions may be localized, multifocal or diffuse, and painful or pruritic. Concurrent fever, depresssion, and/or lameness may be present.

TOP DIFFERENTIALS

Cutaneous drug reactions may mimic many other skin disorders, especially other immune-mediated and autoimmune diseases. Specific differentials depend on the clinical presentation.

DIAGNOSIS

1. Usually based on history of recent drug administration and ruling out other differentials.
2. Hemogram—Anemia, thrombocytopenia, leukopenia, and/or leukocytosis may be present.
3. Serum biochemistry panel—Variable abnormalities reflecting damage to other organs may be present.
4. Dermatohistopathology (nondiagnostic)—Findings are variable and reflect the gross appearance of the lesions.

TREATMENT AND PROGNOSIS

1. Discontinue use of offending medication. Lesions usually resolve within 14 days, but occasionally they persist for several weeks.
2. Give symptomatic and supportive care (i.e., whirlpool baths, systemic antibiotics, fluids) as needed.
3. Glucocorticosteroid therapy may help alleviate

symptoms in some cases. Give prednisone, 1–2 mg/kg (dogs) or 2–4 mg/kg (cats) PO q 24 hours, until lesions resolve (approximately 1–3 weeks). Then taper the dosage over a 2- to 3-week period.

4. Avoid future use of the offending medication.
5. Prognosis is good unless there is multiorgan involvement or extensive epidermal necrosis.

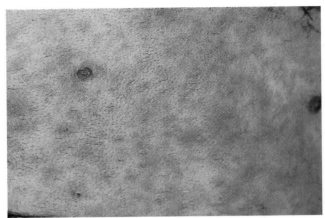

FIGURE 8–33. Cutaneous Drug Reaction. These generalized, erythematous papules developed acutely. (Courtesy of D. Angarano)

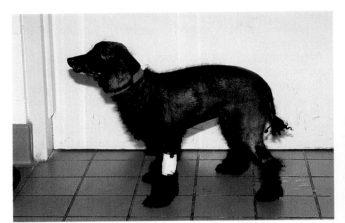

FIGURE 8–31. Cutaneous Drug Reaction. The generalized alopecia in this poodle occurred during chemotherapy. (Courtesy of D. Angarano)

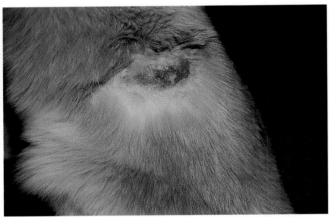

FIGURE 8–34. Cutaneous Drug Reaction. This focal, crusting, ulcerative lesion was believed to be caused by propofol.

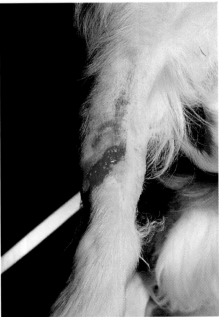

FIGURE 8–32. Cutaneous Drug Reaction. This ulcerative lesion was caused by the injection of a chemotherapy agent.

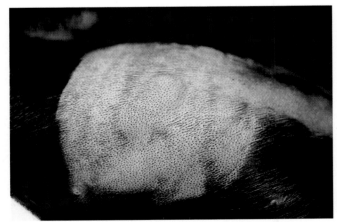

FIGURE 8–35. Cutaneous Drug Reaction. The erythematous lesions on the lumbar region of this dog developed after trimethoprim sulfa administration.

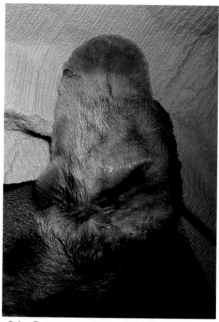

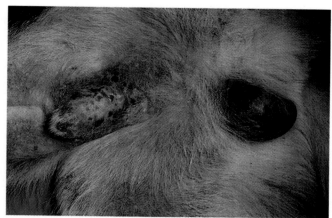

FIGURE 8-37. Cutaneous Drug Reaction. Prepucial and scrotal erosive dermatitis caused by lime sulfur dip. (Courtesy of D. Angarano)

FIGURE 8-36. Cutaneous Drug Reaction. The moist dermatitis in the ear canal of this dog was caused by a topical otic medication. (Courtesy of D. Angarano)

Suggested Readings

Crawford M and Folic C. 1989. Vasculitis: Clinical Syndromes in Small Animals. Compend Cont Edu Pract Vet. 11(4): 400–415.

Fadok V and Barrie J. 1984. Sulfasalazine Responsive Vasculitis in the Dog: A Case Report. JAAHA. 20: 161–167.

Immunologic Skin Diseases, pp. 588–606. In Scott DW, Miller WH Jr, and Griffin CE. 1995. Muller & Kirk's Small Animal Dermatology. Ed. 5. W.B. Saunders, Philadelphia, PA.

Manning T. 1980. Cutaneous Vasculitis in a Dog. JAAHA. 16: 61–67.

Marsella R. 1999. Pentoxyfylline: Drug of the Nineties? TNAVC 1999 Proceedings, pp. 151–152.

Morris D. 1998. Cutaneous Vasculitis. In Proc. 16th ACVIM Forum, San Diego, CA, pp. 452–454.

Parker W and Foster R. 1996. Case Report: Cutaneous Vasculitis in Five Jack Russell Terriers. Vet Derm. 7: 109–115.

Plumb DC. 1999. Veterinary Drug Handbook. Ed. 3. Iowa State University Press, Ames, IA.

Rothstein E, Scott D, and Riis R. 1997. Tetracycline and Niacinamide for the Treatment of Sterile Pyogranuloma/Granuloma Syndrome in a Dog. JAAHA. 33: 540–543.

Vitale C, Gross T, and Magro C. 1999. Case report: Vaccine-induced ischemic dermatopathy in the dog. Vet Derm. 10(2): 131–142.

9

Endocrine Diseases

- **Canine Hyperadrenocorticism** (Cushing's disease)

- **Feline Hyperadrenocorticism**

- **Canine Hypothyroidism**

- **Sex Hormone Dermatosis—Intact Male Dogs**

- **Sex Hormone Dermatosis—Neutered Male Dogs**

- **Sex Hormone Dermatosis—Intact Female Dogs**

- **Sex Hormone Dermatosis—Neutered Female Dogs**

- **Alopecia "X"** (adrenal sex hormone imbalance, hyposomatotropism, growth hormone-responsive dermatosis, pseudo-Cushing's disease)

- **Canine Recurrent Flank Alopecia** (seasonal flank alopecia, cyclic flank alopecia, cyclic follicular dysplasia)

- **Pituitary Dwarfism**

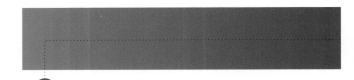

Canine Hyperadrenocorticism

(Cushing's disease) (Figs. 9–1 to 9–10)

FEATURES

Spontaneously occurring disease is caused by excessive production of endogenous glucocorticoids (pituitary microadenoma, pituitary macroadenoma, or adrenal cortical neoplasia). Iatrogenically induced disease is secondary to excessive administration of exogenous glucocorticoids. Iatrogenic hyperadrenocorticism is common especially in chronically pruritic dogs controlled with long-term glucocorticoids and can occur at any age. Spontanously occuring hyperadrenocorticism is also common and tends to occur in middle-aged to older dogs, with an increased incidence in boxers, Boston terriers, dachshunds, poodles, and Scottish terriers.

The haircoat often becomes dry and lusterless, and slowly progressing, bilaterally symmetric alopecia is common. The alopecia may become generalized, but it usually spares the head and limbs. Remaining hairs are easily epilated, and alopecic skin is often thin, hypotonic, and hyperpigmented. Cutaneous stria and comedones may be seen on the ventral abdomen. The skin may be mildly seborrheic (fine, dry scales), bruise easily, and exhibit poor wound healing. Chronic secondary superficial or deep pyoderma, dermatophytosis, or demodicosis is common and may be the client's primary complaint. Calcinosis cutis (whitish, gritty, firm, bone-like papules and plaques) may develop, especially on the dorsal midline of the neck, on ventral abdomen, or in the inguinal areas.

Polyuria and polydipsia (water intake >100 ml/kg/day) and polyphagia are common. Muscle wasting/weakness, a pot-bellied appearance (from hepatomegaly, fat redistribution, and weakened abdominal muscles), increased susceptibility to infections (conjunctival, skin, urinary tract, lung), excessive panting, and variable behavioral or neurologic signs (pituitary macroadenoma) are often present.

TOP DIFFERENTIALS

Other causes of endocrine alopecia.

DIAGNOSIS

1. Hemogram—Neutrophilia, lymphopenia, and eosinopenia are often seen.
2. Serum biochemistry panel—An elevated alkaline phosphatase enzyme level is typical. There may also be mild to markedly elevated alanine trans- aminase activity, as well as elevated cholesterol, triglycerides, and/or glucose levels.
3. Urinalysis—The specific gravity is usually low, and there may be bacteriuria or proteinuria.
4. Urine cortisol/creatinine ratio—Usually elevated. A screening test that is not diagnostic by itself because false-positive, and false-negative results are possible.
5. Dermatohistopathology—Often shows nondiagnostic changes consistent with any endocrinopathy. Dystrophic mineralization (calcinosis cutis), thin dermis, and absent erector pili muscles are highly suggestive of hyperadrenocorticism, but these changes are not always present.
6. Abdominal ultrasonography—May demonstrate adrenal tumor or hyperplasia.
7. Computed tomography/magnetic resonance imaging (CT/MRI) (dogs showing neurologic signs)—May demonstrate a pituitary tumor.
8. Adrenal function tests:

    Adrenocorticotropic hormone (ACTH) stimulation test—An exaggerated post-ACTH cortisol level is highly suggestive of endogenous hyperadrenocortism, but false-negative and false-positive results can occur. In iatrogenic cases, an inadequate response to ACTH stimulation is typical.

    Low-dose (0.01 mg/kg) dexamethasone suppression test—Inadequate cortisol suppression is highly suggestive of endogenous hyperadrenocortism, but false-negative and false-positive results can occur.

    High-dose (0.1 mg/kg) dexamethasone suppression test—Used to help differentiate between adrenal neoplasia and pituitary-dependent hyperadrenocorticism. A lack of cortisol suppression is suggestive of adrenal neoplasia, whereas cortisol suppression suggests pituitary disease.

    Endogenous ACTH assay—Used to help differentiate between adrenal neoplasia and pituitary-dependent hyperadrenocorticism. An elevated ACTH level is suggestive of pituitary disease, whereas a depressed ACTH level is suggestive of adrenal neoplasia.

TREATMENT AND PROGNOSIS

1. Treat any concurrent infections with appropriate therapies.
2. Treatment of choice for iatrogenically induced cases is to progressively taper and then discontinue glucocorticoid therapy.
3. Treatment of choice for adrenal neoplasia is adrenalectomy.
4. Dogs with inoperable adrenal tumors and/or metastases may benefit from mitotane, 50 mg/kg PO q 24 hours with food for 7–14 days. An ACTH stimulation test is performed q 7 days. If inadequate cortisol suppression persists, increase the mitotane dosage to 75–100 mg/kg/day for an additional 7–14 days, monitoring with ACTH

stimulation tests weekly. When adequate adrenal suppression is demonstrated, maintenance mitotane therapy is initiated as described below (#7).

5. Treatment of choice for pituitary macroadenomas (tumor >8 mm in diameter) is radiation therapy.

6. Treatment of choice for pituitary microadenomas is mitotane, 50 mg/kg PO q 24 hours with food. The daily dosage is continued until the basal serum or plasma cortisol level normalizes and does not increase following ACTH stimulation. Control is usually achieved within 5–10 days of initiating therapy, so patient should be closely monitored with ACTH stimulation tests performed q 2–3 days. If signs of adrenal insufficiency develop (anorexia, depression, vomiting, diarrhea, ataxia, disorientation), stop mitotane therapy and give hydrocortisone, 0.5–1.0 mg/kg PO q 12 hours, until symptoms resolve.

7. To maintain remission following mitotane induction, give mitotane PO with food, 50 mg/kg once weekly or 25 mg/kg twice weekly. Dogs that relapse during maintenance therapy should be reinduced with daily mitotane for 5–14 days or until recontrolled, then maintained with 62–75 mg/kg once weekly or 31–37.5 mg/kg twice weekly.

8. Alternative but less successful treatments for pituitary microadenomas include:

Ketoconazole, 15 mg/kg PO with food q 12 hours.

Selegiline (L-deprenyl), 1–2 mg/kg PO q 24 hours.

9. For calcinosis cutis, adjunctive topical treatments with DMSO gel q 24 hours may help resolve the lesions.

10. Prognosis ranges from good to poor, depending on the etiology and severity of the disease.

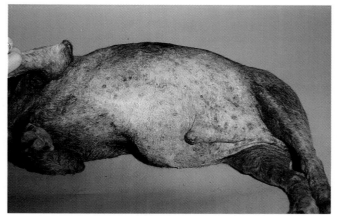

FIGURE 9–2. Canine Hyperadrenocorticism. Close-up of the dog in Figure 9–1. Distended abdomen, ventral alopecia, and papular dermatitis. (Courtesy of J. MacDonald)

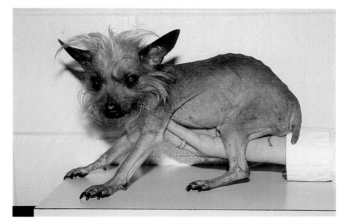

FIGURE 9–3. Canine Hyperadrenocorticism. This Yorkshire terrier gradually developed nearly total alopecia over several months.

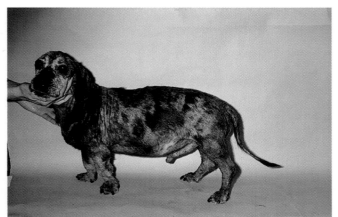

FIGURE 9–1. Canine Hyperadrenocorticism. Generalized alopecia, a secondary bacterial pyoderma, and the distended abdomen (pot belly) are typical of Cushing's disease. (Courtesy of J. MacDonald)

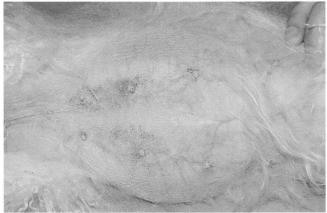

FIGURE 9–4. Canine Hyperadrenocorticism. The generalized alopecia and cutaneous atrophy allow the blood vessels to be visualized through the skin. Note the distended abdomen.

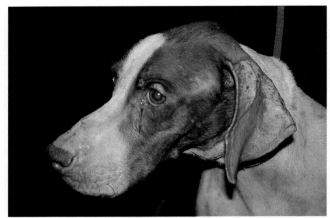

FIGURE 9–5. Canine Hyperadrenocorticism. Multifocal alopecia on the head.

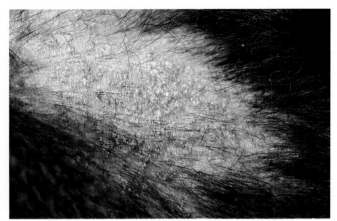

FIGURE 9–8. Canine Hyperadrenocorticism. The multiple lesions on the dorsum of this adult German shepherd were caused by calcium deposition (calcinosis cutis).

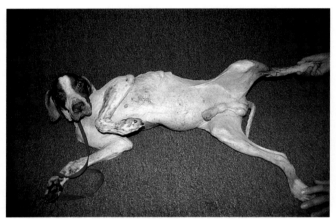

FIGURE 9–6. Canine Hyperadrenocorticism. Close-up of the dog in Figure 9–5. Ventral alopecia with a distended abdomen.

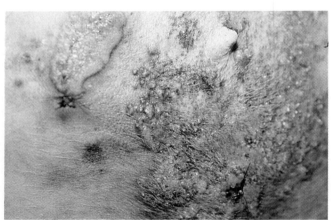

FIGURE 9–9. Canine Hyperadrenocorticism. Calcinosis cutis on the flank of a boxer. The erythema and crusting are caused by the calcium deposits.

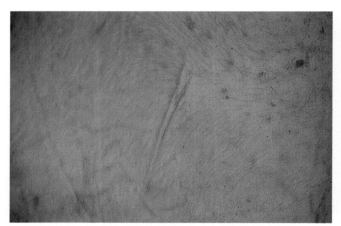

FIGURE 9–7. Canine Hyperadrenocorticism. Same dog as in Figures 9–5 and 9–6. The cutaneous atrophy provides a clear view of the underlying vasculature. The normal resilience of the skin is reduced, causing persistent wrinkling.

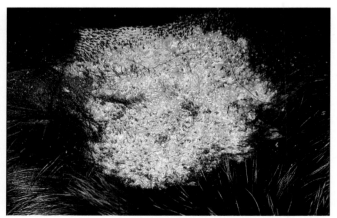

FIGURE 9–10. Canine Hyperadrenocorticism. Calcinosis cutis in a dog. The lesions resolved when the Cushing's disease was controlled.

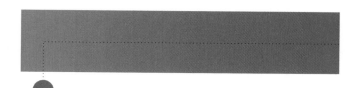

Feline Hyperadrenocorticism
(Figs. 9–11 to 9–14)

FEATURES

Naturally occurring and iatrogenic hyperadrenocorticism are rare in cats, with an increased incidence in middle-aged to older cats.

Polyuria and polydipsia are common symptoms. Depression, anorexia or polyphagia, weight loss, muscle wasting, and a pot-belly appearance may also be present. Skin changes, if present, may include symmetrical alopecia and hyperpigmentation of the trunk, flanks, and/or ventral abdomen. The skin may be thin and fragile, and may tear or bruise easily. Comedones and recurrent abscesses may be seen. Curling of ear tips is often associated with iatrogenic hyperadrenocorticism. Concurrent diabetes mellitus is common.

TOP DIFFERENTIALS

Cutaneous asthenia, paraneoplastic alopecia.

DIAGNOSIS

1. Rule out other differentials.
2. Hemogram, serum biochemistry panel, urinalysis—May show changes associated with concurrent diabetes mellitus but otherwise are nondiagnostic.
3. Dermatohistopathology—Often appears histologically normal, but cat may have decreased amount of dermal collagen.
4. Abdominal ultrasonography—Unilateral or bilateral adrenal enlargement.
5. Adrenal function tests:

   ACTH stimulation test—An exaggerated post-ACTH cortisol level is suggestive of endogenous hyperadrenocorticism, whereas a poor response to ACTH stimulation is suggestive of iatrogenic disease. However, false-negative and false-positive results can occur.

   Low-dose (0.1 mg/kg) dexamethasone suppression test—Inadequate cortisol suppression is suggestive of endogenous hyperadrenocortism, but false-positive and false-negative results can occur.

   High-dose (1 mg/kg) dexamethasone suppression test—Used to help differentiate between adrenal neoplasia and pituitary-dependent hyperadrenocorticism. Lack of cortisol suppression is suggestive of adrenal neoplasia, whereas cortisol suppression suggests pituitary disease.

TREATMENT AND PROGNOSIS

1. Treat diabetes mellitus or secondary infections, if present.
2. Treatment of choice for iatrogenically induced disease is to taper off and stop glucocorticoid therapy.
3. Treatment of choice for adrenal neoplasia is adrenalectomy.
4. Treatment of choice for pitituary-dependent disease is bilateral adrenalectomy followed by life-long supplementation with replacement doses of glucocorticoids and mineralocorticoids. Because the mortality rate from surgical complications is high, presurgical stabilization with metyrapone may be indicated in severely morbid cats.
5. Medical therapies for pituitary-dependent disease that can be considered but have low success rates include:

   Metyrapone, 65 mg/kg PO q 12 hours.

   Ketoconazole, 10–15 mg/kg PO with food q 12 hours.

6. Mitotane treatment does not induce remission when used as directed for canine hyperadrenocorticism, but may be effective after longer induction periods.
7. Prognosis is usually poor. Concurrent diabetes mellitus is difficult to control unless the hyperadrenocorticism is treated.

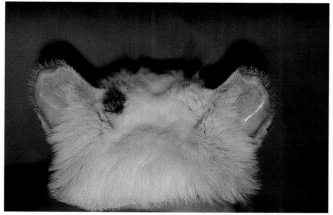

FIGURE 9–11. Feline Hyperadrenocorticism. The alopecia and curling of the ear pinnae are typical of Cushing's syndrome in cats.

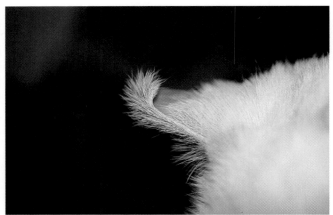

FIGURE 9–12. Feline Hyperadrenocorticism. Close-up of the cat in Figure 9–11. Curling of the ear pinnae.

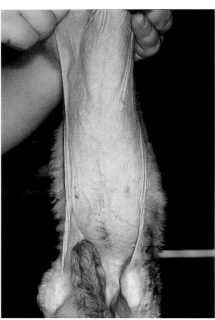

FIGURE 9–14. Feline Hyperadrenocorticism. Close-up of the cat in Figure 9–13. The cutaneous atrophy allows clear visualization of the underlying vessels. The cat's distended abdomen is also apparent. (Courtesy of A. Yu)

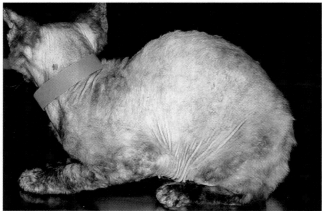

FIGURE 9–13. Feline Hyperadrenocorticism. Generalized alopecia and cutaneous atrophy. (Courtesy of A. Yu)

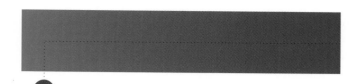

Canine Hypothyroidism

(Figs. 9–15 to 9–22)

FEATURES

This endocrinopathy is most often associated with primary thyroid dysfunction from lymphocytic thyroiditis or idiopathic thyroid atrophy. Common in dogs, with the highest incidence in middle-aged to older dogs. Young adult large and giant-breed dogs are also occasionally affected. Congenital hypothyroidism is extremely rare.

A variety of cutaneous symptoms can be seen. Alopecia on the bridge of the nose occurs in some dogs. The haircoat may be dull, dry, and brittle. There may be bilaterally symmetric alopecia with easily epilated hairs that spares the extremities. The alopecic skin may be hyperpigmented, thickened, and/or cool to the touch. Thickened and droopy facial skin from dermal mucinosis, chronic seborrhea sicca or oleosa, and/or ceruminous otitis externa may be present. Seborrheic skin and ears may be secondarily infected with yeast and/or bacteria. In some dogs, the only symptom is recurrent or antibiotic-resistant pyoderma or adult-onset generalized demodicosis. Pruritus is not a primary feature of hypothyroidism and, if present, reflects secondary pyoderma, *Malassezia* infection, or demodicosis. Noncutaneous symptoms of hypothyroidism are variable and may include lethargy, mental dullness, obesity, thermophilia, neuromuscular disorders, and reproductive problems. Puppies with congenital hypothyroidism are disproportionate dwarfs with short limbs and neck relative to their body length.

TOP DIFFERENTIALS

Other causes of endocrine alopecia and seborrhea, superficial pyoderma, *Malassezia* dermatitis, and demodicosis.

DIAGNOSIS

1. Rule out other differentials.
2. Dermatohistopathology—Usually nonspecific endocrine changes or findings consistent with pyoderma, *Malassezia* dermatitis, or seborrhea are seen. If present, dermal mucinosis is highly suggestive of hypothyroidism, but this can be a normal finding in some breeds (e.g., shar-pei).
3. Serum total thyroxine (TT4), free thyroxine (FT4) by equilibrium dialysis, and thyroid stimulating hormone (TSH) assays—Low TT4, low FT4, and high TSH levels are highly suggestive of hypothyroidism, but false-positive and false-negative results can occur.

TREATMENT AND PROGNOSIS

1. Treat any secondary seborrhea, pyoderma, *Malassezia* dermatitis, or demodicosis with appropriate topical and systemic therapies.
2. Give levothyroxine (Soloxine), 0.02 mg/kg PO q 12 hours, until symptoms resolve (approximately 8–16 weeks). Some dogs can then be maintained with 0.02 mg/kg PO q 24 hours, while others require lifelong twice daily dosing to maintain remission. Because of their variable quality, generic brands of levothyroxine should be avoided.
3. Dogs with concurrent heart disease should be started on levothyroxine more gradually. Begin with 0.005 mg/kg PO q 12 hours and increase dosage by 0.005 mg/kg every 2 weeks until 0.02 mg/kg q 12 hours is being given.
4. After 2–4 months of therapy, the serum TT4 level should be measured 4–6 hours after medication administration and should be in the high normal to supranormal range. If level is low or within normal range and minimal clinical improvement has been seen, increase dosage of levothyroxine and recheck serum TT4 level 2–4 weeks later. If level is >7.5 μg/dl, the levothyroxine dose should be reduced.
5. If signs of thyrotoxicosis from oversupplementation occur (anxiety, panting, polydipsia, and polyuria), the serum TT4 level should be evaluated. If the level is markedly elevated, temporarily stop medication until side effects abate and then reinstitute at a lower level and/or a less frequent dosage schedule.
6. Prognosis is good with lifelong replacement therapy, although hypothyroidism-induced neuromuscular abnormalities may not completely resolve.

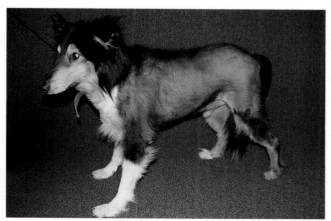

FIGURE 9–15. Canine Hypothyroidism. Generalized truncal alopecia in an adult collie.

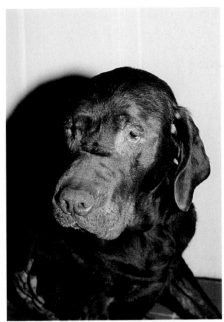

FIGURE 9–16. Canine Hypothyroidism. This "tragic" facial expression is caused by dermal mucinosis (myxedema). (Courtesy of D. Angarano)

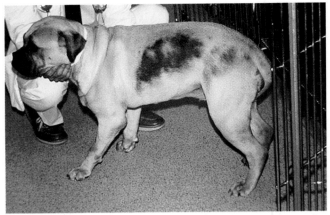

FIGURE 9–18. Canine Hypothyroidism. Well-demarcated alopecia and hyperpigmentation on the lateral flank. Note the similarity to canine recurrent flank alopecia.

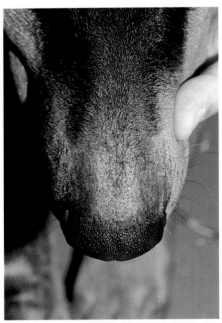

FIGURE 9–17. Canine Hypothyroidism. Mild alopecia on the bridge of the nose of a dog with hypothyroidism.

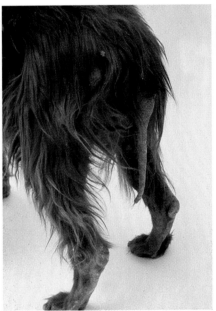

FIGURE 9–19. Canine Hypothyroidism. Alopecia and hyperpigmentation on the tail and distal limbs of an adult Irish setter. (Courtesy of D. Angarano)

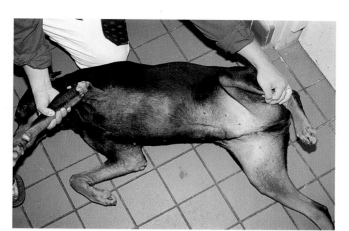

FIGURE 9–20. Canine Hypothyroidism. Generalized ventral alopecia and weight gain were the chief clinical signs affecting this adult Doberman pinscher.

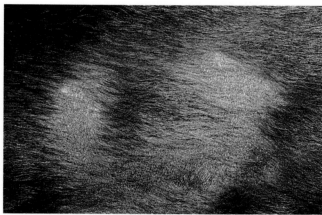

FIGURE 9–21. Canine Hypothyroidism. Close-up of the dog in Figure 9–20. Alopecia and hyperpigmentation, with no evidence of a secondary superficial pyoderma.

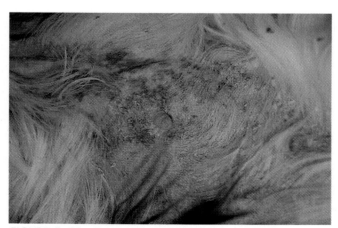

FIGURE 9–22. Canine Hypothyroidism. Crusting papular lesions caused by a secondary superficial pyoderma.

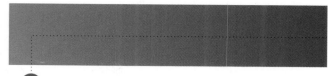

Sex Hormone Dermatosis—Intact Male Dogs (Figs. 9–23 to 9–28)

FEATURES

An endocrinopathy associated with the excessive production of sex hormones and/or precursor sex hormones by the testes or adrenal glands. Common in intact male dogs, with the highest incidence in middle-aged to older dogs.

Bilaterally symmetric alopecia of the neck, rump, perineum, flanks, and/or trunk that may become generalized but spares the head and limbs. Remaining hairs epilate easily. The alopecic skin may become hyperpigmented. Secondary seborrhea and superficial pyoderma may be present. Concurrent gynecomastia, pendulous prepuce, and clinical signs of prostatomegaly and/or prostatitis may be seen. The testicles may be normal, asymmetric, or cryptorchid on palpation. The owner may report that the dog is exhibiting abnormal or overly aggressive sexual behavior toward other dogs and/or humans.

TOP DIFFERENTIALS

Other causes of endocrine alopecia.

DIAGNOSIS

1. Rule out other differentials.
2. Dermatohistopathology—Nonspecific endocrine changes.
3. Sex hormone assays—Usually nondiagnostic.
4. Testicular histopathology (castration)—May be normal, atrophic, or neoplastic (Sertoli cell tumor, interstitial cell tumor, seminoma).
5. Response to castration—Hair regrowth occurs.

TREATMENT AND PROGNOSIS

1. Treatment of choice is castration (both testicles).
2. Treat any seconday pyoderma and prostatitis with appropriate systemic antibiotics.
3. Prognosis is good. Hair regrowth should occur within 3 months following castration. Remission followed by relapse may indicate excessive sex hormone production by the adrenal glands or metastatic testicular neoplasia.

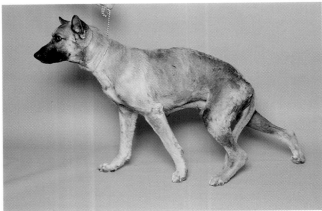

FIGURE 9–23. Sex Hormone Dermatosis. Generalized alopecia with hyperpigmentation in a male dog with a Sertoli cell tumor.

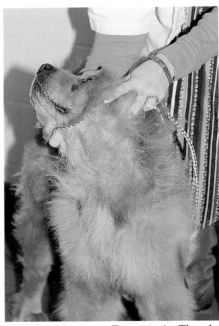

FIGURE 9–26. Sex Hormone Dermatosis. The alopecia and hyperpigmentation on the ventral neck of this intact male chow chow resolved after castration. (Courtesy of D. Angarano)

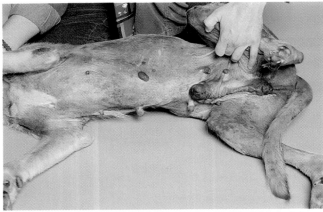

FIGURE 9–24. Sex Hormone Dermatosis. Close-up of the dog in Figure 9–23. Generalized alopecia and hyperfiguration are apparent.

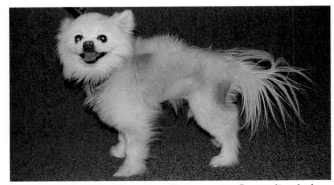

FIGURE 9–27. Sex Hormone Dermatosis. Generalized alopecia in an intact male Pomeranian. The fur coat regrew completely following castration (see Figure 9–28).

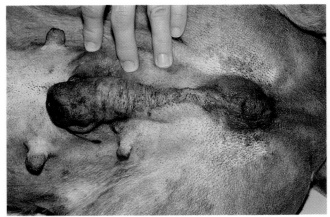

FIGURE 9–25. Sex Hormone Dermatosis. Close-up of the dog in Figures 9–23 and 9–24. Linear preputial hyperpigmentation in a dog with a Sertoli cell tumor.

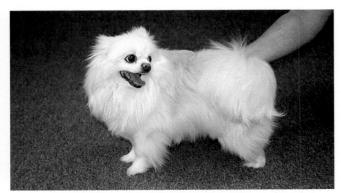

FIGURE 9–28. Sex Hormone Dermatosis. Same dog as in Figure 9–27. Following castration, the fur coat regrew completely.

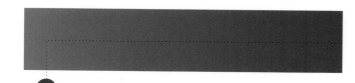

Sex Hormone Dermatosis— Neutered Male Dogs

FEATURES

An endocrinopathy that may be caused by inadequate synthesis or defective metabolism of sex hormones. Rare in neutered male dogs, with the highest incidence in middle-aged to older male dogs castrated at a young age.

Bilaterally symmetric alopecia over the trunk that spares the head and limbs. Remaining hairs epilate easily. The alopecic skin may become hyperpigmented. A coat color change (lightening) may occur. There are no systemic signs of illness.

TOP DIFFERENTIALS

Other causes of endocrine alopecia.

DIAGNOSIS

1. Usually based on ruling out other differentials.
2. Dermatohistopathology—Nonspecific endocrine changes.
3. Sex hormone assays—Usually nondiagnostic.

TREATMENT AND PROGNOSIS

1. Observation without treatment is reasonable because this disease is purely cosmetic and affected dogs are otherwise healthy.
2. Treatment with methyltestosterone may be effective in some cases. Give methyltestosterone, 1 mg/kg (maximum 30 mg) PO q 48 hours, until hair regrowth is seen (approximately 3 months), then taper to 1 mg/kg (maximum 30 mg) once or twice per week for maintenance. Because methyltestosterone is potentially hepatotoxic, clients should be informed of this risk before initiating therapy and serum liver enzyme levels should be monitored periodically.
3. Prognosis for hair regrowth is unpredictable. This is a cosmetic disease that does not affect the dog's quality of life.

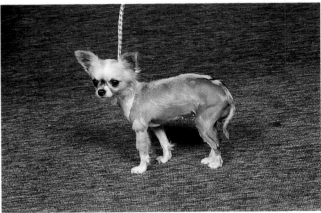

FIGURE 9–29. Sex Hormone Dermatosis. Generalized alopecia in an adult intact female Chihuahua with an ovarian cyst. The hair regrew normally following an ovariohysterectomy.

Sex Hormone Dermatosis— Intact Female Dogs (Figs. 9–29 to 9–32)

FEATURES

An endocrinopathy presumably caused by elevated estrogen levels. Rare in intact female dogs, with the highest incidence in middle-aged to older dogs that have cystic ovaries or ovarian neoplasia. It can also occur in neutered female dogs receiving exogenous estrogen therapy for urinary incontinence.

Bilaterally symmetric, regionalized (flanks, perineum, inguinal) to generalized truncal alopecia that usually spares the head and limbs. Remaining hairs epilate easily. The alopecic skin usually becomes hyperpigmented. There may be secondary lichenification, seborrhea, and superficial pyoderma. Concurrent gynecomastia and vulvar enlargement are usually present. Some dogs have a history of estrus cycle abnormalities, prolonged pseudopregnancies, or nymphomania.

TOP DIFFERENTIALS

Other causes of endocrine alopecia.

DIAGNOSIS

1. Rule out other differentials.
2. Dermatohistopathology—Nonspecific endocrine changes.
3. Sex hormone assays—estrogen levels may be elevated, but results are often nondiagnostic.
4. Response to ovariohysterectomy/cessation of estrogen therapy—Hair regrowth occurs.

TREATMENT AND PROGNOSIS

1. Treat any secondary seborrhea or pyoderma with appropriate therapies.
2. If iatrogenically induced, stop estrogen therapy.
3. Ovariohysterectomy is treatment of choice for intact females.
4. Prognosis is good. Resolution of clinical signs and hair regrowth usually occur in 3–4 months, but in some dogs may take as long as 6 months.

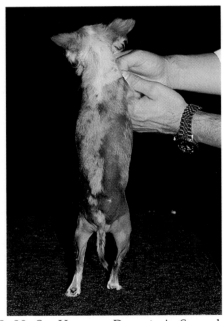

FIGURE 9–30. Sex Hormone Dermatosis. Same dog as in Figure 9–29. The alopecia and hyperpigmentation extend from the neck to the distal rear limbs.

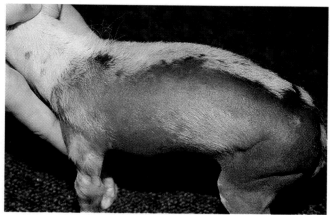

FIGURE 9–31. Sex Hormone Dermatosis. Close-up of the dog in Figures 9–29 and 9–30. Generalized alopecia and hyperpigmentation, with no evidence of a secondary superficial pyoderma.

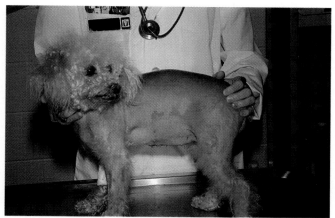

FIGURE 9–32. Sex Hormone Dermatosis. Generalized alopecia in a hermaphrodite poodle with female external genitalia.

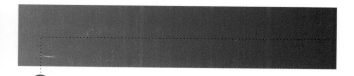

Sex Hormone Dermatosis— Neutered Female Dogs

FEATURES

An endocrinopathy thought to be associated with decreased sex hormone levels. Rare in neutered female dogs, with the highest incidence in those neutered at an early age.

Affected dogs typically develop a bilaterally symmetric alopecia as young adults. Hair loss involves the perineum, flanks, ventral abdomen and thorax, and/or trunk. Remaining hairs epilate easily. Vulva and nipples are usually infantile. There are no systemic signs of illness.

TOP DIFFERENTIALS

Other causes of endocrine alopecia.

DIAGNOSIS

1. Usually based on ruling out other differentials.
2. Dermatohistopathology—Nonspecific endocrine changes.
3. Sex hormone assays—Often nondiagnostic.

TREATMENT AND PROGNOSIS

1. Observation without treatment is reasonable because this disease is purely cosmetic and affected dogs are otherwise healthy.
2. Treatment with diethylstibestrol has been successful in some dogs; however, this drug is no longer available. While Premarin may be an effective substitute, its use has been limited to the treatment of spay incontinence.
3. Alternatively, treatment with methyltestosterone may be effective in some dogs. Give 1 mg/kg (maximum 30 mg) PO q 48 hours until hair regrowth occurs (approximately 1–3 months); then give 1 mg/kg (maximum 30 mg) PO once or twice per week for maintenance. Because methyltestosterone is potentially hepatotoxic, clients should be informed of this risk before initiating therapy, and serum liver enzyme levels should be monitored periodically.
4. Prognosis for hair regrowth is unpredictable. This is a cosmetic disease that does not affect the dog's quality of life.

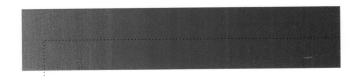

Alopecia "X" (adrenal sex hormone imbalance, hyposomatotropism, growth hormone-responsive dermatosis, pseudo-Cushing's disease) (Figs. 9–33 to 9–36)

FEATURES

The cause of this endocrinopathy is unclear, but it may be due to growth hormone deficiency or excessive production of androgenic steroids by the adrenal glands. Uncommon in dogs, with the highest incidence in adult dogs 2–5 years old, especially chow chows, Pomeranians, keeshonds, Samoyeds, and miniature poodles.

Gradual loss of primary hairs progressing to complete generalized alopecia that spares the head and limbs. The hair loss is bilaterally symmetric, remaining hairs epilate easily, and the alopecic skin may become hyperpigmented, thin, and hypotonic. Mild secondary seborrhea and superficial pyoderma may occur. There are no systemic signs of illness.

TOP DIFFERENTIALS

Other causes of endocrine alopecia.

DIAGNOSIS

1. Rule out other differentials.
2. Dermatohistopathology—Nonspecific endocrine changes.
3. Sex hormone assays (base line and/or post ACTH stimulation)—Sex hormone levels may be elevated, but false-positive and false-negative results can occur.

TREATMENT AND PROGNOSIS

1. Observation without treatment is reasonable because this disease is purely cosmetic and affected dogs are otherwise healthy.
2. Neutering intact dogs may induce permanent or temporary hair regrowth.
3. A variety of medical therapies have been used to stimulate hair regrowth. Treatments that may be effective include:

Melatonin, 3–6 mg/dog PO q 8–12 hours, until maximum hair regrowth occurs (approximately 3–4 months). Then give 3–6 mg PO q 24 hours for 2 months, followed by 3–6 mg q 48 hours for 2 months and then 3–6 mg twice weekly for maintenance.

Cimetidine, 5–10 mg/kg PO q 8 hours.

Methyltestosterone (neutered dogs), 1 mg/kg (maximum 30 mg) PO q 24 hours until hair regrowth occurs (approximately 1–3 months). Then give 1 mg/kg (maximum 30 mg) q 48 hours for 2 months, followed by 1 mg/kg (maximum 30 mg) twice per week for 2 months and then once weekly for maintenance.

Prednisone, 1 mg/kg PO q 24 hours for 1 week, then gradually taper dose to 0.5 mg/kg PO q 48 hours.

Mitotane, 15–25 mg/kg PO with food q 24 hours for 5 days. (An ACTH stimulation test on day 7 should show the post-ACTH cortisol level between 5–7 μg/dl.) Then give mitotane, 15–25 mg/kg PO with food q 1–2 weeks for maintenance.

Porcine growth hormone, 0.15 IU/kg SC twice per week for 6 weeks. Periodic retreatments may be necessary if relapse occurs.

4. Newer therapies that show promise in the treatment of this disorder include:

Leuprolide acetate (Lupron), 100 μg/kg IM q 4–8 weeks, until hair regrowth is seen.

Goserelin (Zoladex), 60 mg/kg SC q 21 days, until hair regrowth occurs.

5. Regardless of the therapy used, hair regrowth may be incomplete or transient. Initial hair regrowth should be seen within 6–8 weeks. If no response is seen after 3 months of treatment, a different therapeutic agent should be considered. The owner should be informed of potential drug risks before any treatment is initiated. For instance, methyltestosterone is potentially hepatotoxic, and serum liver enzyme levels should be monitored periodically. Permanent adrenal insufficiency is a potentially serious complication of mitotane therapy. Growth hormone therapy is potentially diabetogenic, and blood glucose levels should be monitored closely during treatment. Porcine growth hormone is difficult to obtain but is preferable to human growth hormone, which may cause death from anaphylaxis.

6. Prognosis for hair regrowth is unpredictable. This is a cosmetic disease that does not affect the dog's quality of life.

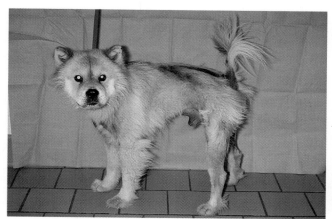

FIGURE 9–33. Alopecia "X." Generalized alopecia and hyperpigmentation in a 3-year-old male chow chow. (Courtesy of D. Angarano)

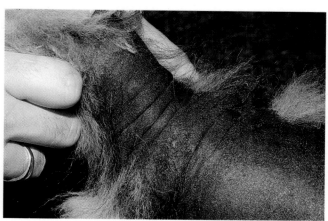

FIGURE 9–35. Alopecia "X." Close-up of the affected dog in Figure 9–34. Alopecia and hyperpigmentation on the dorsal neck. The few remaining hairs are dry and brittle.

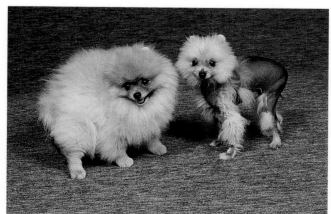

FIGURE 9–34. Alopecia "X." These two related male Pomeranians have alopecia "X." The dog with the normal fur coat previously had generalized alopecia and hyperpigmentation similar to that of the dog on the right. He was treated with growth hormone therapy, which stimulated the fur regrowth.

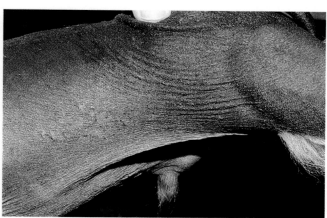

FIGURE 9–36. Alopecia "X." Close-up of the affected dog in Figures 9–34 and 9–35. Alopecia and hyperpigmentation, with no evidence of a secondary bacterial pyoderma.

Canine Recurrent Flank Alopecia (seasonal flank alopecia, cyclic flank alopecia, cyclic follicular dysplasia) (Figs. 9–37 to 9–40)

FEATURES

A seasonally recurring alopecia of unknown etiology. The onset of alopecia in the Northern Hemisphere usually occurs between November and March. Most dogs regrow their hair spontaneously 3–8 months later. The episodes of hair loss may occur sporadically only once or twice, or regularly each year. With repeated episodes, a progressive increase in the amount and duration of hair loss may be seen. Uncommon in dogs, with the highest incidence in boxers, bulldogs, Airedales, and schnauzers.

Nonpruritic, noninflamed, well-demarcated alopecia of flanks that is usually bilaterally symmetric but may be asymmetric or involve only one flank. Occasionally, alopecia may also involve dorsum of nose, perineum, and base of tail or ears. There are no systemic signs of illness.

TOP DIFFERENTIALS

Superficial pyoderma, demodicosis, dermatophytosis, other endocrinopathies, alopecia areata.

DIAGNOSIS

1. Usually based on history and clinical findings, but rule out other differentials.
2. Dermatohistopathology—Dysplastic, keratin-filled hair follicles with finger-like projections into underlying dermis. Increased melanin may be seen in sebaceous ducts and in hair follicles.

TREATMENT AND PROGNOSIS

1. Observation without treatment is reasonable, because this disease is purely cosmetic and affected dogs are otherwise healthy.
2. Treatment with melatonin may be effective. Protocols include:

   Sustained release melatonin, one to four 12 mg implants/dog SC once.
   Melatonin, 3–6 mg/dog PO q 8–12 hours or 9 mg/dog PO q 24 hours for 4–6 weeks.

3. Prognosis for hair regrowth is variable. Spontaneous hair regrowth often occurs within 3–8 months even without treatment. New hairs may have altered pigmentation or regrowth may be incomplete. Reinitiating melatonin therapy each year 4–6 weeks prior to anticipated recurrences may prevent future episodes. This is a cosmetic disease that does not affect the dog's quality of life.

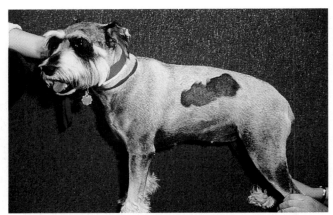

FIGURE 9–37. Canine Recurrent Flank Alopecia. Well-demarcated alopecia and hyperpigmentation on the lateral flank of a 2-year-old schnauzer. The lesion recurred every spring and resolved in the winter.

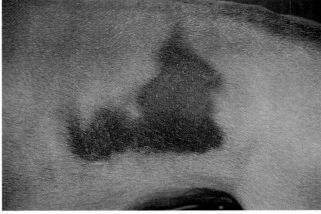

FIGURE 9–38. Canine Recurrent Flank Alopecia. Alopecia and hyperpigmentation on the lateral flank of an adult boxer. This lesion waxed and waned with the seasons but never completely resolved.

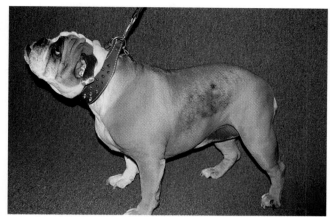

FIGURE 9–39. Canine Recurrent Flank Alopecia. Alopecia on the flank on an adult bulldog.

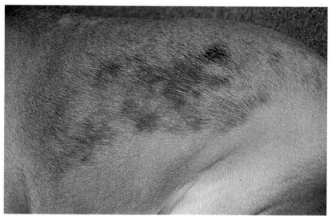

FIGURE 9–40. Canine Recurrent Flank Alopecia. Close-up of the dog in Figure 9–39. Alopecia and hyperpigmentation, with no evidence of a secondary superficial pyoderma.

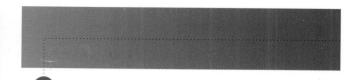

Pituitary Dwarfism (Figs. 9–41 and 9–42)

FEATURES

A hereditary hypopituitarism with variable thyroid, adrenal, and gonadal abnormalities. Rare in dogs, with the highest incidence in German shepherds.

Affected dogs appear to be normal at birth but stop growing at 2–3 months of age. Permanent teeth may fail to erupt. There are no primary hairs over the trunk (only a puppy coat). Progressive, gradual loss of this puppy coat begins during puppyhood and results in a bilaterally symmetric alopecia that spares the head and limbs. Remaining hairs epilate easily. The alopecic skin becomes hyperpigmented, thin, and hypotonic. Secondary seborrhea, superficial pyoderma, and/or *Malassezia* dermatitis are common. Concurrent signs of hypothyroidism, hypoadrenocorticism, and/or gonadal atrophy (testicular atrophy, no estrus) may be present.

TOP DIFFERENTIAL

Congenital hypothyroidism.

DIAGNOSIS

1. Usually based on signalment, history, and clinical signs.
2. Dermatohistopathology—Nonspecific endocrine changes.
3. Skeletal radiographs—Delayed closure of long bone growth plates.
4. Growth hormone assay—Not available for dogs at this writing.
5. Insulin-like growth factor level—Elevated.
6. Thyroid and adrenal function tests—May be abnormal if concurrent hypothyroidism or hypoadrenocorticism is present.

TREATMENT AND PROGNOSIS

1. Treat any secondary seborrhea, superficial pyoderma, or *Malassezia* dermatitis with appropriate topical and systemic therapies.
2. Treat any concurrent hypothyroidism or adrenal insufficiency with appropriate medications.
3. In experimental studies, treatments with bovine growth hormone (10 IU) or porcine growth hormone (2 IU) SC q 48 hours for 4–6 weeks successfully induced hair regrowth, but the dogs remained dwarfs. Growth hormone for use in dogs is not readily available at this writing. Potential

side effects include hypersensitivity reactions and diabetes mellitus.

4. Prognosis is poor. Pituitary dwarfs usually live for only 3–8 years. Because this disease is hereditary, affected dogs should not be bred.

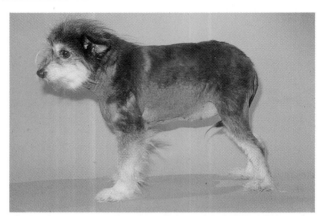

FIGURE 9–41. Pituitary Dwarfism. Alopecia, hyperpigmentation, and a poor-quality fur coat in a stunted 8-year-old female spayed husky. (Courtesy of D. Angarano)

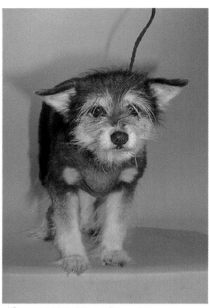

FIGURE 9–42. Pituitary Dwarfism. Same dog as in Figure 9–41. Alopecia, hyperpigmentation, and a poor-quality fur coat. (Courtesy of D. Angarano)

Suggested Readings

Beale K and Morris D. 1998. Treatment of Canine Calcinosis Cutis with Dimethylsulfoxide Gel. 14th Proc AAVD/ACVD Mtg, pp. 97–98.

Bruyette D, Ruehl W, Entriken T, Griffin D, and Darling L. 1997. Management of Canine Pituitary-Dependent Hyperadrenocorticism with l-Deprenyl (Anipryl). Vet Clin North Am Sm Anim Pract. 27(2): 273–286.

Endocrine and Metabolic Diseases, pp. 627–719. In Scott DW, Miller WH Jr, and Griffin CE. 1995. Muller & Kirk's Small Animal Dermatology. Ed. 5. W.B. Saunders Philadelphia, PA.

Ferguson DC. 1994. Update on Diagnosis of Canine Hypothyroidism. Vet Clin North Am Sm Anim Pract. 24:515–539.

Paradis M. 2000. Melatonin Therapy for Canine Alopecia. In Kik's Current Veterinary Therapy, XIII, Small Animal Practice. W.B. Saunders, Philadelphia, PA.

Plumb DC. 1999. Veterinary Drug Handbook. Ed. 3. Iowa State University Press, Ames, IA.

Schmeitzel L, Lothrop C, and Rosenkrantz W. 1995. Congenital Adrenal Hyperplasia Like Syndrome, pp. 600–604. In Bonagwa JD (ed). Kirk's Current Veterinary Therapy, XII, Small Animal Practice. W.B. Saunders, Philadelphia, PA.

Zerbe CA. 2000. Screening Tests to Diagnose Hyperadrenocorticism in Dogs and Cats. Compend Cont Edu Pract Vet. 22: 17–18.

Zerbe CA. 2000. Differentiating Tests to Evaluate Hyperadrenocorticism in Dogs and Cats. Compend Cont Edu Pract Vet. 22: 149–158.

10

Hereditary, Congenital, and Acquired Alopecias

- **Alopecic Breeds**
- **Congenital Hypotrichosis**
- **Color Dilution Alopecia** (color mutant alopecia)
- **Black Hair Follicular Dysplasia**
- **Canine Pattern Baldness**
- **Idiopathic Bald Thigh Syndrome of Greyhounds**
- **Feline Preauricular and Pinnal Alopecias**
- **Anagen and Telogen Defluxion**
- **Excessive Shedding**
- **Postclipping Alopecia**
- **Traction Alopecia**
- **Injection Reaction**

Alopecic Breeds (Figs. 10-1 and 10-2)

FEATURES

These dogs and cats are bred deliberately to produce hairless offspring. Alopecic breeds include the Mexican hairless dog, Chinese crested dog, Inca hairless dog, American hairless terrier, and sphinx cat.

Generalized truncal alopecia at birth is typical. Mild secondary pyodermas and/or seborrhea may develop in dogs. Sphinx cats, because of reluctance to groom, often become greasy, seborrheic, and malodorous.

DIAGNOSIS

1. Based on signalment, history, and clinical findings.
2. Dermatohistopathology—Atrophic, decreased numbers, or complete absence of hair follicles. Adnexae are often similarly affected.

TREATMENT AND PROGNOSIS

1. Use antiseborrheic and antibacterial shampoo baths and conditioners as needed for secondary seborrhea and pyoderma.
2. Prognosis is good. These animals are meant to be hairless.

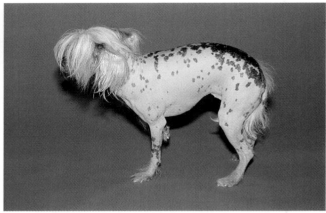

FIGURE 10-1. Alopecic Breeds. This Chinese crested demonstrates the characteristic pattern of alopecia typical of this breed.

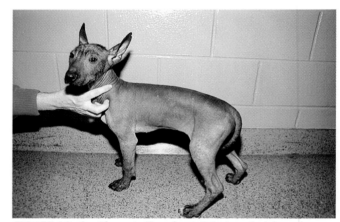

FIGURE 10-2. Alopecic Breeds. A Mexican hairless dog with generalized alopecia.

Congenital Hypotrichosis

(Figs. 10–3 and 10–4)

FEATURES

A developmental non-color-linked alopecic disorder. Rare in dogs and cats. One or more animals in the litter may be affected.

Affected animals are either born with alopecia or appear normal at birth but begin losing hair at around 1 month of age. Hair loss is symmetric and usually involves the head, trunk, or ventrum. Regionalized or generalized alopecia may be seen. The alopecic skin often becomes secondarily hyperpigmented and seborrheic. Abnormal dentition may be present.

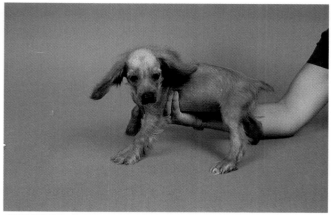

FIGURE 10–3. Congenital Hypotrichosis. This young puppy was born with alopecia on the head and trunk. (Courtesy of D. Angarano)

TOP DIFFERENTIALS

Demodicosis, dermatophytosis, superficial pyoderma.

DIAGNOSIS

1. Based on history, clinical findings, and ruling out other differentials.
2. Dermatohistopathology—Hair follicles are completely absent or atrophic and decreased in number in affected skin.

TREATMENT AND PROGNOSIS

1. No treatment is known.
2. Prognosis is good; this is a cosmetic problem that does not affect the animal's quality of life. Affected animals should not be bred.

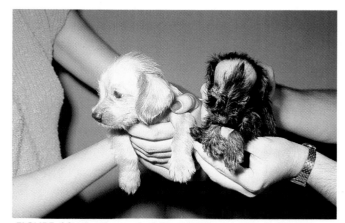

FIGURE 10–4. Congenital Hypotrichosis. Focal alopecia on the face and ears of two puppies from the same litter. (Courtesy of D. Angarano)

Color Dilution Alopecia (color mutant alopecia) (Figs. 10–5 to 10–8)

FEATURES

A developmental alopecic disorder associated with abnormal melanin distribution in hair shafts. Common in dogs bred to be blue (dilution of black) or fawn (dilution of brown), especially Doberman pinschers.

Affected dogs appear normal at birth but usually begin losing hair over the dorsum of the trunk between 6 months and 2 years of age. Although the haircoat thinning often progresses to partial or complete alopecia, only the color-diluted hairs are lost. The dog's normal-colored markings are not affected. Secondary superficial pyoderma is common.

TOP DIFFERENTIALS

Dermatophytosis, demodicosis, superficial pyoderma, causes of endocrine alopecia (hypothyroidism, hyperadrenocorticism, sex hormone dermatosis).

DIAGNOSIS

1. Usually based on signalment, history, clinical findings, and ruling out other differentials.
2. Dermatohistopathology—Dilated, cystic, keratin-filled hair follicles. Abnormal clumps of melanin are present in epidermal and follicular basal cells, hair, and peribulbar melanophages.

TREATMENT AND PROGNOSIS

1. No specific treatment is known that reverses or prevents further hair loss.
2. Treat symptomatically with mild antiseborrheic or antibacterial shampoos and conditioners as needed.
3. Give appropriate systemic antibiotics for 3–4 weeks if secondary pyoderma is present.
4. Prognosis is good. Although hair loss is irreversible and routine symptomatic skin care may be needed, this is a cosmetic problem that does not affect the dog's quality of life.

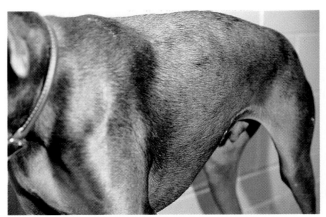

FIGURE 10–5. Color Dilution Alopecia. The thin haircoat on this blue Doberman pinscher was caused by abnormal clumping of melanin within the hair.

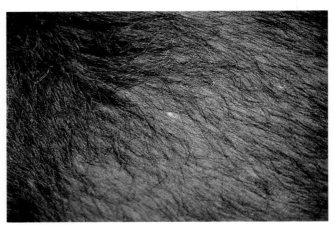

FIGURE 10–6. Color Dilution Alopecia. Close-up of the dog in Figure 10–5. Partial alopecia on the trunk, with no evidence of a secondary superficial pyoderma.

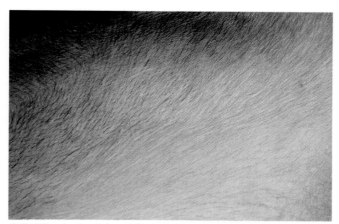

FIGURE 10–7. Color Dilution Alopecia. The areas of color-diluted hair were partially alopecic in this Doberman pinscher. The adjacent area of normal colored hair was unaffected.

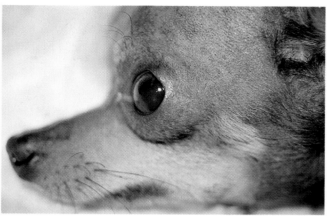

FIGURE 10–8. Color Dilution Alopecia. The areas of color-diluted hair were partially alopecic in this Chihuahua. The adjacent area of normal colored hair was unaffected.

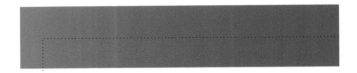

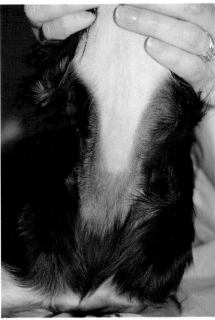

FIGURE 10–9. Black Hair Follicular Dysplasia. Partial alopecia affecting only the areas of black hair.

Black Hair Follicular Dysplasia (Figs. 10–9 and 10–10)

FEATURES

A developmental alopecic disorder associated with defective hair pigmentation and formation. Rare in dogs.

Affected puppies appear normal at birth but begin losing hair at around 1 month of age. Only black hairs are affected, with the alopecia progressing until all the black hairs have been lost.

TOP DIFFERENTIALS

Dermatophytosis, demodicosis, superficial pyoderma, and causes of endocrine alopecia.

DIAGNOSIS

1. Based on history, clinical findings, and ruling out other differentials.
2. Dermatohistopathology—Non-black-haired skin is normal. Black-haired skin has dilated hair follicles filled with keratin, hair shaft fragments, and free melanin. Abnormal clumps of melanin are present in follicular and epidermal basal cells and in hair matrix cells.

TREATMENT AND PROGNOSIS

1. No treatment is known.
2. Prognosis is good. Although the alopecia is irreversible, this is a cosmetic problem that does not affect the dog's quality of life.

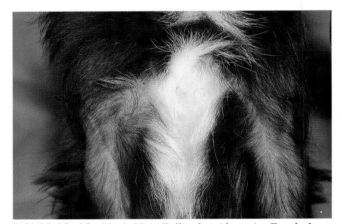

FIGURE 10–10. Black Hair Follicular Alopecia. Focal alopecia on the forearms of a young dog. Only the black hairs were affected. (Courtesy of J. MacDonald)

Canine Pattern Baldness

(Figs. 10–11 and 10–12)

FEATURES

An idiopathic alopecic disorder that is most common in dachshunds but can occur in other short-coated breeds such as Chihuahuas, whippets, and Manchester terriers. A clinically distinct pattern baldness also occurs in American water spaniels and Portuguese water dogs. Pattern baldness often begins during late puberty or early adulthood.

There is a gradual thinning of hairs that usually progresses to complete alopecia as the dog grows older. The hair loss is symmetric, but remaining hairs do not epilate easily. The alopecic skin becomes secondarily hyperpigmented over time. In short-coated dogs, the alopecia may involve the lateral ear pinnae, postauricular skin, caudomedial thighs, and/or ventral aspect of the neck, chest, and abdomen. The pattern baldness of American water spaniels and Portuguese water dogs involves the ventral neck, caudomedial thighs, and tail.

TOP DIFFERENTIALS

Dermatophytosis, demodicosis, superficial pyoderma, causes of endocrine alopecia (hyperadrenocorticism, hypothyroidism, sex hormone dermatosis).

DIAGNOSIS

1. Rule out other differentials.
2. Dermatohistopathology—Hair follicles are smaller than normal.

TREATMENT AND PROGNOSIS

1. Melatonin, 3–6 mg PO q 8–12 hours may be effective in some dogs.
2. Prognosis is good. Although the hair loss is often irreversible, this is a cosmetic problem that does not affect the dog's quality of life.

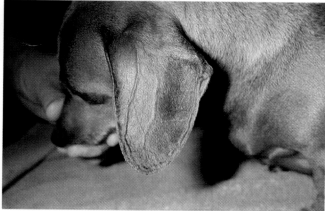

FIGURE 10–11. Canine Pattern Baldness. The complete alopecia on this dachshund's ear pinnae is typical of this syndrome. (Courtesy of J. MacDonald)

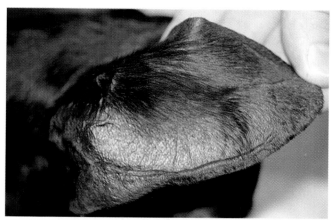

FIGURE 10–12. Canine Pattern Baldness. Diffuse alopecia on the ear pinnae of an adult dachshund.

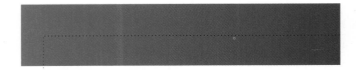

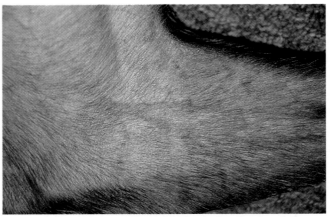

FIGURE 10–13. Idiopathic Bald Thigh Syndrome of Greyhounds. Diffuse alopecia on the rear legs of an adult greyhound. There is no evidence of secondary infection.

Idiopathic Bald Thigh Syndrome of Greyhounds

(Figs. 10–13 and 10–14)

FEATURES

An alopecic disorder of unknown etiology that is common in greyhound dogs. The alopecia may begin during late puberty or early adulthood and often progresses slowly as the dog ages.

There is a gradual, bilaterally symmetrical thinning of hairs on the lateral and caudal aspects of the thighs that often extends to the ventral abdomen. Remaining hairs do not epilate easily. Except for the alopecia, affected skin appears otherwise normal. There are no systemic signs of illness.

TOP DIFFERENTIALS

Demodicosis, dermatophytosis, superficial pyoderma, and causes of endocrine alopecia (hypothyroidism, hyperadrenocorticism, sex hormone dermatosis).

DIAGNOSIS

1. Based on signalment, history, clinical findings, and ruling out other differentials.
2. Dermatohistopathology (nondiagnostic)—Findings are nonspecific and similar to those seen with endocrinopathies.

TREATMENT AND PROGNOSIS

1. There is no specific treatment that will reverse or prevent further hair loss.
2. Prognosis is good. Although the hair loss is usually permanent, this is a cosmetic disease that does not affect the dog's quality of life.

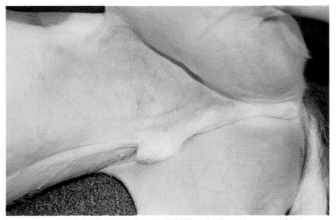

FIGURE 10–14. Idiopathic Bald Thigh Syndrome of Greyhounds. Complete alopecia on the abdominal and inguinal regions of an adult greyhound. There is no evidence of a secondary infection.

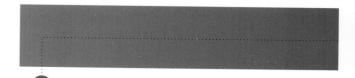

Feline Preauricular and Pinnal Alopecias (Figs. 10–15 and 10–16)

FEATURES

Preauricular alopecia is a common and normal finding in cats. It is characterized by sparsely haired skin on the head between the ears and eyes that is not usually noticeable in long-haired cats but is more readily apparent in short-haired cats. No skin lesions are present.

Pinnal alopecia is uncommon in cats and is characterized by periodic episodes of nonpruritic pinnal alopecia. Siamese cats are predisposed. The alopecia may be patchy or involve most of the pinna, and both ears are usually involved. Except for the alopecia, the skin is otherwise normal.

TOP DIFFERENTIALS

Dermatophytosis, demodicosis.

DIAGNOSIS

1. Based on history, clinical findings, and ruling out other differentials.

TREATMENT AND PROGNOSIS

1. No treatment is known.
2. Prognosis is good. Preauricular alopecia is a normal finding in cats. Cats with pinnal alopecia usually regrow hair within several months.

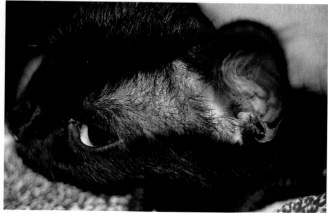

FIGURE 10–15. Feline Preauricular and Pinnal Alopecia. Diffuse alopecia on the preauricular skin of this adult cat.

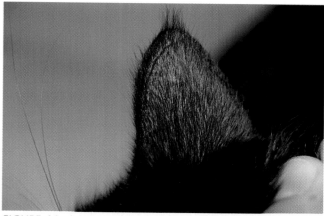

FIGURE 10–16. Feline Preauricular and Pinnal Alopecia. Close-up of the cat in Figure 10–15. Partial alopecia on the ear pinnae, with no evidence of infection.

Anagen and Telogen Defluxion (Figs. 10–17 to 10–20)

FEATURES

Alopecia develops when the normal hair growth and hair cycle are adversely affected by underlying disease or stress such as chemotherapy drug administration, infections, metabolic disease, fever, pregnancy, shock, surgery, and anesthesia. Rare in dogs and cats.

There is an acute onset of hair loss within days of the insult (anagen defluxion) or 1–3 months after the insult (telogen defluxion). Except for the alopecia, affected skin appears otherwise normal. In telogen defluxion the hair loss is usually widespread, progresses rapidly over a few to several days, and tends to spare the head. In anagen defluxion, the hair loss is less dramatic and is characterized by excessive shedding.

TOP DIFFERENTIALS

Hyperadrenocorticism, hypothyroidism, sex hormone imbalance, alopecia "X," seasonal flank alopecia, excessive shedding.

DIAGNOSIS

1. Based on history, clinical findings, and ruling out other differentials.
2. Dermatohistopathology (rarely diagnostic)—Usually reveals normal skin, but hairs diffusely in telogen may be seen in telogen defluxion and findings in anagen defluxion may include abnormal hair matrix cells with dysplastic hair shafts.

TREATMENT AND PROGNOSIS

1. Identify and address the underlying cause.
2. Prognosis is good. Spontaneous hair regrowth occurs after resolution or cessation of inciting cause.

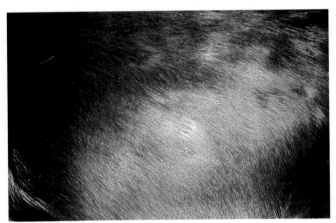

FIGURE 10–17. Telogen Defluxion. The moth-eaten alopecia on this dog's body was caused by telogen defluxion. (Courtesy of A. Yu)

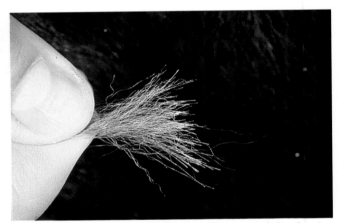

FIGURE 10–18. Telogen Defluxion. Close-up of the dog in Figure 10–17. The large clump of hair was epilated easily. (Courtesy of A. Yu)

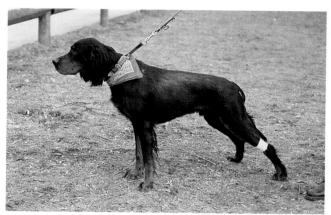

FIGURE 10–19. Telogen Defluxion. Generalized alopecia in an adult dog caused by telogen defluxion. (Courtesy of M. Austel)

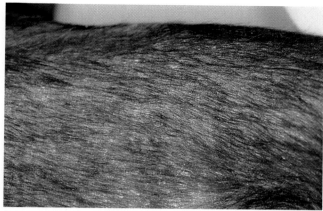

FIGURE 10–20. Telogen Defluxion. Close-up of the dog in Figure 10–19. Partial alopecia, with no evidence of infection. (Courtesy of M. Austel)

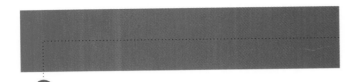

Excessive Shedding (Figs. 10–21 and 10–22)

FEATURES

Shedding is a normal phenomenon in dogs and cats, but some animals shed more than others. A common owner complaint. Some animals shed more in spring and fall, while others shed excessively year round. In spite of continual hair loss, there is no alopecia or skin abnormalities. While hairs may epilate easily, focal areas of alopecia cannot be created.

TOP DIFFERENTIALS

Superficial pyoderma, dermatophytosis, demodicosis, anagen or telogen defluxion, causes of endocrine alopecia.

DIAGNOSIS

1. Based on history, clinical findings, and ruling out other differentials.

TREATMENT AND PROGNOSIS

1. Groom the animal every day to remove shed hairs before they fall off.
2. Make sure the diet is balanced.
3. Daily fatty acid supplementation may be helpful.
4. Sometimes outdoor animals improve when brought indoors and vice versa.
5. Prognosis is good. Although excessive shedding is annoying to owners, affected animals are otherwise healthy.

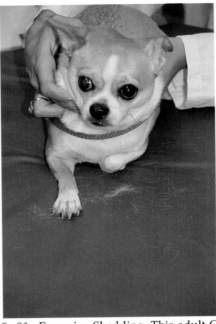

FIGURE 10–21. Excessive Shedding. This adult Chihuahua presented with excessive shedding. There were no cutaneous or systemic abnormalities.

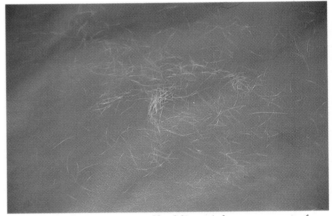

FIGURE 10–22. Excessive Shedding. A large amount of hair was shed in just a few minutes from the dog in Figure 10–21.

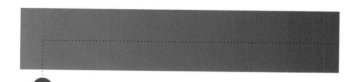

Postclipping Alopecia (Figs. 10–23 to 10–25)

FEATURES

Hairs fail to regrow in areas that have been clipped. It may occur following clipping for a surgical procedure or for grooming purposes. Uncommon in dogs.

Several months postclipping, the affected areas looks as if it has just been clipped. The rest of the haircoat is normal.

TOP DIFFERENTIALS

Hyperadrenocorticism, hypothyroidism, sex hormone imbalance, alopecia "X."

DIAGNOSIS

1. Based on history, clinical findings, and ruling out other differentials.
2. Dermatohistopathology—May show predominantly catagen hair follicles.

TREATMENT AND PROGNOSIS

1. Spontaneous hair regrowth usually occurs, but can take up to 2 years.
2. Short-term treatment with levothyroxine, 0.02 mg/kg PO q 12 hours for 4–6 weeks, is usually effective in stimulating hair regrowth within 2–3 months.
3. Prognosis is good.

FIGURE 10–24. Post-Clipping Alopecia. Close-up of the dog in Figure 10–23. The clipper marks remain visible due to the lack of new hair growth.

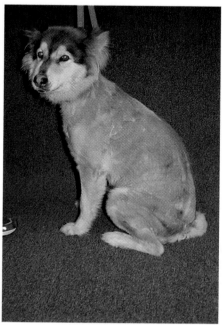

FIGURE 10–23. Post-Clipping Alopecia. This 6-year-old Alaskan malamute was clipped for summer 5 months earlier. There is minimal evidence of hair regrowth.

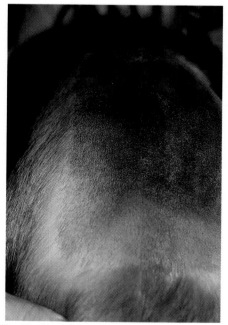

FIGURE 10–25. Post-Clipping Alopecia. This area was clipped for surgery 3 months earlier. There is minimal evidence of new hair growth.

Traction Alopecia (Fig. 10-26)

FEATURES

Alopecia that occurs when hair clips or rubber bands used to hold hair in place are fastened too tightly or for too long. Uncommon in dogs.

Initially, an erythematous plaque appears at the site of the hair device. It may progress to a localized patch of scarred alopecia. The lesion occurs most commonly on top of or on the lateral aspect of the head.

TOP DIFFERENTIALS

Demodicosis, dermatophytosis, superficial pyoderma, alopecia areata.

DIAGNOSIS

1. Usually based on the history and clinical findings.
2. Dermatohistopathology—Variable mononuclear cell infiltrates, edema, vasodilatation, pilosebaceous atrophy, fibrosing dermatitis, and/or scarring alopecia.

TREATMENT AND PROGNOSIS

1. Remove the hair device.
2. As a preventive measure, hair devices should be applied properly to avoid excessive traction on hairs.
3. Prognosis depends on the duration of the lesion. Early lesions should resolve spontaneously after the hair device is removed. Chronic, scarred lesions may be permanent.

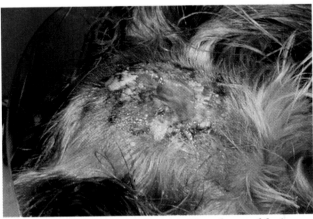

FIGURE 10-26. Traction Alopecia. The ulcerated lesion on the head of this 4-year-old female Yorkshire terrier was caused by excessive traction from a hair bow. (Courtesy of T. DeManuelle)

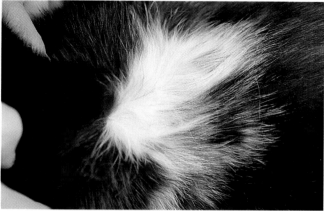

FIGURE 10–27. Injection Reaction. The leukotrichia (whiting of the hair) developed shortly after a steroid injection.

Injection Reaction (Figs. 10–27 to 10–30)

FEATURES

A focal area of alopecia that occurs at the site where a subcutaneous injection of rabies vaccine, Droncit, glucocorticoids, or progestational compounds have been administered. Uncommon in dogs and cats.

A focal, circumscribed to ovoid area of alopecia develops at injection site (over the shoulder, back, posterolateral thigh) 2–4 months later. In dogs, affected skin is usually thin, atrophic, and hypopigmented if the lesion is glucocorticoid or progesterone induced. With the canine rabies vaccine, the lesion may initially be thickened, plaque-like, and erythematous, later becoming mildly scaly, shiny, and hyperpigmented. In cats, both pruritic, ulcerative, plaque-like to nodular lesions and lesions similar to those seen in dogs after rabies vaccination have been described. Pigmentary changes may occur.

TOP DIFFERENTIALS

Dogs. Localized demodicosis, dermatophytosis, superficial pyoderma, alopecia areata.

Cats. Localized demodicosis, dermatophytosis, idiopathic ulcerative dermatosis, neoplasia.

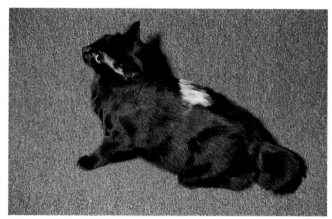

FIGURE 10–28. Injection Reaction. Distant view of the same cat in Figure 10–27. The focal area of white hair is apparent.

DIAGNOSIS

1. Based on history, clinical findings, and ruling out other differentials.
2. Dermatohistopathology—With rabies vaccine reactions, varying degrees of panniculitis are usually present. Vasculitis and atrophic hair follicles may also be seen. With glucocorticoid or progesterone injection reactions, varying degrees of dermal and pilosebaceous atrophy are usually seen.

TREATMENT AND PROGNOSIS

1. For dogs, no treatment is usually needed. Spontaneous hair regrowth is typical, but can take as long as a year to occur.
2. For dogs whose lesions remain permanently alopecic, surgical excision is curative.
3. Cats with pruritic lesions may be difficult to manage medically. Systemic antibiotics for secondary pyoderma may be indicated.
4. For cats with chronic lesions, surgical excision should be considered.
5. Prognosis is usually good, but regrown hair may have altered pigmentation.

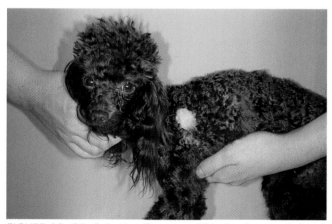

FIGURE 10–29. Injection Reaction. This focal area of alopecia developed after a routine vaccination injection. (Courtesy of A. Yu)

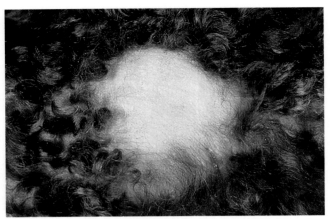

FIGURE 10-30. Injection Reaction. Close-up of the dog in Figure 10–29. The alopecia at the injection site is apparent. (Courtesy of A. Yu)

Suggested Readings

Acquired Alopecias, pp. 720–735. In Scott DW, Miller WH Jr, and Griffin CE. 1995. Muller & Kirk's Small Animal Dermatology. Ed. 5. W.B. Saunders, Philadelphia, PA.

Congenital and Hereditary Defects, pp. 771–781. In Scott DW, Miller WH Jr, and Griffin CE. 1995. Muller & Kirk's Small Animal Dermatology. Ed. 5. W.B. Saunders, Philadelphia, PA.

Lewis CJ. 1995. Black Hair Follicular Dysplasia in UK Bred Salukis. Veterinary Record. 137:294–295.

Plumb DC. 1999. Veterinary Drug Handbook. Ed. 3. Iowa State University Press, Ames, IA.

Shanley KJ. 1995. Acquired, Non-endocrine Alopecias of the Dog and Cat, pp. 606–610. In Bonagura JD (ed). Kirk's Current Veterinary Therapy, XII, Small Animal Practice. W.B. Saunders, Philadelphia, PA.

11

Congenital and Hereditary Defects

- **Epidermolysis Bullosa**

- **Familial Canine Dermatomyositis**

- **Ehlers-Danlos Syndrome** (cutaneous asthenia, dermatosparaxis)

- **Cutaneous Mucinosis**

- **Dermoid Sinus**

- **Familial Footpad Hyperkeratosis**

Epidermolysis Bullosa (Figs. 11–1 and 11–2)

FEATURES

A group of hereditary mechanobullous diseases in which minor trauma results in blister formation. Structural defects in the basement membrane zone are responsible for incomplete cohesion between the epidermis and dermis. Rare in dogs and cats, with affected animals usually developing lesions shortly after birth.

Vesicles, bullae, erosions, crusts, and ulcers appear at sites of frictional trauma such as on the footpads, lips, gingiva, tongue, and palate and over bony prominences of the limbs. Lesions may also involve the face, trunk, tail, and/or ventral abdomen. Claw sloughing and secondary bacterial paronychia may be seen.

TOP DIFFERENTIALS

Dermatomyositis, pemphigus vulgaris, bullous pemphigoid, systemic lupus erythematosus, erythema multiforme/toxic epidermal necrolysis, drug eruption, vasculitis.

DIAGNOSIS

1. Rule out other differentials.
2. Dermatohistopathology—Subepidermal clefting and vesicle formation with minimal inflammation.
3. Electron microscopy (skin biopsy specimens)—Depending on the subtype of epidermolysis bullosa, clefting may be intraepidermal from cytolysis of basal cells, below the lamina densa, or within the lamina lucida of the basement membrane zone.

TREATMENT AND PROGNOSIS

1. No specific treatment is known.
2. Avoid trauma by keeping the affected animal indoors, away from other animals, and handling it carefully.
3. Give appropriate systemic antibiotics for secondary bacterial paronychia as needed.
4. Prognosis for severely affected animals is poor. With proper environmental management, mildly affected animals may enjoy a reasonable quality of life. Affected animals should not be bred.

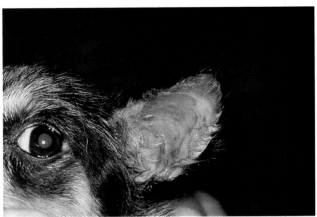

FIGURE 11–1. Epidermolysis Bullosa. Ulceration of the ventral ear pinnae. (Courtesy of P. Rakich)

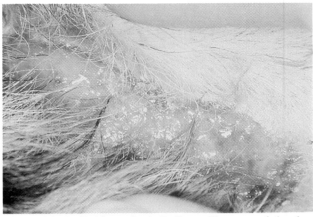

FIGURE 11–2. Epidermolysis Bullosa. Close-up of the dog in Figure 11–1. An ulcerated skin lesion with a purulent exudate. (Courtesy of P. Rakich)

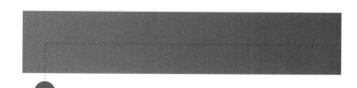

Familial Canine Dermatomyositis

(Figs. 11–3 to 11–10)

FEATURES

An inherited inflammatory disorder of skin, muscles, and occasionally blood vessels. The cause is unclear, but a genetic predisposition followed by a trigger (infection or other environmental factor) that initiates the clinical signs or an immune-mediated process has been proposed. Uncommon in dogs, with the highest incidence in collies, Shetland sheepdogs, and their crossbreeds. Lesions usually first appear in puppies between 2 and 6 months of age. Several litter mates may be affected, but the severity of the disease often varies significantly among the puppies.

Skin lesions are nonpruritic, vary in severity, and may wax and wane. They are characterized by papules and vesicles (rare) and by variable degrees of erythema, alopecia, scaling, crusting, erosions, ulceration, and scarring. Lesions occur on the bridge of the nose, around the eyes and lips, in the inner ear pinnae, on the tail tip, and over bony prominences of the distal extremities. Rarely, footpad ulcers are seen. Signs of myositis are variable. Dogs may be asymptomatic, have bilaterally symmetric atrophy of the masseter and/or temporalis muscles, or have generalized symmetric muscle atrophy. Dogs with masseter muscle involvement may have difficulty eating, drinking, and swallowing. Severely affected dogs may be stunted, lame, and infertile. If the esophageal muscles are affected, megaesophagus may develop.

TOP DIFFERENTIALS

Demodicosis, dermatophytosis, superficial pyoderma, autoimmune skin diseases, vasculitis, polymyositis.

DIAGNOSIS

1. Rule out other differentials.
2. Dermatohistopathology (may be nondiagnostic)—Scattered epidermal basal cell degeneration, perifollicular inflammatory infiltrates of lymphocytes, histiocytes, and variable numbers of mast cells and neutrophils, follicular basal cell degeneration, and follicular atrophy are highly suggestive findings but may not be present, especially in chronic or scarred lesions.
3. Electromyography—Fibrillation potentials, bizarre high-frequency discharges, and sharp waves are seen in affected muscles.
4. Histopathology (abnormal muscles)—Variable multifocal accumulations of inflammatory cells including lymphocytes, macrophages, plasma cells, neutrophils, and eosinophils; myofibril degeneration; and myofiber atrophy and regeneration.

TREATMENT AND PROGNOSIS

1. Symptomatic shampoo therapy to remove crusts may be helpful.
2. Treat any secondary superficial pyoderma with appropriate systemic antibiotics.
3. Avoid activities that may traumatize the skin.
4. Keep the dog indoors during the day to avoid exposure to sunlight, which may exacerbate the skin lesions.
5. Spay intact females because estrus, pregnancy, and lactation exacerbate the disease.
6. Supplementation with essential fatty acids and treatment with vitamin E, 400–800 IU PO q 24 hours, may be beneficial for the skin lesions. Improvement should be seen after 1–2 months of therapy.
7. Treatment with pentoxifylline, 10 mg/kg PO q 8–12 hours with food, may be beneficial in some dogs. Improvement should be seen after 1–2 months of therapy.
8. Prednisone, 1 mg/kg PO q 24 hours, then tapered, may be used for acute flare-ups; however, prolonged steroid usage may exacerbate muscle atrophy.
9. Prognosis is variable, depending on the severity of disease. Skin lesions in minimally affected dogs tend to resolve spontaneously, with no scarring. Skin lesions in mildly to moderately affected dogs usually resolve eventually, but residual scarring is common. In severely affected dogs, the dermatitis and myositis do not resolve and the prognosis for long-term survival is poor. Regardless of disease severity, affected dogs should not be bred.

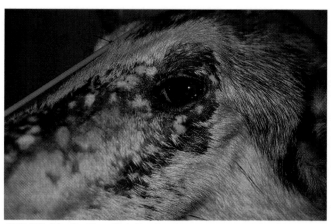

FIGURE 11–3. Familial Canine Dermatomyositis. Alopecia and scarring on the face of an adult collie. The erythematous macules were active lesions.

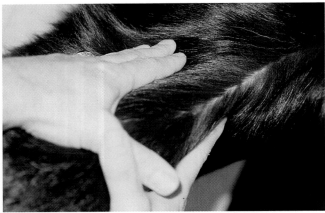

FIGURE 11–4. Familial Canine Dermatomyositis. Severe muscle atrophy of the lumbar musculature in an affected dog. The lateral processes of the vertebrae were easily palpated. (Courtesy of D. Angarano)

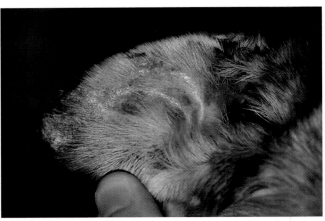

FIGURE 11–7. Familial Canine Dermatomyositis. Crusting, erosive lesions on the ear pinnae of an adult collie with chronic lesions.

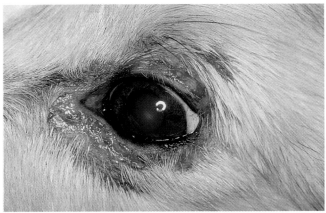

FIGURE 11–5. Familial Canine Dermatomyositis. Erosive lesions of the periocular skin are characteristic of active lesions. As the dog ages and the active lesions resolve, the skin may become scarred and remain alopecic (see Figure 11–6). (Courtesy of M. Mahaffey)

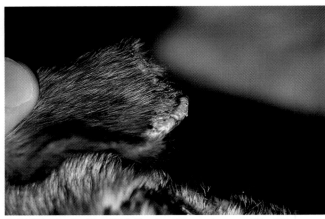

FIGURE 11–8. Familial Canine Dermatomyositis. Close-up of the dog in Figure 11–7. The crusting lesions on the ear margin waxed and waned for several years. Note the similarity to vasculitis and other autoimmune skin diseases.

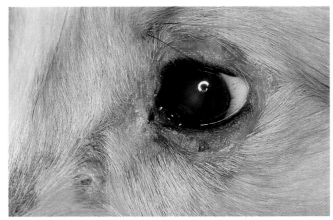

FIGURE 11–6. Familial Canine Dermatomyositis. The same dog as in Figure 11–5. The active lesions have resolved, leaving alopecic, scarred skin. (Courtesy of M. Mahaffey)

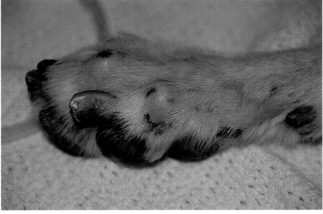

FIGURE 11–9. Familial Canine Dermatomyositis. Alopecia and scarring typical of chronic lesions.

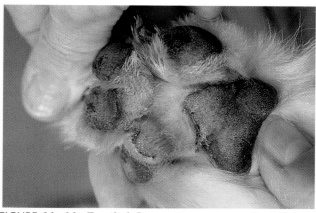

FIGURE 11–10. Familial Canine Dermatomyositis. Ulcerative lesions on the footpad of a Sheltland sheepdog. Note the similarity to autoimmune skin diseases. (Courtesy of M. Mahaffey)

Ehlers-Danlos Syndrome
(cutaneous asthenia, dermatosparaxis)
(Figs. 11–11 to 11–14)

FEATURES

A group of hereditary disorders in which defective collagen synthesis or fiber formation results in abnormal skin extensibility and fragility. Rare in dogs and cats.

Cutaneous signs are characterized by skin hyperextensibility and/or skin that is thin and fragile. Hyperextensible skin is loosely attached to the underlying tissues, can be stretched to extreme lengths, and may hang in folds, especially on the limbs and ventral aspect of the neck. Minimal trauma may create large tears with little to no bleeding that heal by scarring. Concurrent widening of the bridge of the nose, hygromas, joint laxity, corneal changes, lens luxation, and/or cataracts may be present.

TOP DIFFERENTIALS

None. This is a clinically distinct syndrome.

DIAGNOSIS

1. Usually based on history and clinical findings.
2. Skin extensibility index—Divide the maximum height that a dorsal lumbar skin fold can be stretched by the body length from the base of the tail to the occipital crest and convert into a percentage. Affected dogs and cats have values above 14.5% and 19%, respectively.
3. Dermatohistopathology (often nondiagnostic)— Dermal collagen may appear to be architecturally normal or may be fragmented, disoriented, and abnormally organized.
4. Electron microscopy (skin biopsy)—Abnormal structure and/or amount of collagen.

TREATMENT AND PROGNOSIS

1. No specific treatment is known.
2. Avoid trauma by keeping the affected animal indoors and away from other animals. Pad or remove objects with sharp or rough edges and surfaces. Leash-walk dogs in well-groomed areas.
3. Handle and restrain the animal carefully to avoid tearing the skin.
4. Declaw cats to prevent self-trauma from scratching.

5. Bedding and resting areas should be well padded to prevent hygromas.
6. Practice routine flea control, and promptly address and treat other skin conditions to prevent self-trauma from pruritus.
7. Surgically repair lacerations as they occur.
8. Prognosis is poor, especially for animals with joint laxity. Affected animals should not be bred.

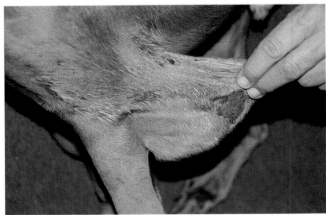

FIGURE 11–13. Ehlers-Danlos Syndrome. Close-up of the dog in Figures 11–11 and 11–12. The remarkable elasticity of the skin is demonstrated on the elbow.

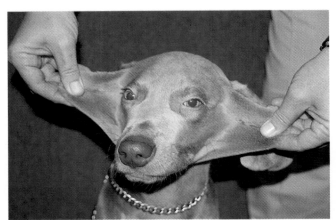

FIGURE 11–11. Ehlers-Danlos Syndrome. This 5-month-old weimaraner has the characteristic skin elasticity associated with this syndrome.

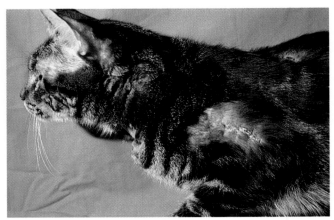

FIGURE 11–14. Ehlers-Danlos Syndrome. A healing laceration on the lateral shoulder of a cat. Wound prevention and management are the most significant clinical concerns for these patients. (Courtesy of J. MacDonald)

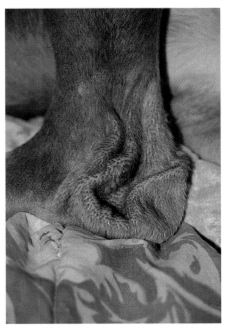

FIGURE 11–12. Ehlers-Danlos Syndrome. Close-up of the dog in Figure 11–11. The collagen defect caused the skin to loosen, producing these wrinkles.

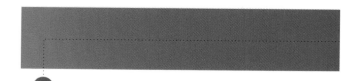

Cutaneous Mucinosis (Figs. 11–15 to 11–17)

FEATURES

An idiopathic condition characterized by an excessive accumulation or deposition of dermal mucin. Rare in dogs except for Chinese shar pei dogs.

Mild, moderate, or severe exaggeration of skin folds, especially on the head, ventrum, and distal extremities. Affected skin is puffy, thickened, and nonpitting. Clear vesicles and bullae that contain a viscous, sticky fluid (mucin) may be present. If the oropharynx is involved, upper respiratory stridor may be present.

TOP DIFFERENTIALS

For vesicular lesions—autoimmune and immune-mediated skin disorders.

DIAGNOSIS

1. Usually based on signalment, history, clinical findings, and ruling out other differentials.
2. Cytology (vesicle, bulla)—Amorphous, acellular, basophilic substance (mucin).
3. Dermatohistopathology—Excessive dermal mucin, with no other histologic abnormalities.

TREATMENT AND PROGNOSIS

1. Observation with no treatment is reasonable because the skin changes resolve spontaneously in most Chinese shar pei dogs by 2–5 years of age.
2. For severely affected dogs, treatment with prednisone 2 mg/kg PO q 24 hours for 7 days, followed by a gradual reduction in dosage over 30 days, may reduce mucin accumulation. Most dogs need only one course of treatment, but some may require repeated treatments or continuous low-dose maintenance therapy.
3. Prognosis is good. This is primarily a cosmetic problem which most dogs eventually outgrow. Dogs with oropharyngeal mucinosis are anesthetic risks and must be monitored carefully during anesthesia to prevent respiratory arrest.

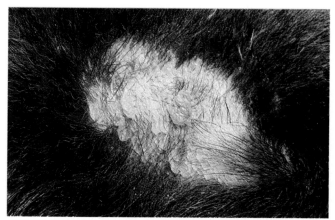

FIGURE 11–16. Cutaneous Mucinosis. Multiple mucin-filled vesicles on the neck of an adult shar pei.

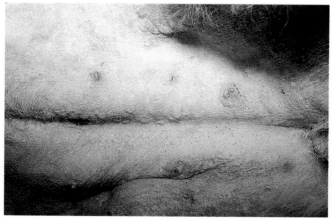

FIGURE 11–15. Cutaneous Mucinosis. Numerous vesicles filled with mucin on the abdomen of an adult shar pei.

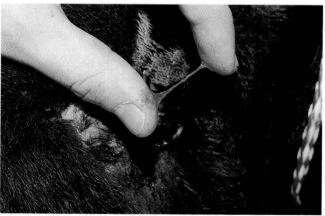

FIGURE 11–17. Cutaneous Mucinosis. Same dog as in Figure 11–16. The vesicle has been ruptured. Note the viscosity of the mucin.

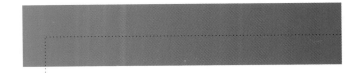

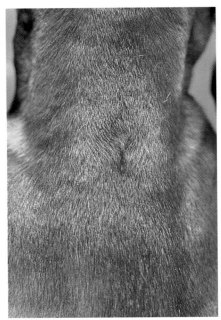

Dermoid Sinus (Figs. 11–18 and 11–19)

FEATURES

A defect in embryonic development that results in an incomplete separation between the skin and the neural tube. A sinus forms that may extend from the skin to the dura mater of the spinal cord or may end as a blind sac in the subcutaneous tissue. Rare in dogs, with the highest incidence in Rhodesian ridgebacks.

The sinus has single or multiple small openings that may have tufts of hair protruding from them. The sinus may be found anywhere along the dorsal midline but is most common over the cervical spine. A cord of tissue that extends from the cutaneous opening toward the spinal cord may be palpable. The sinus may contain sebum, keratin, debris, and hair. Sinuses may become inflamed, secondarily infected, cystic, and drain and, if they extend to the spinal cord, lead to bacterial meningoencephalitis.

FIGURE 11–18. Dermoid Sinus. The sinus on the back of a Rhodesian ridgeback appears as a small cutaneous defect.

TOP DIFFERENTIALS

Foreign body, deep infection (bacterial, fungal).

DIAGNOSIS

1. Usually based on signalment, history, and clinical findings.
2. Fistulogram—Delineates a tract extending from the skin toward the spine.

TREATMENT AND PROGNOSIS

1. For quiescent sinuses, observation without treatment is acceptable.
2. For draining or cystic tracts, surgical removal of the sinus is the treatment of choice.
3. Give appropriate treatment for bacterial meningoencephalitis, if present.
4. Prognosis is good. Affected dogs should not be bred.

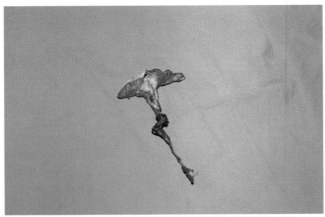

FIGURE 11–19. Dermoid Sinus. The sinus has been surgically removed from the dog in Figure 11–18. The deep extension of the lesion is apparent.

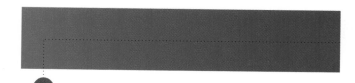

Familial Footpad Hyperkeratosis (Figs. 11–20 and 11–21)

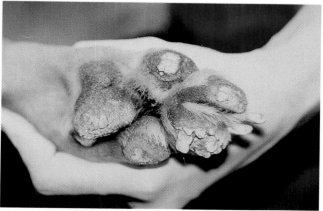

FIGURE 11–20. Familial Footpad Hyperkeratosis. Severe hyperkeratosis and crusting of the pads is characteristic of this disorder. (Courtesy of M. Paradis; Paradis M: Footpad hyperkeratosis in a family of Dogues de Bordeaux. Vet Dermatol. 3: 75, 1992. Blackwell Science Ltd.)

FEATURES

A familial disorder that results in severe digital hyperkeratosis by 6 months of age. Rare in dogs, with the highest incidence in Irish terriers and Dogue de Bordeaux dogs.

There is marked hyperkeratosis and horn formation that involves the entire surface of all the footpads. Fissures and secondary bacterial infection may result in lameness. There is no other skin involvement.

TOP DIFFERENTIALS

Distemper, zinc-responsive dermatosis, pemphigus foliaceus, systemic or discoid lupus erythematosus.

DIAGNOSIS

1. Rule out other differentials.
2. Dermatohistopathology—Marked orthokeratotic hyperkeratosis with mild to severe epidermal hyperplasia.

TREATMENT AND PROGNOSIS

1. No specific treatment is known.
2. Symptomatically treat with daily foot soaks in 50% propylene glycol. Significant improvement should be seen within 5 days, but lifelong maintenance therapy is required for control.
3. Give appropriate systemic antibiotics for 3–4 weeks if footpads are secondarily infected.
4. Prognosis for cure is poor, but most dogs enjoy a good quality of life with routine symptomatic therapy. Affected dogs should not be bred.

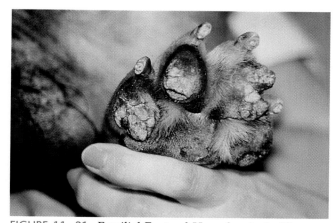

FIGURE 11–21. Familial Footpad Hyperkeratosis. The severe hyperkeratosis has resulted in footpad disfigurement. (Courtesy of M. Paradis; Paradis M: Footpad hyperkeratosis in a family of Dogues de Bordeaux. Vet Dermatol. 3: 75, 1992. Blackwell Science Ltd.)

Suggested Readings

Congenital and Hereditary Defects, pp. 755, 756–764, 785–790, 800–801. In Scott DW, Miller WH Jr, and Griffin CE. 1995. Muller & Kirk's Small Animal Dermatology. Ed. 5. W.B. Saunders, Philadelphia, PA.

Fatone G, Brunetti A, Lamagna F, and Potena A. 1995. Dermoid Sinus and Spinal Malformations in a Yorkshire Terrier: Diagnosis and Follow-up. JSAP. 36: 178–180.

Hargis A and Mundell A. 1992. Familial Canine Dermatomyositis. Compend Cont Edu Pract Vet. 14(7): 855–863.

Knottenbelt C and Knottenbelt M. 1996. Black Hair Follicular Dysplasia in a Tricolor Jack Russell Terrier. Vet Rec. 138: 475–476.

Penrith M and van Schouwenburg S. 1994. Dermoid Sinus in a Boerboel Bitch. Tydskr S Afr vet Ver. 65(2): 38–39.

Plumb DC. 1999. Veterinary Drug Handbook. Ed. 3. Iowa State University Press, Ames, IA.

Schoning P and Cowan L. 2000. Bald Thigh Syndrome of Greyhound Dogs: Gross and Microscopic Findings. Vet Derm. 11: 49–51.

Wallin-Hakanson B and Wallin-Hakanson N. 2000. Palmoplantar Hyperkeratosis in Irish Terriers: Evidence of Autosomal Recessive Inheritance. JSAP. 41: 52–55.

12

Pigmentary Abnormalities

- **Lentigo**
- **Postinflammatory Hyperpigmentation**
- **Nasal Depigmentation** (Dudley nose, Snow nose)
- **Vitiligo**

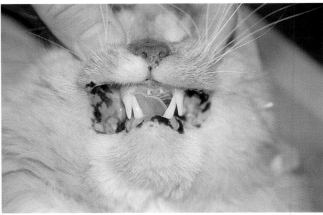

FIGURE 12–1. Lentigo. Multiple pigmented macules on the lip of a young adult cat.

Lentigo (Figs. 12–1 and 12–2)

FEATURES

An asymptomatic condition characterized by one (lentigo) or more (lentigines) flat macule(s) or patch(es) of black skin. Common in dogs, with the highest incidence in middle-aged to older dogs. Uncommon in cats, with the highest incidence in young orange cats.

Dogs. One or more macular to patchy areas of hyperpigmented skin. Lesions are most commonly found on the ventral abdomen and chest.

Cats. Multiple 1–10 mm diameter black macules that may coalesce on lips, gingiva, and/or eyelids.

TOP DIFFERENTIAL

Melanoma.

DIAGNOSIS

1. Usually based on history and clinical findings.
2. Dermatohistopathology—Epidermal hyperplasia, hyperpigmentation, and increased numbers of melanocytes.

TREATMENT AND PROGNOSIS

1. No medical treatment is known.
2. Cosmetically unacceptable lesions can be surgically excised.
3. Prognosis is good. Lentigines are benign skin changes.

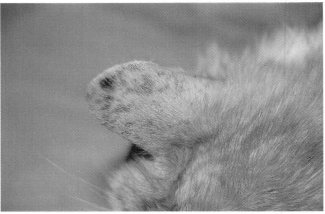

FIGURE 12–2. Lentigo. Multiple pigmented macules on the ear pinnae of a young adult cat.

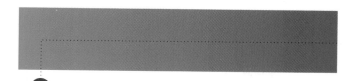

Postinflammatory Hyperpigmentation (Figs. 12–3 to 12–6)

FEATURES

Skin (melanoderma) and/or hairs (melanotrichia) become hyperpigmented as a sequela to an underlying skin disease such as pyoderma, demodicosis, dermatophytosis, or hypersensitivity. The hyperpigmentation may be focal and circumscribed, patchy, or diffuse. Common in dogs. Uncommon in cats.

DIAGNOSIS

1. Usually based on history, clinical findings, and identification of an underlying disease.

TREATMENT AND PROGNOSIS

1. Identify and treat the underlying cause.
2. Prognosis is good. Melanoderma usually resolves slowly after the underlying cause is treated. Melanotrichia usually resolves at the next shedding cycle.

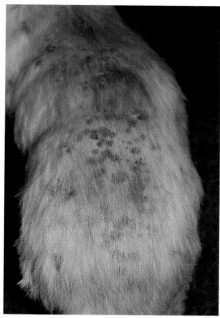

FIGURE 12–5. Postinflammatory Hyperpigmentation. Multiple pigmented macules on the dorsal lumbar region of a flea-allergic dog.

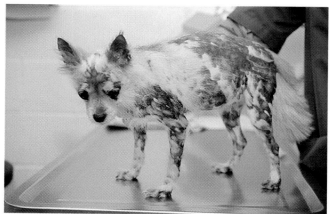

FIGURE 12–3. Postinflammatory Hyperpigmentation. Generalized hyperpigmentation associated with resolving erythema multiforme.

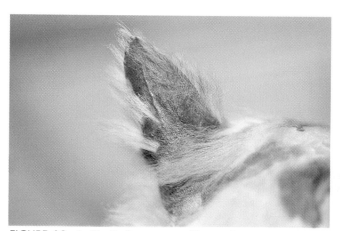

FIGURE 12–4. Postinflammatory Hyperpigmentation. Close-up of the dog in Figure 12–3. The pigmented macules on the ear pinnae occurred after the initial lesions healed.

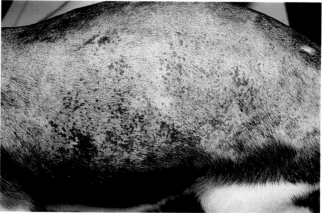

FIGURE 12–6. Postinflammatory Hyperpigmentation. Multiple pigmented macules on the lateral flank of a dog. The initial papular dermatitis was caused by contact dermatitis.

Nasal Depigmentation (Dudley nose, Snow nose) (Figs. 12–7 and 12–8)

FEATURES

An idiopathic disorder in which affected dogs are born with pigmented noses which later in life lighten to a light brown or whitish color. The nasal depigmentation may wax and wane, be seasonal, resolve spontaneously, or be a permanent change. Only the nose is affected. Common in dogs, with the highest incidence in golden retrievers, yellow Labrador retrievers, Siberian huskies, and Alaskan malamutes.

TOP DIFFERENTIALS

Vitiligo, nasal solar dermatitis, discoid lupus erythematosus, pemphigus erythematosus.

DIAGNOSIS

1. Usually based on history and clinical findings.
2. Dermatohistopathology—Marked reduction of epidermal melanocytes and melanin.

TREATMENT AND PROGNOSIS

1. No treatment is known.
2. Prognosis is good, as this is a cosmetic problem only. However, it is considered a defect in show dogs.

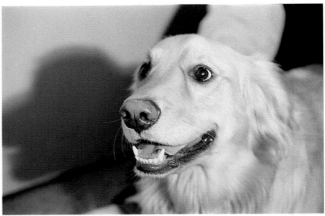

FIGURE 12–7. Nasal Depigmentation. Nasal depigmentation in a golden retriever.

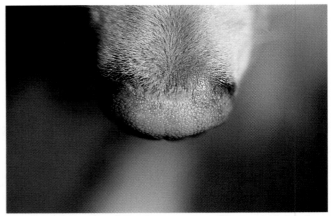

FIGURE 12–8. Nasal Depigmentation. Close-up of the dog in Figure 12–7. Seasonal depigmentation on the nose of a golden retriever. The nose repigmented completely during the spring and summer.

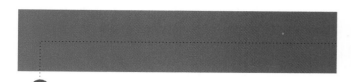

Vitiligo (Figs. 12–9 and 12–12)

FEATURES

An asymptomatic condition characterized by one or more macular areas of depigmented skin (leukoderma) and/or depigmented hair (leukotrichia). Uncommon in dogs, with the highest incidence in Belgian Tervurens, German shepherds, rottweilers, and Doberman pinschers. Rare in cats, with the highest incidence in Siamese cats. Lesions are usually first noted in young adulthood and often affect the nose, lips, face, buccal mucosa, and/or footpads.

TOP DIFFERENTIALS

Uveodermatologic syndrome, nasal depigmentation, autoimmune skin diseases.

DIAGNOSIS

1. Dermatohistopathology—Essentially normal skin except that no melanocytes are seen.

TREATMENT AND PROGNOSIS

1. No treatment is known.
2. Prognosis is good. This is a cosmetic disease that does not affect the animal's quality of life. The depigmentation is usually permanent, but in some animals spontaneous repigmentation may eventually occur.

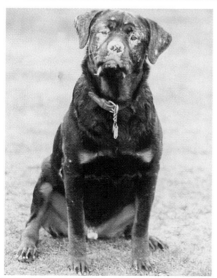

FIGURE 12–9. Vitiligo. Multiple areas of macular depigmentation affecting an adult rottweiler. (Courtesy of D. Angarano)

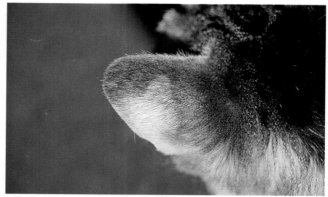

FIGURE 12–10. Vitiligo. Well-demarcated depigmentation on the ear pinnae of a cat.

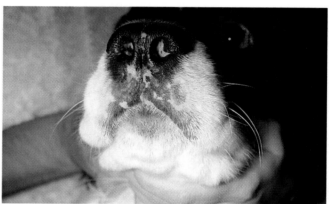

FIGURE 12–11. Vitiligo. Macular depigmentation on the muzzle of a mixed-breed dog. (Courtesy of D. Angarano)

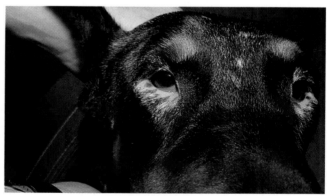

FIGURE 12–12. Vitiligo. Depigmentation around the eye of an adult Doberman pinscher.

Suggested Readings

Pigmentary Abnormalities, pp. 806–823. In Scott DW, Miller WH Jr, and Griffin CE. 1995. Muller & Kirk's Small Animal Dermatology. Ed. 5. W.B. Saunders, Philadelphia, PA.

13

Keratinization and Seborrheic Disorders

- **Canine Primary Seborrhea**

- **Vitamin A-Responsive Dermatosis**

- **Ichthyosis**

- **Epidermal Dysplasia of West Highland White Terriers**

- **Sebaceous Adenitis**

- **Zinc-Responsive Dermatosis**

- **Superficial Necrolytic Migratory Erythema** (hepatocutaneous syndrome, superficial necrolytic dermatitis)

- **Schnauzer Comedo Syndrome**

- **Canine Ear Margin Dermatosis**

- **Idiopathic Nasodigital Hyperkeratosis**

- **Tail Gland Hyperplasia** (stud tail)

- **Feline Acne**

- **Facial Dermatitis of Persian Cats**

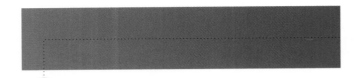

Canine Primary Seborrhea
(Figs. 13–1 to 13–8)

FEATURES

A hereditary disorder of keratinization. Common in dogs, with the highest incidence in American cocker spaniels, English springer spaniels, West Highland white terriers, and basset hounds. Clinical symptoms initially appear during puppyhood and may be mild at first but worsen with age.

Clinical signs include dull, dry, lusterless haircoat, excessive scaling (dandruff), follicular casts, scaly and crusty seborrheic patches and plaques, and/or greasy, malodorous skin. Most of the body is involved to some degree, with interdigital areas, perineum, face, axillae, ventral neck, abdomen, and skin folds usually the most severely affected. Pruritus is mild to intense, and ceruminous otitis externa is common. Secondary skin and ear infections with bacteria and *Malassezia* are often present.

TOP DIFFERENTIALS

Ichthyosis, epidermal dysplasia, vitamin A-responsive dermatosis, sebaceous adenitis, and causes of secondary seborrhea (Table 13–1).

DIAGNOSIS

1. Based on early age of onset and ruling out other causes of seborrhea.
2. Dermatohistopathology (nonspecific)—Hyperplastic, superficial, perivascular dermatitis with orthokeratotic and/or parakeratotic hyperkeratosis, follicular keratosis, and variable dyskeratosis. Bacteria and yeast may be seen within surface and follicular keratin. Secondary bacterial folliculitis and dermatitis are common.

TREATMENT AND PROGNOSIS

1. Ensure good nutrition. Feed a commercially balanced dog food that meets Association of American Feed Control Officials (AAFCO) requirements.
2. Treat any secondary bacterial and *Malassezia* skin and ear infections with appropriate topical and systemic therapies. Periodic retreatments or long-term, low-dose maintenance therapy may be needed because these dogs are susceptible to recurring infections.
3. For symptomatic control of ceruminous otitis, long-term maintenance ear care is necessary. Institute once or twice weekly ear cleaning and instill a topical otic preparation containing an astringent and/or steroid AU q 1–7 days to control cerumen accumulation.
4. For symptomatic control of seborrhea, use antiseborrheic shampoos and emollients q 2–7 days until skin condition is improved (approximately 2–3 weeks), then decrease bathing frequency to q 1–2 weeks or as needed for maintenance (Table 13–2).
5. Daily fatty acid supplementation may be helpful as an adjunctive therapy.
6. For dogs with severe greasy, malodorous, pruritic seborrhea, treatment with systemic corticosteroids may be helpful. Give prednisone 1–2 mg/kg PO q 24 hours, until symptoms are controlled (approximately 2 weeks), then taper to the lowest possible alternate-day dosage if maintenance therapy is needed. However, unacceptable steroid side effects and recurrent skin and ear infections are potential sequelae if long-term steroid therapy is used.

TABLE 13–1 Causes of Secondary Seborrhea

Infection	Pyoderma
	Dermatophytosis
	Malassezia dermatitis
Allergic	Flea allergy dermatitis
	Atopy
	Food hypersensitivity
	Contact dermatitis
Endocrine	Hypothyroidism
	Hyperadrenocorticism
	Sex hormone imbalance
	Diabetes mellitus
Parasitic	Demodicosis
	Scabies
	Cheyletiellosis
	Pediculosis
	Otodectes spp.
Nutritional	Vitamin A-responsive dermatosis
	Zinc-responsive dermatosis
	Dietary imbalance
Immune-mediated	Pemphigus foliaceous
	Pemphigus erythematosus
	Systemic lupus erythematosus
	Cutaneous drug reaction
	Sebaceous adenitis
Metabolic	Malabsorption/maldigestion
	Superficial necrolytic migratory erythema
Neoplasia	Cutaneous epitheliotropic lymphoma

TABLE 13–2 Antiseborrheic Shampoo Therapy

Ingredient	Therapeutic Effect	Usage	Disadvantages
Benzoyl peroxide	Antibacterial Follicular flushing Degreasing Keratolytic	A potent degreasing, follicular flushing topical ingredient with excellent antibacterial effects. Mildly antiseborrheic. Good for crusting and oily seborrheic disorders.	Drying Skin irritation May bleach fabrics
Ethyl lactate	Antibacterial Decreases skin pH Degreasing Comedolytic	A mild degreasing, antiseborrheic shampoo with good antibacterial activity. Good for dry, scaling seborrhea.	
Sulfur/salicylic acid	Keratolytic Keratoplastic	A moderately well-tolerated shampoo with good antiseborrheic activity. Good for crusting or dry, seborrheic disorders.	
Tar	Keratolytic Keratoplastic Degreasing Antipruritic Vasoactive	A potent degreasing and antiseborrheic shampoo. Good for severe oily, seborrheic disorders.	Toxic to cats Drying Skin irritation Staining Photosensitization Superficial migratory necrolytic dermatitis
Selenium sulfide	Keratolytic Keratoplastic Degreasing	A potent degreasing shampoo with good antiseborrheic activity. Good for oily seborrheic disorders. Moderate activity against yeast.	Drying Skin irritation

7. Retinoids may be helpful in some dogs. Etretinate, 1 mg/kg PO q 24 hours, has been used successfully but is no longer available. A newer retinoid, Acitretin, may also be effective (0.5–1 mg/kg PO q 24 hours).

8. Calcitriol (vitamin D), 10 mg/kg/day PO, may be helpful in some cases. Serum calcium levels should be closely monitored.

9. Prognosis is variable, depending on the severity of the seborrhea. This is an incurable condition that requires lifelong therapy to control. Do not breed affected dogs.

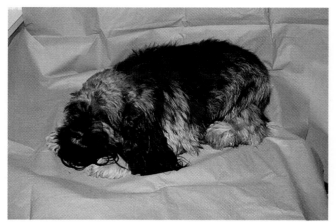

FIGURE 13–1. Canine Primary Seborrhea. Greasy, poor-quality fur coat in a 4-year-old female spayed cocker spaniel. (Courtesy of A. Yu)

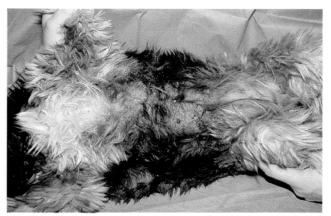

FIGURE 13–2. Canine Primary Seborrhea. Close-up of the dog in Figure 13–1. Partial alopecia and seborrheic dermatitis on the ventral abdomen. (Courtesy of A. Yu)

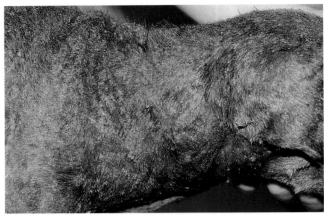

FIGURE 13–3. Canine Primary Seborrhea. Close-up of the dog in Figures 13–1 and 13–2. The fur coat has been clipped, revealing the generalized seborrhea, scales, crusts, and erythema. (Courtesy of A. Yu)

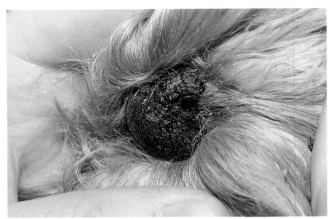

FIGURE 13–6. Canine Primary Seborrhea. Close-up of the dog in Figures 13–1 to 13–5. Hyperkeratosis of the footpad. (Courtesy of A. Yu)

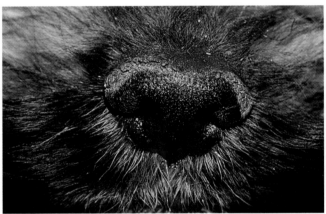

FIGURE 13–4. Canine Primary Seborrhea. Close-up of the dog in Figures 13–1 to 13–3. The crusting around the nose is characteristic of this disease. (Courtesy of A. Yu)

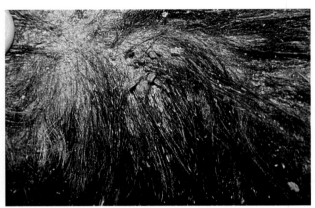

FIGURE 13–7. Canine Primary Seborrhea. Alopecia, erythema, scale, and crusts are typical of this disease. The lesions may be focal or generalized. (Courtesy of A. Yu)

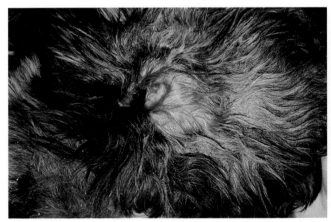

FIGURE 13–5. Canine Primary Seborrhea. Close-up of the dog in Figures 13–1 to 13–4. Inflammation of the ear pinnae and canal with a secondary otitis externa. The hair on the ear pinnae was clumping from the abnormal oily secretions. (Courtesy of A. Yu)

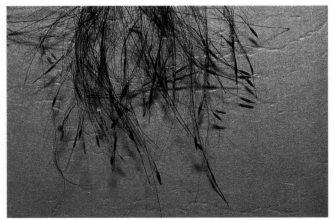

FIGURE 13–8. Canine Primary Seborrhea. The follicular casts are apparent after the hair is epilated. Follicular casts are characteristic findings in several primary keratinization disorders.

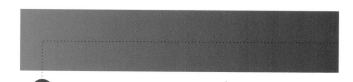

Vitamin A-Responsive Dermatosis (Figs. 13–9 to 13–12)

FEATURES

An incompletely understood disorder of keratinization that responds to treatment with high doses of vitamin A. Rare in dogs, with the highest incidence in young (2- to 3-year-old) American cocker spaniels.

There is marked follicular plugging, focal areas of crusting, and hyperkeratotic plaques that have keratinaceous frond-like plugs. Lesions are most commonly found on the ventral and lateral aspects of the chest and abdomen. Mild to moderate pruritus, a dull, dry haircoat that epilates easily, a rancid body odor, and generalized scaling may be present. Concurrent ceruminous otitis externa is common.

TOP DIFFERENTIALS

Primary seborrhea, sebaceous adenitis, zinc-responsive dermatosis, and causes of secondary seborrhea (Table 13–1).

DIAGNOSIS

1. Rule out other differentials.
2. Dermatohistopathology—Marked, disproportionate follicular orthokeratotic hyperkeratosis with minimal epidermal hyperkeratosis.

TREATMENT AND PROGNOSIS

1. Give vitamin A, 10,000 IU PO with a fatty meal q 24 hours. Improvement should be seen within 4–6 weeks and complete clinical remission within 8–10 weeks.
2. For symptomatic control of seborrhea, use antiseborrheic shampoos and emollients q 2–7 days until skin condition is improved (approximately 2–3 weeks), then decrease bathing frequency to q 1–2 weeks or as needed for maintenance (Table 13–2).
3. Prognosis is good, but lifelong vitamin A therapy is usually necessary to maintain remission.

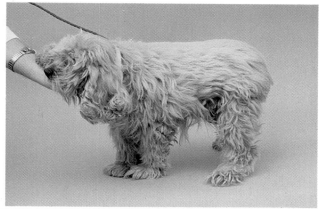

FIGURE 13–9. Vitamin A-Responsive Dermatosis. Greasy, poor-quality fur coat in an adult cocker spaniel. Note the similarity to canine primary seborrhea. (Courtesy of A. Yu)

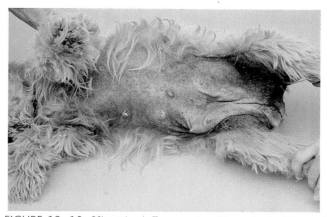

FIGURE 13–10. Vitamin A-Responsive Dermatosis. Close-up of the dog in Figure 13–9. Alopecia and seborrheic dermatitis on the ventral abdomen. The papular dermatitis was caused by a secondary superficial pyoderma. (Courtesy of A. Yu)

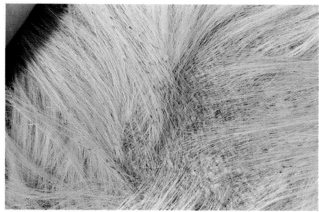

FIGURE 13–11. Vitamin A-Responsive Dermatosis. Close-up of the dog in Figures 13–9 and 13–10. Scale and follicular casts. These skin lesions were generalized. (Courtesy of A. Yu)

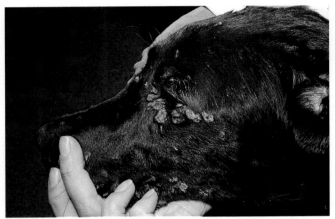

FIGURE 13–12. Vitamin A-Responsive Dermatosis. Focal seborrheic plaques on the face of a Labrador.

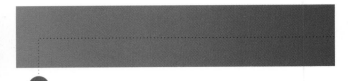

Ichthyosis (Figs. 13–13 and 13–14)

FEATURES

A congenital keratinization disorder. Rare in dogs, with West Highland white terriers possibly predisposed. Dogs are abnormal at birth, and one or more puppies in the litter may be affected.

Most of the body is covered with tightly adhering scales which may flake off in large sheets or accumulate as seborrheic debris on the surface of the skin. The skin may be erythematous and alopecic. Marked hyperkeratosis of the nasal planum and footpads, especially at the margins of the pads, is typical. The feet may be swollen and painful.

TOP DIFFERENTIALS

Primary seborrhea, epidermal dysplasia.

DIAGNOSIS

1. Dermatohistopathology—Marked orthokeratotic hyperkeratosis, hypergranulosis, and numerous mitotic figures in keratinocytes are usually seen. Follicular keratosis and plugging are common. Reticular degeneration may be seen.

TREATMENT AND PROGNOSIS

1. No specific treatment is known.
2. Therapeutic trials with isotretinoin (1–2 mg/kg PO q 12 hours) have not been effective.
3. For symptomatic treatment, frequent bathing with salicylic acid and sulfur-containing shampoos followed by emollient rinses or sprays may be helpful in some cases.
4. Prognosis is poor. This is a chronic and incurable disease that is difficult to manage symptomatically. Affected dogs should not be bred.

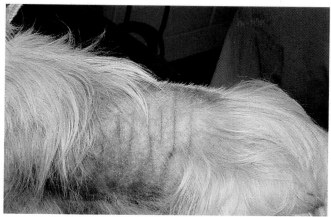

FIGURE 13–13. Ichthyosis. Alopecia, erythema, and scaling in a female spayed West Highland white terrier.

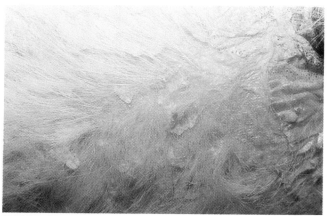

FIGURE 13–14. Ichthyosis. Alopecia and large, tightly adherent scales are typical. (Courtesy of K. Credille and R. Dunstan)

Epidermal Dysplasia of West Highland White Terriers (Figs. 13–15 to 13–18)

FEATURES

An uncommon inherited disorder of keratinization in West Highland white terriers. Clinical signs usually appear when the dog is between 6 and 12 months of age. Secondary *Malassezia* dermatitis is a complicating factor in this disease.

The development of a greasy haircoat is followed by mild to moderate pruritus of the face, ears, limbs, feet, and ventrum. With chronicity the pruritus becomes intense, and widespread areas of erythema, alopecia, crusting, lichenification, and hyperpigmentation develop.

TOP DIFFERENTIALS

Primary seborrhea, ichthyosis, causes of secondary seborrhea (Table 13–1).

DIAGNOSIS

1. Rule out other differentials.
2. Cytology (skin imprints)—Yeast organisms are seen. Bacterial cocci may also be present.
3. Dermatohistopathology—Epidermal hyperplasia and dysplasia (frequent keratinocytic mitotic figures, crowding of epidermal basal cells, and loss of polarity). Parakeratotic hyperkeratosis, follicular hyperkeratosis, and surface yeasts are usually seen.

TREATMENT AND PROGNOSIS

1. There is no specific treatment.
2. Treat any secondary pyoderma with appropriate systemic antibiotics for at least 3–4 weeks.
3. Treat secondary *Malassezia* infection for 30–45 days with ketoconazole, 10 mg/kg PO with food q 12–24 hours; itraconazole, 10 mg/kg PO with food q 24 hours; or enilconazole, 0.2% solution applied topically q 3–4 days. After the *Malassezia* infection is resolved, continue the ketoconazole (10 mg/kg PO q 48 hours) or 0.2% enilconazole solution (applied periodically as needed) to prevent yeast reinfections. Treatment with other topical antifungal therapies may also be beneficial.

4. Treatment with prednisone, 1 mg/kg PO q 12–24 hours, until skin is improved, then tapered to the lowest possible alternate-day dosage for long-term maintenance, may control symptoms in some dogs if the steroid therapy is begun early in the course of the disease.

5. Alternatively, anecdotal reports suggest that cyclosporin A administration may be helpful in some dogs. Give cyclosporin A (Neoral), 5 mg/kg PO q 24 hours for 6 weeks, then slowly taper to the lowest dose/frequency that controls clinical signs.

6. Topical antiseborrheic therapy may be somewhat beneficial (Table 13–2).

7. Prognosis is poor. This condition is incurable and often minimally controllable. Do not breed affected dogs.

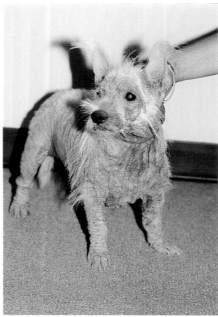

FIGURE 13–15. Epidermal Dysplasia of West Highland White Terriers. Generalized alopecia, lichenification, and hyperpigmentation are characteristic of this disorder. Secondary *Malassezia* dermatitis worsens the lichenification.

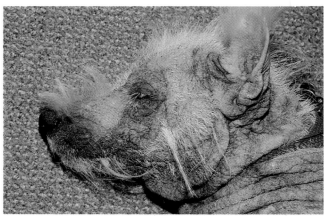

FIGURE 13–17. Epidermal Dysplasia of West Highland White Terriers. Close-up of the dog in Figures 13–15 and 13–16. Generalized alopecia, lichenification, and hyperpigmentation affecting the face. Secondary *Malassezia* and bacterial infections worsen the pruritus, alopecia, and lichenification.

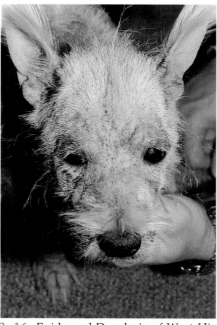

FIGURE 13–16. Epidermal Dysplasia of West Highland White Terriers. Close-up of the dog in Figure 13–15. Alopecia, lichenification, and hyperpigmentation affecting the face. The crusting papular dermatitis was caused by a secondary superficial pyoderma.

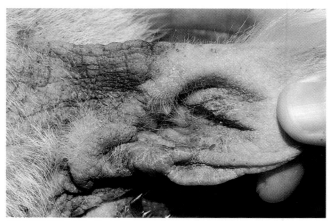

FIGURE 13–18. Epidermal Dysplasia of West Highland White Terriers. Close-up of the dog in Figures 13–15 to 13–17. Alopecia, lichenification, and hyperpigmentation on the ear.

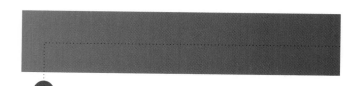

Sebaceous Adenitis (Figs. 13–19 to 13–24)

FEATURES

A poorly understood, destructive, inflammatory disease of sebaceous glands. Genetic factors may be involved. Uncommon in dogs, with the highest incidence in young to middle-aged standard poodles, Hungarian vizslas, Akitas, and Samoyeds.

There is mild to severe scaling that most often involves the dorsum of the back and neck, top of the head, face, and ear pinnae. In short-coated dogs, the scales are usually fine and nonadherent. In longer-coated dogs, the scales adhere tightly to the hairs. The haircoat may be dull, dry, and/or matted, and follicular casts may be present. Patchy to diffuse alopecia is common. Pruritus is not usually seen unless there is a secondary bacterial or *Malassezia* infection. Subclinical disease (histologic lesions without clinical symptoms) has also been documented in standard poodles.

TOP DIFFERENTIALS

Primary seborrhea, causes of secondary seborrhea (Table 13–1).

DIAGNOSIS

1. Rule out other differentials.
2. Dermatohistopathology (from dorsum of neck in suspected subclinical cases)—In early lesions there are discrete granulomas in areas where sebaceous glands should be, with no involvement of other adnexa. In chronic lesions, the sebaceous glands are absent and are replaced by fibrosis. Follicular plugging and hyperkeratosis may also be seen.

TREATMENT AND PROGNOSIS

1. Treat any secondary bacterial or *Malassezia* skin infections with appropriate systemic medications.
2. For mild cases, daily essential fatty acid supplementation and topical therapy with antiseborrheic shampoos, emollient rinses, and humectants q 2–4 days or as needed may effectively control symptoms.
3. For more severe cases, daily treatments with high doses of fatty acids and topical spray applications of 50–75% propylene glycol in water may be helpful.

4. Systemic therapy may be effective in preventing further sebaceous gland destruction in some dogs. Drugs that have been used with variable results include:

   Prednisone, 2 mg/kg PO q 24 hours until lesions controlled, then tapered to the lowest possible alternate-day dosage that controls signs.

   Isotretinoin, 1 mg/kg PO q 24 hours.

   Etretinate, 1–2 mg/kg PO q 24 hours (no longer available, but a newer retinoid, Acitretin, may also be effective at a dose of 0.5–1 mg/kg PO q 24 hours).

   Cyclosporin (Neoral), 5 mg/kg PO q 12 hours.

   Asparaginase, 10,000 IU IM q 7 days for two or three treatments, then as needed.

   Vitamin A, 10,000 IU PO q 24 hours plus tetracycline and niacinamide (as described in Table 7–2).

5. Prognosis is variable, depending on disease severity. This is an incurable disease, but early diagnosis and treatment improve the prognosis for long-term control. Short-coated dogs, which tend to have milder symptoms, may have a more favorable prognosis than longer-coated dogs. Standard poodles and Akitas have the greatest tendency to develop progressive, refractory disease. Affected dogs should not be bred.

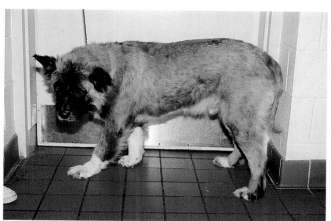

FIGURE 13–19. Sebaceous Adenitis. Generalized scaling with adherent crusts on an adult Akita.

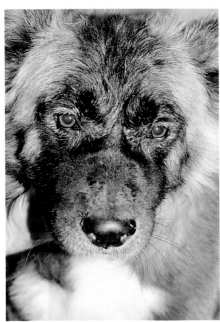

FIGURE 13-20. Sebaceous Adenitis. Close-up of the dog in Figure 13-19. The crusts on the bridge of the nose and the clumping of the fur on the face are apparent.

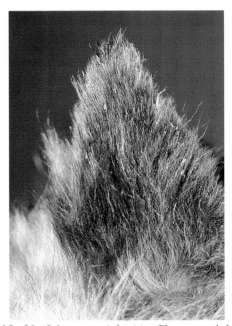

FIGURE 13-21. Sebaceous Adenitis. Close-up of the dog in Figures 13-19 and 13-20. The poor-quality hair coat with adherent scale and crusts on the ear pinnae is typical of this disease.

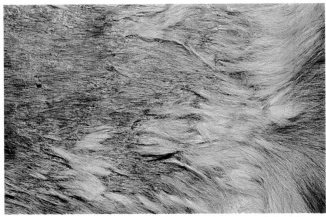

FIGURE 13-22. Sebaceous Adenitis. Close-up of the dog in Figures 13-19 to 13-21. Scales and adherent crusts on the trunk. The hair forms clumps, which are easily epilated.

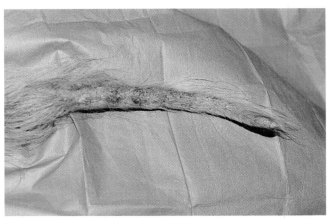

FIGURE 13-23. Sebaceous Adenitis. Close-up of the dog in Figures 13-19 to 13-22. Alopecia and crusting of the distal tail.

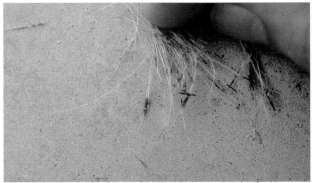

FIGURE 13-24. Sebaceous Adenitis. When the hair is epilated, the follicular casts are apparent. Follicular casts are characteristic of several primary keratinization disorders.

Zinc-Responsive Dermatosis

(Figs. 13–25 to 13–28)

FEATURES

A zinc deficiency-induced disorder of keratinization. An inherent diminished ability to absorb zinc from the intestinal tract, a zinc-deficient diet, or interference with zinc absorption from excessive calcium supplementation or from phytates in cereal-based diets can cause zinc deficiency. Rare in dogs, with the highest incidence in young adult Siberian huskies and Alaskan malamutes and in young, rapidly growing puppies of any breed.

Hyperkeratotic or thick, crusty plaques usually develop on the elbows, stifles, and other pressure points and at sites of trauma. The footpads may be hyperkeratotic and fissured. In some dogs, erythema, alopecia, crusting, and scaling develop around the mouth and eyes, as well as on the chin, ears, and genitalia. Secondary bacterial and *Malassezia* skin infections are common. Concurrent depression, anorexia, lymphadenomegaly, and pitting edema of the distal extremities may be seen. Severely affected puppies may have stunted growth.

TOP DIFFERENTIALS

Primary seborrhea, other causes of secondary seborrhea (Table 13–1).

DIAGNOSIS

1. Rule out other differentials.
2. Dermatohistopathology—Marked, diffuse epidermal and follicular parakeratosis and superficial perivascular dermatitis. Papillomatosis, spongiosus, and evidence of secondary infection (intraepidermal pustules, folliculitis) are common.

TREATMENT AND PROGNOSIS

1. Treat any secondary bacterial or *Malassezia* skin infection with appropriate medical therapy for at least 3–4 weeks.
2. For dogs with dietary-induced zinc deficiency, identify and correct the dietary imbalance. Discontinue any mineral and vitamin supplements. Feed only AAFCO-approved dog foods. Skin lesions should resolve within 2–6 weeks of the diet change.
3. Zinc supplementation may be needed in some dogs, either initially for the first few weeks of the diet change or lifelong if there is diminished ability to absorb zinc. Give zinc methionine, 1.7 mg/kg/day PO with food. Signs of zinc toxicosis include depression, anorexia, vomiting, and diarrhea.
4. Concurrent symptomatic therapy with warm water soaks, antiseborrheic shampoo baths, and topical applications of petrolatum or ointments on the lesions may be helpful.
5. Prognosis is good for most dogs, although lifelong zinc supplementation is sometimes needed. In rare cases, zinc supplementation is not effective.

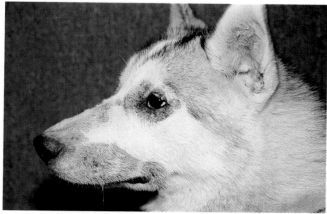

FIGURE 13–25. Zinc-Responsive Dermatosis. Alopecia and hyperkeratotic plaques on the face of a young adult Siberian husky.

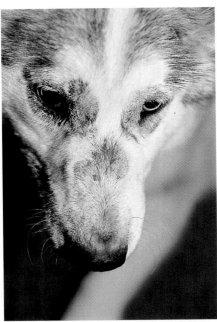

FIGURE 13–26. Zinc-Responsive Dermatosis. Close-up of the dog in Figure 13–25. The alopecia and crusting around the nose and eyes resolved with zinc supplementation.

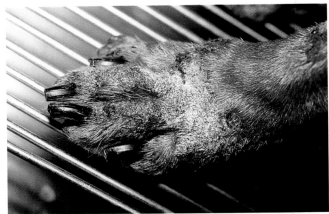

FIGURE 13–28. Zinc-Responsive Dermatosis. Alopecia with scale and crust formation of the foot of a dog with dietary zinc deficiency.

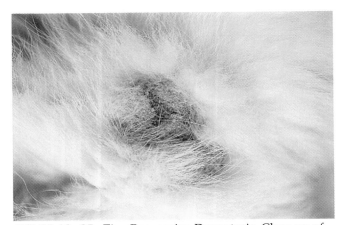

FIGURE 13–27. Zinc-Responsive Dermatosis. Close-up of the dog in Figures 13–25 and 13–26. An alopecic, seborrheic plaque on the abdomen.

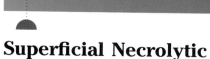

Superficial Necrolytic Migratory Erythema

(hepatocutaneous syndrome, superficial necrolytic dermatitis)

(Figs. 13–29 to 13–32)

FEATURES

A unique skin disease in animals that have chronic liver disease or glucagon-secreting pancreatic tumors. Its exact pathogenesis is unknown, but skin lesions may reflect a nutritional deficiency or imbalance. Uncommon in dogs and rare in cats, with the highest incidence in older animals.

Skin lesions are characterized by minimally to intensely pruritic erythema, scaling, crusting, and erosions on the distal limbs and around the mouth and eyes. Lesions may also involve the ear pinnae, elbows, hocks, external genitalia, ventrum, and oral cavity. The footpads are usually mildly to markedly hyperkeratotic. Systemic signs of the underlying metabolic disease are rarely evident at initial presentation but usually become apparent a few to several months later.

TOP DIFFERENTIALS

Demodicosis, dermatophytosis, pyoderma, pemphigus foliaceus, systemic lupus erythematosus, zinc-responsive dermatosis, drug eruption, cutaneous epitheliotrophic lymphoma.

DIAGNOSIS

1. Hemogram—neutrophilia and/or normocytic, normochromic, nonregenerative anemia may be present.
2. Serum biochemistry panel—Findings usually include mild to moderate increases in serum alkaline phosphatase (ALP) and alanine aminotransferase (ALT) activities, total bilirubin, and bile acids. Hypoalbuminemia and decreased blood urea nitrogen (BUN) are also common. Hyperglycemia may be present.
3. Ultrasonography—Evidence of chronic hepatitis, cirrhosis, or pancreatic tumor.
4. Histopathology (liver biopsy)—Chronic hepatitis or cirrhosis.
5. Dermatohistopathology—Early lesions show the characteristic findings of diffuse parakeratotic hyperkeratosis overlying an upper-level band of epidermal edema and a lower-level band of epidermal hyperplasia. Mild, superficial perivascular dermatitis with evidence of secondary bacterial, dermatophyte, or yeast infection may be present. Chronic lesions usually have nonspecific changes that are rarely diagnostic.

TREATMENT AND PROGNOSIS

1. Treat any secondary bacterial, dermatophyte, or yeast infection with appropriate antimicrobial therapies.
2. If the underlying cause is a resectable glucagonoma, surgical excision of the tumor should be curative.
3. Parenteral amino acid supplementation is the symptomatic treatment of choice for animals with liver disease and may prolong survival time by several months. Give a 10% crystalline amino acid solution (Aminosyn, Abbott Labs), 25 ml/kg IV via jugular catheterization over 6–8 hours. Repeat treatments q 7–10 days. Marked improvement in skin lesions should be seen within 1 week.
4. Alternatively, oral supplementation with three to six egg yolks per day, zinc, and essential fatty acids may help improve skin lesions in some animals, but these treatments are usually not as effective as intravenous amino acid therapy.
5. Treatment with anti-inflammatory doses of prednisone may temporarily improve skin lesions, but some dogs with superficial necrolytic migratory erythema are susceptible to diabetes following glucocorticoid use.
6. Symptomatic topical therapies (keratolytic or moisturizing shampoos) may help improve skin lesions.
7. Prognosis for animals with chronic hepatic insufficiency is poor, and survival time after the onset of skin lesions may be only a few months.

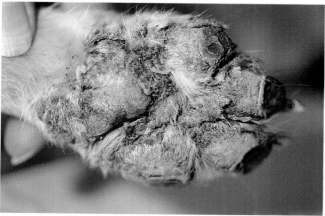

FIGURE 13–29. Superficial Necrolytic Migratory Erythema. Severe crusting and hyperkeratosis of the footpads is typical of this disease.

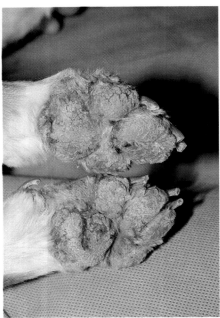

FIGURE 13–30. Superficial Necrolytic Migratory Erythema. The severe crusting and hyperkeratosis of the footpads developed over several months in this aged mixed breed dog. (Courtesy of A. Yu)

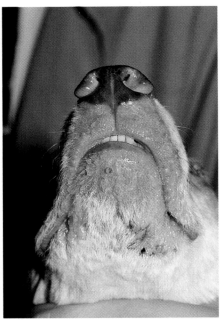

FIGURE 13–32. Superficial Necrolytic Migratory Erythema. Close-up of the dog in Figures 13–30 and 13–31. Moist, alopecic, erosive dermatitis on the muzzle. (Courtesy of A. Yu)

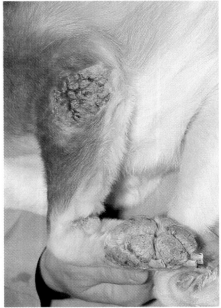

FIGURE 13–31. Superficial Necrolytic Migratory Erythema. Close-up of the dog in Figure 13–30. Hyperkeratosis and crusting of the footpads and elbows. (Courtesy of A. Yu)

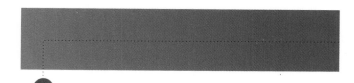

Schnauzer Comedo Syndrome
(Figs. 13–33 and 13–34)

FEATURES

A common acne-like disorder of follicular keratinization in miniature schnauzers.

A few to many nonpainful, nonpruritic comedones (blackheads) and crusted papules are found on the dorsal midline of the back between the shoulders and sacrum. If lesions become secondarily infected, a widespread papular eruption and pruritus may develop.

TOP DIFFERENTIALS

Demodicosis, superficial pyoderma, dermatophytosis.

DIAGNOSIS

1. Usually based on signalment, history, clinical findings, and ruling out other differentials.
2. Dermatohistopathology—The superficial portion of the hair follicle is distended with keratin. The keratin-dilated infundibulum may have a cystic appearance. A secondary bacterial folliculitis and furunculosis with comedone rupture may be present.

TREATMENT AND PROGNOSIS

1. For any secondary pyoderma, give appropriate systemic antibiotics for 3–4 weeks.
2. For mild to moderate lesions, cleanse affected areas with human acne pads, isopropyl alcohol, or 2 1/2% benzoyl peroxide gel q 1–2 days until comedones have resolved (approximately 1–3 weeks). Then cleanse areas q 2–7 days or as needed for maintenance control.
3. For moderate to severe lesions, cleanse affected areas with a sulfur and salicylic acid, ethyl lactate, tar and sulfur, or benzoyl peroxide and sulfur-containing shampoo q 2–3 days until comedones have resolved (approximately 1–3 weeks). Then cleanse areas as needed for long-term control.
4. Alternatively for severe lesions, treatment with isotretinoin, 1 mg/kg PO q 12–24 hours, may be effective in some dogs. Response should be seen within 4 weeks.

5. Alternatively, etretinate, 0.5 mg/kg PO q 12 hours or 1 mg/kg PO q 24 hours, has been used successfully but is no longer available. A newer retinoid, Acitretin, may also be effective (0.5–1 mg/kg PO q 24 hours).
6. Prognosis is good. Unless lesions are secondarily infected, this is a cosmetic disease that does not affect the dog's quality of life and is usually readily controlled with routine symptomatic therapy.

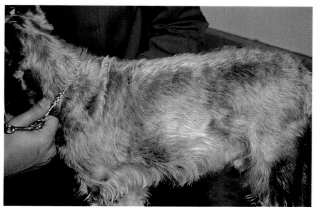

FIGURE 13–33. Schnauzer Comedo Syndrome. When viewed from a distance, a thin fur coat over the dorsum may be the only evidence of this disorder. When the skin is closely examined, the comedones are apparent (see Figure 13–34). (Courtesy of W. Miller)

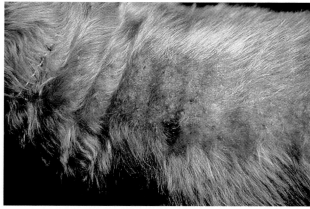

FIGURE 13–34. Schnauzer Comedo Syndrome. Close-up of the dog in Figure 13–33. The comedones are visible through the partial alopecia. (Courtesy of W. Miller)

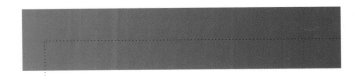

Canine Ear Margin Dermatosis (Figs. 13–35 and 13–36)

FEATURES

An idiopathic seborrheic condition of ear margins in dogs that have pendulous ears. Most common in dachshunds.

Initially, there is an asymptomatic accumulation of soft, greasy, keratinaceus debris along the edges of the ears. With chronicity, the ear margins may become alopecic, crusted, cracked, ulcerated, and fissured. Fissured lesions may be painful and induce head shaking, which further exacerbates the fissuring and pain. Except for the ear margins, the skin is normal.

TOP DIFFERENTIALS

Scabies, vasculitis, neoplasia, other causes of secondary seborrhea (Table 13–1).

DIAGNOSIS

1. Usually based on signalment, history, clinical findings, and ruling out other differentials.
2. Dermatohistopathology—Marked orthokeratotic and/or parakeratotic hyperkeratosis and follicular keratosis.

TREATMENT AND PROGNOSIS

1. No specific treatment is known.
2. Keep dog away from dry heat sources (i.e., wood stoves, fireplaces, forced air ducts), which will aggravate the dermatosis.
3. To remove the accumulated debris, gently cleanse ear margins with a sulfur and salicylic acid or benzoyl peroxide-containing shampoo q 1–2 days until all debris is eliminated (approximately 5–14 days, depending on severity). Then continue cleansing regime on an as-needed basis for maintenance control.
4. If accumulated crusts are tightly adherent and hardened, precede the first few shampoo applications with a 5- to 10-minute warm water soak.
5. Apply a moisturizer to ear margins after each shampoo therapy.

6. If ear margins are mildly to moderately inflamed, add topical therapy with a steroid-containing cream or ointment q 24 hours for the first 5–10 days.
7. If ear margins are severely inflamed, give prednisone, 1 mg/kg PO q 24 hours for 7–10 days.
8. If ear margins are extensively fissured and respond poorly to topical therapy, a cosmetic ear crop to remove the fissured tissue should be considered.
9. Prognosis is variable, depending on severity. This condition is incurable, but most cases can be controlled symptomatically.

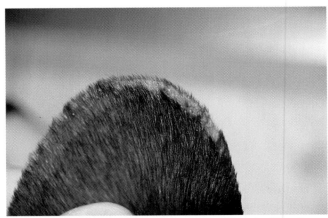

FIGURE 13–35. Canine Ear Margin Dermatosis. The alopecia and scaling affected only the distal margin of this adult dachshund's ear pinnae. The lesions were not pruritic.

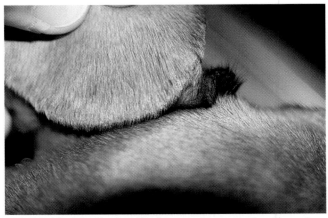

FIGURE 13–36. Canine Ear Margin Dermatosis. Alopecia and crusting on the distal ear margin of a young adult dachshund.

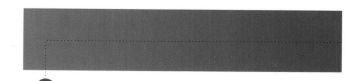

5. For fissured lesions, apply a combination antibiotic/ glucocorticoid ointment to lesions q 8–12 hours until healed.
6. Prognosis is good. Although incurable, this is a cosmetic disease which can usually be symptomatically managed.

Idiopathic Nasodigital Hyperkeratosis (Figs. 13–37 to 13–40)

FEATURES

An idiopathic condition characterized by the excessive formation of nasal and/or footpad keratin. Common in older dogs.

There is thickened, hard, dry keratin accumulation on the nasal planum, footpads, or both. The accumulated keratin is usually most prominent on the dorsum of the nose and at the edges of the footpads. Secondary erosions, ulcers, and fissures may develop. Excessive digital hyperkeratosis may result in horny growths, which can cause pain from pressure against adjacent footpads. Affected dogs are otherwise healthy and have no other skin signs.

TOP DIFFERENTIALS

Distemper, zinc-responsive dermatosis, pemphigus foliaceus, systemic or discoid lupus erythematosus.

DIAGNOSIS

1. Usually based on history, clinical findings, and ruling out other differentials.
2. Dermatohistopathology—Epidermal hyperplasia with marked ortho- and/or parakeratotic hyperkeratosis.

TREATMENT AND PROGNOSIS

1. The intensity of therapy depends on the severity of the lesions.
2. For mild, asymptomatic cases, benign neglect and observation without treatment may be appropriate.
3. For moderate to severe cases, hydrate affected areas with a warm water soak or compress for 5–10 minutes. Then apply a softening agent q 24 hours until excessive keratin has been removed (approximately 7–10 days). Continue treatments on an as-needed basis for control. Effective softening agents include:

Petroleum jelly.

Ichthammol ointment.

Salicylic acid/sodium lactate/urea gel.

Tretinoin gel.

4. For horny growths, excessive keratin should be trimmed away prior to beginning hydration and softening therapy.

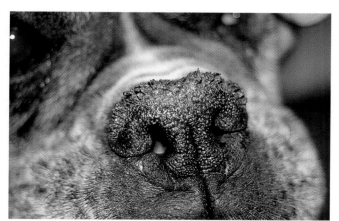

FIGURE 13–37. Idiopathic Nasodigital Hyperkeratosis. Frond-like hyperkeratosis and crusting on the nose of this 6-year-old boxer.

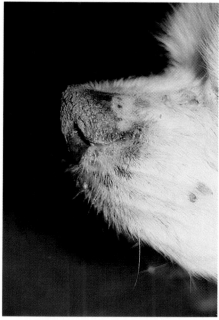

FIGURE 13–38. Idiopathic Nasodigital Hyperkeratosis. Crusting and hyperkeratosis on the nose of a 12-year-old cocker spaniel.

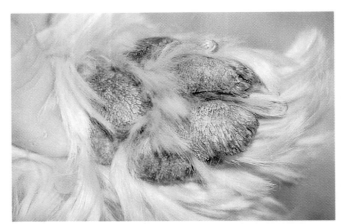

FIGURE 13–39. Idiopathic Nasodigital Hyperkeratosis. The digital hyperkeratosis formed frond-like projections on the feet of this aged cocker spaniel.

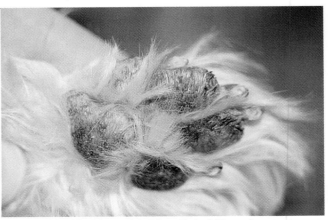

FIGURE 13–40. Idiopathic Nasodigital Hyperkeratosis. Same dog as in Figure 13–39. Hyperkeratotic lesions on the footpads. All four feet were affected.

Tail Gland Hyperplasia (stud tail) (Figs. 13–41 and 13–42)

FEATURES

A seborrheic condition associated with hyperplastic sebaceous glands in the tail gland area (dogs, cats) and/or the perianal region (dogs). In cats it occurs as a localized idiopathic condition. In dogs it may be localized or may be associated with a generalized primary or secondary seborrheic disorder. Common in dogs, with intact males possibly predisposed. Uncommon in cats, with the highest incidence in cage-confined cattery cats or cats with poor grooming habits. Intact male cats may be predisposed.

Dogs. Lesion is a slowly enlarging, asymptomatic, oval, raised area of hair loss on the dorsum of the tail approximately 2.5–5.0 cm distal to the tailhead. Affected skin may be scaly, greasy, and hyperpigmented. Pustules from secondary bacterial infection may be seen. In dogs with primary or secondary seborrhea, other skin lesions are present.

Cats. A band-like strip of matted hair and/or accumulation of waxy, seborrheic debris occurs along the dorsum of the tail. Affected skin may become hyperpigmented or partially alopecic. Lesions are asymptomatic, and there is no other skin involvement.

TOP DIFFERENTIALS

Dogs. Demodicosis, dermatophytosis, superficial pyoderma, neoplasia.

Cats. Demodicosis, dermatophytosis.

DIAGNOSIS

1. Usually based on history, clinical findings, and ruling out other differentials.
2. Dermatohistopathology—Sebaceous gland hyperplasia.

TREATMENT AND PROGNOSIS

1. In dogs, if generalized skin disease is present, identify and address the possible causes of the seborrhea (Table 13–1).
2. In dogs, give appropriate systemic antibiotics for 3–4 weeks if lesion is secondarily infected.
3. Clinical improvement in dogs and cats may be seen with localized topical antiseborrheic therapy on an as-needed basis.
4. In cats, encourage self-grooming by minimizing cage confinement. Regular grooming and combing by owner may be necessary in cats that are poor groomers.
5. In intact male dogs, castration may induce partial to complete lesion regression and/or prevent further lesion enlargement. Improvement should be seen within 2 months of castration. In intact male cats, castration does not cause the lesions to resolve but may help prevent further progression.
6. For cosmetically unacceptable lesions in dogs, excess glandular tissue can be surgically resected. Without castration, however, lesion recurrence within 1–3 years is likely.
7. Prognosis is good. This is a cosmetic disease that does not affect the animal's quality of life.

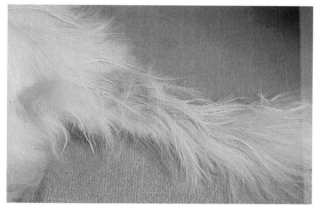

FIGURE 13–41. Tail Gland Hyperplasia. Partial alopecia with a focal, greasy, poor-quality fur coat on the dorsal tail region is characteristic of this disorder. (Courtesy of D. Angarano)

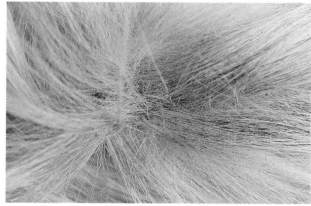

FIGURE 13–42. Tail Gland Hyperplasia. Close-up of the cat in Figure 13–41. The discoloration of the skin and hair is due to abnormal glandular secretion. (Courtesy of D. Angarano)

Feline Acne (Figs. 13–43 to 13–46)

FEATURES

An idiopathic disorder of follicular keratinization. Common in cats.

Asymptomatic comedones (blackheads) form on the chin, the lower lip, and occasionally the upper lip. Papules and pustules and, rarely, furunculosis and cellulitis may develop if lesions become secondarily infected. In severe cases, the affected skin may become edematous, thickened, cystic, or scarred.

TOP DIFFERENTIALS

Demodicosis, dermatophytosis, *Malassezia* dermatitis, and eosinophilic granuloma complex (if edematous).

DIAGNOSIS

1. Usually based on history, clinical findings, and ruling out other differentials.
2. Dermatohistopathology—Follicular keratosis, plugging, and dilation. Perifolliculitis, folliculitis, furunculosis, and/or cellulitis may be seen if secondary bacterial infection is present.

TREATMENT AND PROGNOSIS

1. Treat any secondary bacterial infection with appropriate systemic antibiotics for at least 2–3 weeks.
2. Clip hairs around lesions, apply warm water compresses, and cleanse affected area with human acne pads, or with benzoyl peroxide, sulfursalicylic acid, or ethyl lactate-containing shampoo q 1–2 days until lesions resolve, then as needed for maintenance control.
3. Alternative topical products that may be effective when used q 1–3 days or on an as-needed basis include:

Mupirocin ointment or cream.
2.5% Benzoyl peroxide gel.
0.01–0.025% Tretinoin cream or lotion.
0.75% Metronidazole gel.
Clindamycin, erythromycin, or tetracycline-containing topicals.

4. For refractory cases, systemic isotretinoin therapy may be effective. Give 2 mg/kg or 10 mg/cat PO q 24 hours until lesions resolve (approximately 30 days), then continue same dose q 2–3 days as needed for control.
5. Prognosis is good, but lifelong symptomatic treatment is often necessary for control. Unless secondary infection occurs, this is a cosmetic disease that does not affect the animal's quality of life.

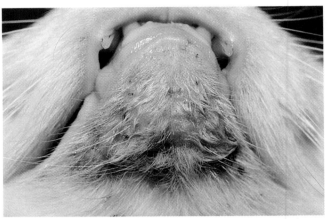

FIGURE 13–43. Feline Acne. Moist, draining papular lesions on the chin of an adult cat. The furunculosis and cellulitis caused the tissue swelling and exudate.

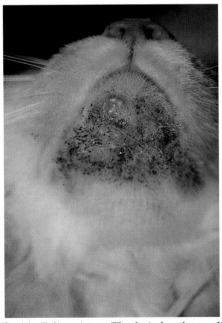

FIGURE 13–44. Feline Acne. The hair has been clipped, allowing better visualization of the comedones, papules, and draining lesions.

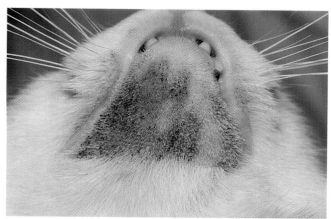

FIGURE 13–45. Feline Acne. The hair has been clipped to provide better visualization of the erythema, hyperpigmentation, and comedones.

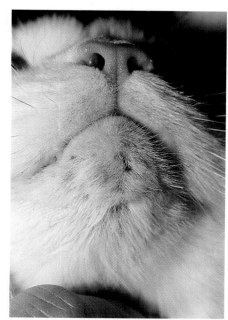

FIGURE 13–46. Feline Acne. Alopecia and scarring remained as sequelae after the treatment with topical mupirocin ointment.

Facial Dermatitis of Persian Cats (Figs. 13–47 and 13–48)

FEATURES

A facial skin disease of unclear etiology. Uncommon to rare in Persian cats, with highest incidence in older kittens and young adult cats.

Black, waxy debris that mats the hair accumulates symmetrically around the eyes, mouth, and/or on the chin. Initially, lesions are not pruritic, but as they progress and become inflamed, moderate to severe pruritus develops. Exudative and erythematous facial folds, a mucoid ocular discharge, erythema of the preauricular skin, and/or otitis externa with black, waxy debris in the ear canals may also be present. Secondary bacterial and *Malassezia* skin infection are common. Submandibular lymphadenomegaly may be seen.

TOP DIFFERENTIALS

Acne, dermatophytosis, and causes of secondary seborrhea (Table 13–1).

DIAGNOSIS

1. Usually based on signalment, history, clinical findings, and ruling out other differentials.
2. Cytology (skin imprints, ear swab)—Waxy debris. Bacteria and/or yeast may be seen.
3. Dermatohistopathology—Findings include marked acanthosis, superficial crusts that often contain sebum, hydropic degeneration of basal cells, and occasional dyskeratotic keratinocytes. Dyskeratoses are most marked in the follicular epithelium. Sebaceous hyperplasia and a superficial dermal infiltrate of eosinophils, neutrophils, mast cells, histiocytes, and occasional melanophages are also typical.

TREATMENT AND PROGNOSIS

1. No specific therapy is known.
2. Treat any secondary bacterial or *Malassezia* skin infections with appropriate systemic medications for at least 3–4 weeks. However, response to antimicrobial therapies is often partial at best.
3. Treatments with methylprednisolone acetate, 4 mg/kg SC q 4–8 weeks or as infrequently as needed, or prednisone, 1–3 mg/kg/day PO for 2–4 weeks, then 1–3 mg/kg PO q 48 hours, may partially control pruritus in some cats.
4. Prognosis is guarded because most cats respond poorly to symptomatic therapy. Do not breed affected cats.

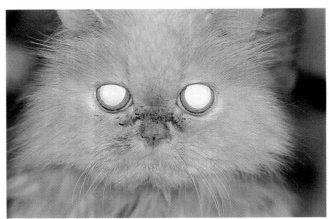

FIGURE 13–47. Facial Dermatitis of Persian Cats. Black, greasy exudate on the face of a young cat.

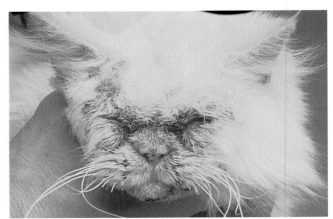

FIGURE 13–48. Facial Dermatitis of Persian Cats. The crusting seborrheic dermatitis on the face of this adult Persian cat resolved with steroid therapy. (Courtesy of C. Martin)

Suggested Readings

Bond R, Curtis CF, Ferguson EA, Mason IS, and Rest J. 2000. An Idiopathic Facial Dermatitis of Persian Cats. Vet. Dermatol. 11: 35–41.

Byrne K. 1999. Metabolic Epidermal Necrosis-Hepatocutaneous Syndrome. Vet Clin North Am, Sm Ani Pract. 29(6): 1337–1355.

Dunstan RW and Hargis AM. 1995. The Diagnosis of Sebaceous Adenitis in Standard Poodle Dogs, pp. 619–621. In Bonagura JD (ed). Kirk's Current Veterinary Therapy, XII, Small Animal Practice. W.B. Saunders, Philadelphia, PA.

Godfrey DR and Rest JR. 2000. Suspected Necrolytic Migratory Erythema Associated with Chronic Hepatopathy in a Cat. J Sm. Anim. Sci. 41: 324–328.

Keratinization Defects, pp. 824–844, 894–898. In Scott DW, Miller WH Jr, and Griffin CE. 1995. Muller & Kirk's Small Animal Dermatology. Ed. 5. W.B. Saunders, Philadelphia, PA.

Patel A, Whitbread T, and McNeil P. 1996. A Case of Metabolic Epidermal Necrosis in a Cat. Vet Dermatol. 7: 221–226.

Plumb DC. 1999. Veterinary Drug Handbook. Ed. 3. Iowa State University Press, Ames, IA.

14

Miscellaneous Cutaneous Disorders of the Dog

- **Acral Lick Dermatitis** (lick granuloma, acral pruritic nodule)

- **Callus**

- **Hygroma**

- **Canine Subcorneal Pustular Dermatosis**

- **Sterile Eosinophilic Pustulosis**

- **Canine Eosinophilic Granuloma**

- **Canine Nasal Solar Dermatosis**

- **Canine Truncal Solar Dermatosis**

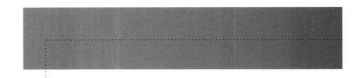

Acral Lick Dermatitis (lick granuloma, acral pruritic nodule)

(Figs. 14–1 to 14–4)

FEATURES

A slowly progressive self-trauma-induced skin lesion that is created from excessively licking or chewing at a focal area on the limb. The pruritus is a response to some underlying stimulus (Table 14–1). Common in dogs, with the highest incidence in middle-aged to older, large-breed dogs.

A pruritic, alopecic, firm, raised, thickened plaque or nodule that may become eroded or ulcerated. Lesions are usually single but may be multiple. They are most often found on the anterior aspect of the carpus, but the metacarpus, tarsus, or metatarsus is sometimes involved. With chronicity, hyperpigmentation and secondary bacterial infection (papules, cellulitis, exudation) are common.

TOP DIFFERENTIALS

Demodicosis, dermatophyte kerion, fungal or bacterial granuloma, neoplasia.

DIAGNOSIS

1. Usually based on history, clinical findings, and ruling out other differentials.
2. Dermatohistopathology—Ulcerative and hyperplastic epidermis, mild neutrophilic and mononuclear perivascular dermatitis, and varying degrees of dermal fibrosis.
3. Bacterial culture (exudates, biopsy specimen)—*Staphylococcus* is often isolated. Mixed gram-positive and gram-negative infections are common.

TABLE 14–1 Underlying Causes of Acral Lick Dermatitis

Hypersensitivity (atopy, food)
Fleas
Demodicosis
Trauma (cut, bruise)
Foreign body reaction
Infection (bacterial, fungal)
Hypothyroidism
Psychogenic (e.g., boredom)
Neuropathy
Osteopathy

TABLE 14–2 Drugs for Psychogenic Dermatoses in Dogs

Drug	Dose
Anxiolytics	
Phenobarbitol	2–6 mg/kg PO q 12 hours
Diazepam (Valium)	0.2 mg/kg PO q 12 hours
Tricyclic Antidepressants	
Fluoxetine (Prozac)	1 mg/kg PO q 24 hours
Amitriptyline (Elavil)	1–3 mg/kg PO q 12 hours
Imipramine (Tofranil)	2–4 mg/kg PO q 24 hours
Clomipramine (Anafranil)	1–3 mg/kg PO q 24 hours
Doxepin (Sinequan)	3–5 mg/kg PO q 12 hours: maximum dose is 150 mg/dog q 12 hours
Endorphin Blocker	
Naltrexone (ReVia)	2 mg/kg PO q 24 hours
Endorphin Substitute	
Hydrocodone (Hycodan)	0.25 mg/kg PO q 8 hours
Topical Products	
Synotic + Banamine	
Deep Heet + Bitter Apple	

TREATMENT AND PROGNOSIS

1. Identify and correct the underlying cause.
2. Treat any secondary bacterial infection with long-term systemic antibiotics (minimum 6–8 weeks), continued at least 2 weeks beyond complete resolution of the infection. Select the antibiotic based on bacterial culture and sensitivity results.
3. Topical applications of analgesic, steroidal, or bad-tasting medications q 8–12 hours may help stop the pruritus.
4. Mechanical barriers such as bandaging, Elizabethan collars, and side braces are also helpful.
5. For early and small lesions, an intralesional injection of triamcinolone acetonide or methylprednisolone acetate may help stop the pruritus.
6. When no underlying cause can be found, treatment with behavior-modifying drugs may be beneficial in some dogs (Table 14–2). Trial treatment periods of up to 4 weeks should be used to find the most effective drug. Lifelong treatment is often necessary.
7. Surgical excision is not recommended because postoperative wound dehiscence is common.
8. Prognosis is variable. Chronic, extensively fibrotic lesions and those for which no underlying cause can be found have the poorest prognosis. Although this disease is rarely life-threatening, its course may be intractable.

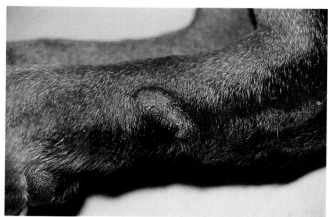

FIGURE 14–1. Acral Lick Dermatitis. This focal area of alopecia and erosion developed on the rear leg of an adult Doberman pinscher after several weeks of chronic licking. This dog had neurologic abnormalities that may have induced this granuloma.

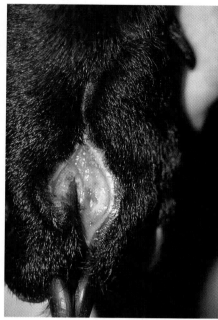

FIGURE 14–3. Acral Lick Dermatitis. This erosive lesion was caused by a traumatic degloving injury, which did not heal normally because of constant licking.

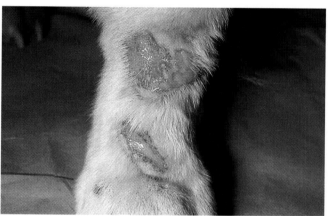

FIGURE 14–2. Acral Lick Dermatitis. Multiple moist, erosive plaques developed on the front leg of an adult dog after several months of licking and chewing. This dog had atopy, which initiated the pruritus. (Courtesy of D. Angarano)

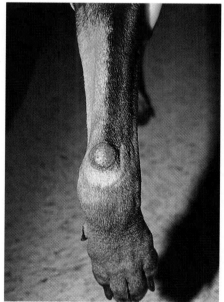

FIGURE 14–4. This focal erosive lesion on the front leg of an adult Doberman pinscher was caused by blastomycosis. Deep infections and neoplasia can mimic acral lick dermatitis. (Courtesy of D. Angarano)

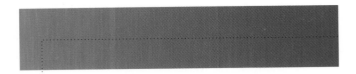

Callus (Figs. 14–5 and 14–6)

FEATURES

A localized, hyperplastic skin reaction to trauma from pressure or friction. Common in dogs, with the highest incidence in large and giant-breed dogs.

A round to oval, alopecic, hyperpigmented, hyperkeratotic, hyperplastic plaque forms over a bony pressure point. The elbow, hock, or sternum (deep-chested dogs) is most commonly affected. Lesions may become ulcerated, fistulated, and exudative from secondary bacterial infection.

TOP DIFFERENTIALS

Dermatophytosis, demodicosis, pyoderma.

DIAGNOSIS

1. Usually based on history and clinical findings.
2. Cytology (exudate)—Purulent or pyogranulomatous inflammation, free hair shafts, and bacteria may be seen.
3. Dermatohistopathology—Marked epidermal hyperplasia, orthokeratotic to parakeratotic hyperkeratosis, follicular keratosis, and dilated follicular cysts.

TREATMENT AND PROGNOSIS

1. Observation without treatment is appropriate for noninfected lesions.
2. If lesion is secondarily infected, give long-term systemic antibiotics (minimum 4–6 weeks).
3. Pad bedding and other sleeping/resting areas and/or use padded bandages to prevent trauma to affected area.
4. In conjunction with padding, apply moisturizers to affected area q 12–24 hours to soften the skin. However, secondary infections are likely to occur if moisturizers are used without implementing protective padding measures.
5. Surgical excision is usually not recommended because wound dehiscence is a possible postoperative complication.
6. The prognosis is good for noninfected lesions. This is a cosmetic disease that does not affect the dog's quality of life.

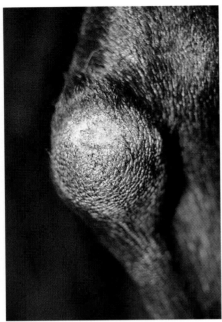

FIGURE 14–5. Callus. This callus developed on the rear leg of an adult labrador over several years. The focal erosion waxed and waned, depending on the bedding material used.

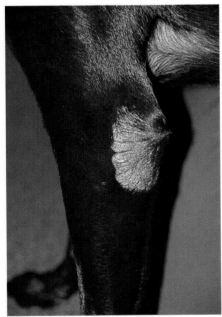

FIGURE 14–6. Callus. Same dog as in Figure 14–5. Alopecic callus on the elbow.

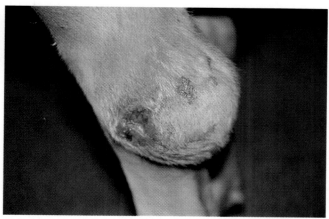

Hygroma (Figs. 14–7 and 14–8)

FEATURES

A cyst-like bursa filled with fluid that develops over a pressure point in response to repeated trauma. Uncommon in dogs, with the highest incidence in large and giant-breed dogs.

A soft to fluctuant, fluid-filled subcutaneous swelling forms over a bony pressure point. Lesions most commonly develop over the elbow or hock or on the sternum (deep-chested dogs). Lesions may become abscessed, granulomatous, and/or fistulate from secondary bacterial infection.

FIGURE 14–7. Hygroma. This large hygroma developed over several weeks on the elbow of a 4-month-old weimaraner with Ehlers-Danlos syndrome. The ulcerated areas drained periodically.

TOP DIFFERENTIALS

Bacterial or fungal granuloma, cyst, neoplasia.

DIAGNOSIS

1. Usually based on history and clinical findings.
2. Cytology (aspirate)—Acellular or blood-tinged fluid if lesion is not infected. Infected lesions may contain purulent to pyogranulomatous inflammation and bacteria.
3. Dermatohistopathology—Cystic spaces are surrounded by walls of granulation tissue.

TREATMENT AND PROGNOSIS

1. Give long-term systemic antibiotics (minimum 4–6 weeks) based on bacterial culture and sensitivity results if lesion is secondarily infected.
2. For early lesions, using loose, padded bandages for 2–3 weeks and implementing protective padding measures in the environment to prevent further trauma are often effective in resolving the hygroma.
3. For severe or chronic lesions, surgical drainage and/or excision may be indicated.
4. Prognosis is good if protective padding measures are instituted. Without corrective padding, persistent lesions and chronic, recurring bacterial infections are likely.

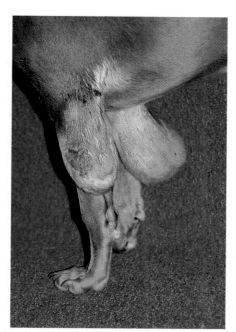

FIGURE 14–8. Hygroma. Same dog as in Figure 14–7. The hygromas enlarged progressively over several weeks.

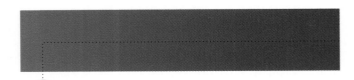

2. Prognosis is good if response to dapsone is seen. In some dogs the dapsone therapy can eventually be discontinued, whereas others require lifelong therapy for control.

Canine Subcorneal Pustular Dermatosis (Figs. 14–9 and 14–10)

FEATURES

A sterile, superficial, pustular skin disease of unknown etiology. Rare in dogs, with miniature schnauzers possibly predisposed.

There are multifocal to generalized pustules with secondary crusts, circumscribed areas of alopecia, epidermal collarettes, and/or scaling. Lesions usually involve the head and trunk. Footpads may be scaly. Lesions may wax and wane, and pruritus varies from none to intense. Peripheral lymphadenomegaly may be present. Concurrent systemic signs of illness (fever, anorexia, depression) are rare.

TOP DIFFERENTIALS

Demodicosis, dermatophytosis, superficial pyoderma, pemphigus foliaceus, systemic lupus erythematosus, drug eruption. If lesion is pruritic, also include scabies, hypersensitivity (flea bite, food, atopy), and sterile eosinophilic pustulosis.

DIAGNOSIS

1. Rule out other differentials.
2. Cytology (pustule)—Numerous neutrophils are seen. An occasional acantholytic keratinocyte may also be present, but no bacteria are found.
3. Dermatohistopathology—Subcorneal pustules containing nondegenerative neutrophils. Acantholytic keratinocytes may also be seen.
4. Bacterial culture (pustule)—No growth.

TREATMENT AND PROGNOSIS

1. Give dapsone, 1 mg/kg PO q 8 hours, until lesions resolve (approximately 2–4 weeks). Gradually taper dosage to 1 mg/kg PO q 24–72 hours, or as infrequently as possible to maintain remission.

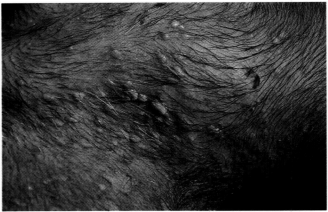

FIGURE 14–9. Canine Subcorneal Pustular Dermatosis. These large, nonfollicular pustules are characteristic of this disease. (Courtesy of D. Angarano)

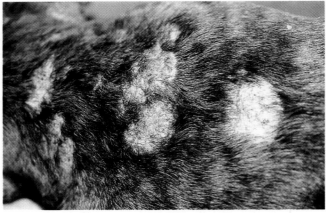

FIGURE 14–10. Canine Subcorneal Pustular Dermatosis. These alopecic, crusting plaques developed after the initial pustular lesions. The generalized lesions resolved when treated with dapsone.

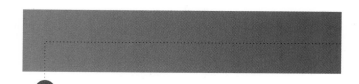

Sterile Eosinophilic Pustulosis
(Figs. 14–11 and 14–12)

FEATURES

A sterile, superficial, pustular skin disease of unknown etiology. Rare in dogs.

Usually there is an acute eruption of multifocal to generalized erythematous papules and pustules over the trunk, with secondary erosions, circumscribed areas of alopecia and hyperpigmentation, epidermal collarettes, and scaling. Lesions are pruritic. Concurrent peripheral lymphadenomegaly, depression, anorexia, and/or fever may occasionally be present.

TOP DIFFERENTIALS

Superficial pyoderma, dermatophytosis, demodicosis, pemphigus foliaceus, systemic lupus erythematosus, drug eruption, subcorneal pustular dermatosis.

DIAGNOSIS

1. Rule out other differentials.
2. Cytology (pustule)—Numerous eosinophils are seen. Neutrophils and occasional acantholytic keratinocytes may also be present, but no bacteria are found.
3. Dermatohistopathology—Eosinophilic intraepidermal pustules, folliculitis, and furunculosis.
4. Hemogram—Peripheral eosinophilia is common.
5. Bacterial culture (pustule)—No growth.

TREATMENT AND PROGNOSIS

1. Give prednisone, 2–4 mg/kg PO q 24 hours, until lesions resolve (approximately 2–4 weeks). Then give prednisone, 2–4 mg/kg PO q 48 hours, tapering to the lowest alternate-day dosage possible for maintenance therapy.
2. Alternatively, treatment with dapsone (as described for subcorneal pustular dermatosis in this chapter), or with a combination of antihistamine and fatty acid supplementation (as described for canine atopy in Chapter 6), may be effective in some dogs.

3. Prognosis for cure is poor, but most dogs can be kept in remission with maintenance medical therapy.

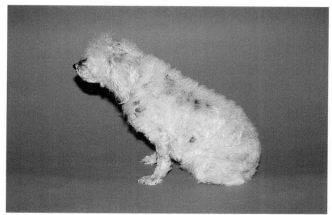

FIGURE 14–11. Sterile Eosinophilic Pustulosis. Multifocal pustules, crusts, alopecia, and hyperpigmentation affecting an adult female poodle.

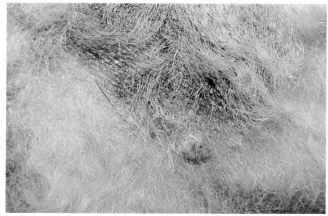

FIGURE 14–12. Sterile Eosinophilic Pustulosis. Close-up of the dog in Figure 14–11. Alopecia, erythema, crusts, and hyperpigmentation on the trunk.

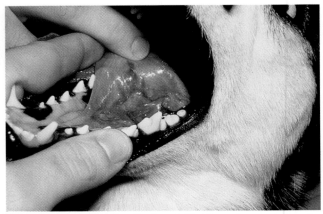

Canine Eosinophilic Granuloma (Figs. 14–13 and 14–14)

FEATURES

An eosinophilic disease characterized by nodules and plaques in the mouth or on the skin. The exact etiology is unknown, but skin lesions may represent a hypersensitivity reaction to arthropod bites or stings. Rare in dogs, with the highest incidence in young Siberian huskies.

Oral lesions are characterized by plaques or proliferative masses. They are most commonly found on the palate and lateral or ventral aspect of the tongue. Oral lesions may be painful. Halitosis is usually the presenting complaint.

Cutaneous lesions are papules, plaques, and nodules. They are neither painful nor pruritic and most commonly occur on the ventral abdomen and flanks.

FIGURE 14–13. Canine Eosinophilic Granuloma. An eosinophilic plaque on the tongue of a Siberian husky. (Courtesy of J. Noxon)

TOP DIFFERENTIALS

Bacterial and fungal granulomas, neoplasia.

DIAGNOSIS

1. Rule out other differentials.
2. Dermatohistopathology—Eosinophilic and histiocytic granulomas with foci of collagen degeneration.
3. Microbial cultures (tissue)—Negative for anaerobic and aerobic bacteria, mycobacteria, and fungi.

TREATMENT AND PROGNOSIS

1. Solitary lesions may regress spontaneously without therapy.
2. Systemic glucocorticoid therapy is usually curative. Give prednisone, 0.5–2.0 mg/kg PO q 24 hours, until lesions resolve (approximately 2–3 weeks) and then taper off.
3. Prognosis is good.

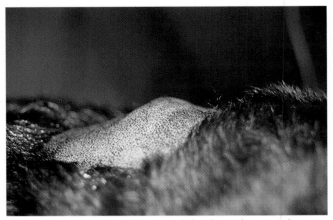

FIGURE 14–14. Canine Eosinophilic Granuloma. A large, eosinophilic granuloma on the lateral chest of a mixed-breed dog. The dog had multiple nodules covering its entire body, which recurred every spring.

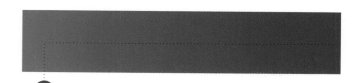

Canine Nasal Solar Dermatosis (Fig. 14–15)

FEATURES

A dermatosis caused by actinic damage to lightly pigmented or nonpigmented nasal skin. With repeated exposure to ultraviolet light, preneoplastic lesions (actinic keratoses, squamous cell carcinoma in situ) may develop. Uncommon in dogs, with the highest incidence in outdoor dogs.

Initially, the nose and adjacent nonpigmented, sparsely haired skin become erythematous and scaly (sunburned). Continued exposure to sunlight leads to alopecia, crusting, erosions, ulceration, and scarring.

TOP DIFFERENTIALS

Nasal pyoderma, demodicosis, dermatophytosis, discoid lupus erythematosus, pemphigus erythematosus, neoplasia.

DIAGNOSIS

1. Usually based on a history of prolonged sun exposure, clinical findings, and ruling out other differentials.
2. Dermatohistopathology—In early lesions, there is epidermal hyperplasia and superficial perivascular dermatitis. Vacuolated epidermal cells, dyskeratotic keratinocytes, and/or basophilic degeneration of elastin (solar elastosis) may be seen. In advanced lesions, the epidermis may be hyperplastic and dysplastic, without invasion through the basement membrane (actinic keratosis).

TREATMENT AND PROGNOSIS

1. Prevent further exposure to sunlight, especially between 9 A.M. and 4 P.M.
2. If some sun exposure is unavoidable, apply sun block (zinc oxide) or sunscreen twice daily to protect area. For sunscreens, use waterproof products with a sun protection factor (SPF) of at least 30.
3. To reduce inflammation, give prednisone, 1 mg/kg PO q 24 hours for 7–10 days.
4. If lesions are secondarily infected, give appropriate systemic antibiotics for 2–3 weeks.
5. Prognosis is variable, depending on lesion chronicity. With sun avoidance early lesions usually heal completely, but chronic ulcerative lesions often heal by scarring. With continued sun exposure, lesions may progress to squamous cell carcinoma.

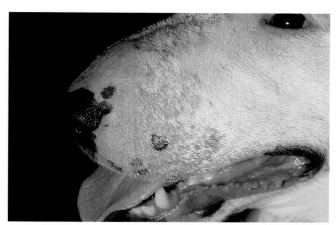

FIGURE 14–15. Canine Nasal Solar Dermatosis. Alopecia and erythema with a papular dermatitis on the muzzle. (Courtesy of D. Angarano)

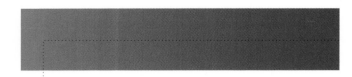

Canine Truncal Solar Dermatosis (Figs. 14–16 to 14–18)

FEATURES

A dermatosis caused by actinic damage to nonpigmented, sparsely haired skin. Initially, the skin becomes sunburned, but with continued exposure to excessive ultraviolet light, preneoplastic lesions (actinic keratoses, squamous cell carcinoma in situ), or neoplasia may develop. Uncommon in dogs, with the highest incidence in outdoor dogs that are avid sunbathers or kept in unshaded areas. Predisposed breeds include white boxers and bull terriers, American Staffordshire terriers, beagles, dalmations, and German shorthaired pointers.

Initially, affected skin becomes erythematous and scaly (sunburned). With continued sun exposure, erythematous macules, papules, plaques, and nodules develop. These lesions may be crusted, eroded, and ulcerated. Palpable irregular thickenings of what appears to be visually normal skin may be detected. The ventral and lateral aspects of the abdomen and inner thighs are most frequently affected, but lesions may also develop on the flanks, tail tip, or distal extremities. Secondary pyoderma is common.

TOP DIFFERENTIALS

Demodicosis, dermatophytosis, pyoderma, drug reaction, neoplasia.

DIAGNOSIS

1. Based on signalment, history, clinical findings, and ruling out other differentials.
2. Dermatohistopathology—In early lesions there is epidermal hyperplasia and superficial perivascular dermatitis. Vacuolated epidermal cells, dyskeratotic keratinocytes, and/or basophilic degeneration of elastin (solar elastosis) may be seen. In advanced lesions the epidermis may be hyperplastic and dysplastic, without invasion through the basement membrane (actinic keratosis).

TREATMENT AND PROGNOSIS

1. Prevent further exposure to sunlight, especially between 9 A.M. and 4 P.M.
2. If some sun exposure is unavoidable, apply sun block (zinc oxide) or waterproof sunscreen with an SPF of at least 30 to susceptible areas twice daily.
3. If inflammation is severe, give prednisone, 1 mg/kg PO q 24 hours for 7–10 days.
4. If lesions are secondarily infected, give appropriate systemic antibiotics for 2–3 weeks.
5. Treatment with etretinate, 0.5 mg/kg PO q 12 hours or 1 mg/kg PO q 24 hours, has been shown to be effective in resolving lesions in some dogs, but this product is no longer available. Alternatively, acitretin may possibly be effective (0.5–1 mg/kg PO q 24 hours).
6. Prognosis is variable. In early cases, prognosis is good if further exposure to sunlight is avoided. With continued exposure to sunlight, the likelihood of developing squamous cell carcinoma is high. Sun-damaged skin is also more predisposed to developing hemangiomas or hemangiosarcomas.

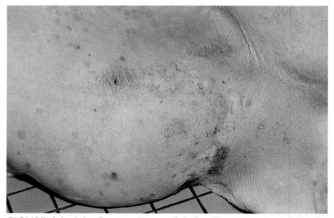

FIGURE 14–16. Canine Truncal Solar Dermatosis. Multiple erythematous papules and plaques on the abdomen of an aged dog.

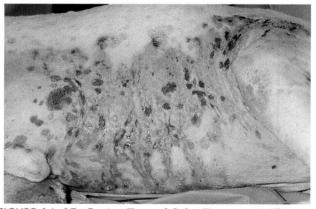

FIGURE 14–17. Canine Truncal Solar Dermatosis. This large, erythematous plaque on the abdomen of this American Staffordshire terrier is a combination of chronic solar dermatitis and squamous cell carcinoma. The pigmented areas of skin were protected and thus not affected.

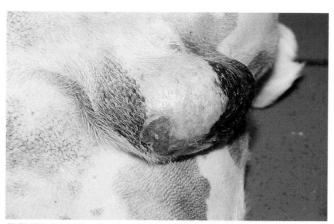

FIGURE 14-18. Canine Truncal Solar Dermatosis. The erythematous papular lesions on the scrotum are typical of solar dermatitis. The ulcerated lesion has progressed to squamous cell carcinoma.

Suggested Readings

Frank L and Calderwood-Mays MB. 1994. Solar Dermatitis in Dogs. Compend Cont Edu Prac Vet. 16: 465–472.

Goldberger E and Rapoport J. Canine Acral Lick Dermatitis: Response to the Antiobsessional Drug Clomipramine. J Am Anim Hosp Assoc. 27:179–182.

Miscellaneous Diseases, pp. 902–955. In Scott DW, Miller WH Jr, and Griffin CE. 1995. Muller & Kirk's Small Animal Dermatology. Ed. 5. W.B. Saunders, Philadelphia, PA.

Overall K. 1997. Pharmacologic Treatments for Behavior Problems. Vet Clin North Am Small Anim Pract. 27(3, May):637–665. Review.

Plumb DC. 1999. Veterinary Drug Handbook. Ed. 3. Iowa State University Press, Ames, IA.

15

Miscellaneous Cutaneous Disorders of the Cat

- **Feline Psychogenic Alopecia** (neurodermatitis)
- **Feline Eosinophilic Plaque**
- **Feline Eosinophilic Granuloma** (linear granuloma)
- **Indolent Ulcer** (rodent ulcer, eosinophilic ulcer)
- **Feline Plasma Cell Pododermatitis**
- **Feline Idiopathic Ulcerative Dermatosis**
- **Feline Solar Dermatosis**
- **Paraneoplastic Alopecia**

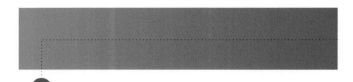

Feline Psychogenic Alopecia

(neurodermatitis) (Figs. 15–1 to 15–4)

FEATURES

A self-induced alopecia from excessive grooming (licking, chewing, and/or pulling hairs out). The overgrooming is a manifestation of anxiety, but the owners may be unaware of this behavior if the cat does not do it in their presence. Uncommon in cats, with Siamese, Burmese, and Abyssinian cats possibly predisposed.

Alopecia is produced when the cat grooms hard enough to remove hairs but not vigorously enough to damage the skin. There is regional, multifocal, or generalized hair loss. The alopecia may occur anywhere on the body where the cat can lick, but it most commonly involves the medial forelegs, inner thighs, perineum, and/or ventral abdomen. The hair loss is often bilaterally symmetrical, but remaining hairs do not epilate easily. Close inspection of the alopecic skin reveals that the hairs have not actually fallen out; they are still present and broken off near the surface of the skin. Rarely, overly aggressive grooming may result in an area of abraded skin. Hair in the feces and/or vomited hairballs may be seen.

TOP DIFFERENTIALS

Dermatophytosis, ectoparasites (demodicosis, cheyletiellosis, fleas), hypersensitivity (atopy, flea bite, food).

DIAGNOSIS

1. Usually based on history, clinical findings, and ruling out all other differentials.
2. Trichogram (microscopic examination of plucked hairs)—Hairs are broken off.
3. Dermatohistopathology—Normal, noninflamed skin.

TREATMENT AND PROGNOSIS

1. Identify and correct the underlying cause of the psychological stress, if possible.
2. Initiate a good flea control program to prevent fleas from aggravating the pruritus.
3. Using a mechanical barrier (Elizabethan collar, T-shirt) for 1–2 months to prevent grooming may help break the habit.

4. Behavior-modifying drugs may help stop the abnormal grooming behavior. In some cases, treatment may be discontinued after 30–60 days of therapy; in others, lifelong therapy is required for control. Drugs that may be effective include:

   Amitryptiline, 5–10 mg/cat PO q 12–24 hours.
   Clomiprimine, 0.5 mg/kg PO q 24 hours.
   Phenobarbital, 4–8 mg/cat PO q 12 hours.
   Diazepam, 1–2 mg/cat PO q 12–24 hours.
   Naloxone, 1 mg/kg SC q several weeks as needed.

5. If skin is secondarily excoriated, short-term treatment with prednisone, 0.5–1.0 mg/kg PO q 12 hours for 2–4 weeks, or methylprednisolone acetate, 4 mg/kg SC once or twice 2 weeks apart, is often beneficial. However, if long-term steroid treatment is required, an underlying allergic or ectoparasitic disease should be suspected and ruled out.

6. Prognosis for hair regrowth is variable, depending on whether the underlying cause can be identified and corrected. Some cats respond completely to behavior-modifying drugs. Psychogenic alopecia is essentially a cosmetic disease, so observation without treatment may be reasonable, because use of long-term behavioral-modifying drugs may result in serious side effects.

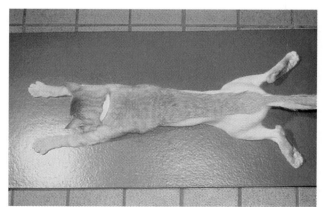

FIGURE 15–1. Feline Psychogenic Alopecia. Symmetrical alopecia caused by excessive grooming. (Courtesy of T. Manning)

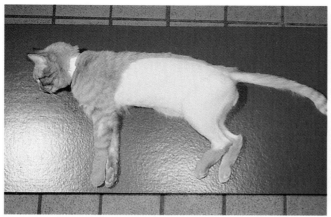

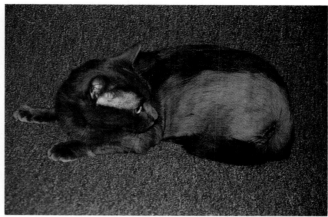

FIGURE 15–2. Feline Psychogenic Alopecia. Same cat as in Figure 15–1. Alopecia on the lateral flank caused by excessive grooming. The hair on the dorsal midline was difficult for the cat to reach and remained normal. (Courtesy of T. Manning)

FIGURE 15–4. Alopecia on the lateral trunk caused by excessive grooming in a food allergic cat. Note the similarity to Figure 15–2.

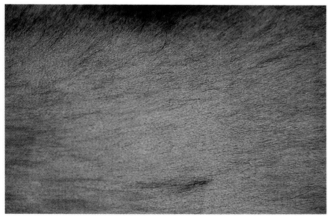

FIGURE 15–3. Feline Psychogenic Alopecia. Alopecia with no evidence of a secondary infection.

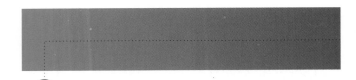

Feline Eosinophilic Plaque
(Figs. 15–5 to 15–7)

FEATURES

An inflammatory skin disease that is usually associated with an underlying hypersensitivity (flea bite, food, atopy). Common in cats, with the highest incidence in young adult to middle-aged cats.

Single to multiple well-circumscribed, raised, erythematous, eroded or ulcerated plaques. Lesions are usually intensely pruritic and may be anywhere on the body, but are most commonly found on the ventral abdomen and medial thighs. Regional lymphadenomegaly may be present.

TOP DIFFERENTIALS

Bacterial or fungal granulomas, neoplasia.

DIAGNOSIS

1. Usually based on history, clinical findings, and ruling out other differentials.
2. Cytology (impression smear)—Eosinophils are usually seen, but neutrophils and bacteria may predominate if lesion is secondarily infected.
3. Dermatohistopathology—Hyperplastic, superficial and deep perivascular to diffuse eosinophilic dermatitis. Eosinophilic microabscesses may be seen.
4. Hemogram—Peripheral eosinophilia is common.

TREATMENT AND PROGNOSIS

1. Identify and manage any underlying allergies.
2. To induce remission, give methylprednisolone acetate, 20 mg/cat or 4 mg/kg SC q 2–3 weeks, or give prednisone, 2 mg/kg PO q 12 hours until lesions resolve (approximately 2–8 weeks). Significant improvement should be seen within 2–4 weeks. Once lesions have resolved, oral prednisone therapy should be gradually tapered to the lowest possible alternate-day dosage possible or methylprednisolone acetate given SC q 2–3 months as needed.
3. Alternative steroids for prednisone- or methylprednisolone acetate-refractory cases include:

   Triamcinolone (induction dose), 0.8 mg/kg PO q 24 hours.

   Dexamethasone (induction dose), 0.4 mg/kg PO q 24 hours.

   Once lesions have resolved, triamcinolone or dexamethasome therapy should be gradually tapered to the lowest possible dosage q 2–3 days.

4. For glucocorticoid-refractory lesions, alternative therapies that may be effective include:

   Chlorambucil, 0.2 mg/kg PO q 24–48 hours.

   Aurothioglucose, 1 mg/kg IM q 7 days until remission occurs (8–14 weeks), then 1 mg/kg IM q 4 weeks.

5. Treatment with systemic antibiotics for 2–3 weeks may be helpful.
6. Other treatments that may be effective in some cats include surgical excision, laser therapy, and radiation therapy.
7. Prognosis is variable. Cats with underlying allergies that are successfully managed have a good prognosis. Cats with recurring lesions for which no underlying cause can be found usually require long-term symptomatic therapy to keep lesions in remission. These cats have a poorer prognosis, as they may become refractory to or develop unacceptable side effects from medical therapy.

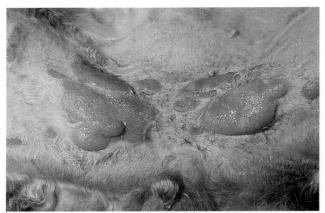

FIGURE 15–5. Feline Eosinophilic Plaque. These multifocal erosive plaques on the abdomen were intensely pruritic.

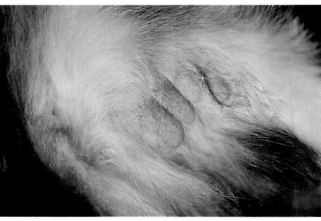

FIGURE 15–6. Feline Eosinophilic Plaques. These focal areas of alopecia and erythema on the abdomen are typical of early eosinophilic plaques. The lesions on this cat were caused by a combination of flea and food allergy.

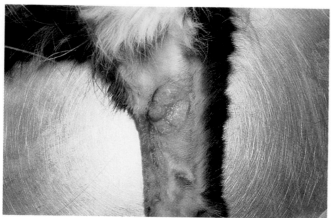

FIGURE 15–7. Feline Eosinophilic Plaque. Focal erosive plaque on the front leg of an allergic cat. The distal limb is an atypical location.

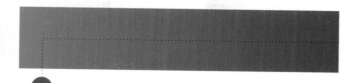

Feline Eosinophilic Granuloma (linear granuloma)
(Figs. 14–8 to 14–14)

FEATURES

An inflammatory cutaneous and/or oral mucosal disease that is usually associated with an underlying hypersensitivity (flea bite, food, atopy). Common in cats.

Cutaneous lesions usually occur singly and may be raised, firm, linear plaques or papular to nodular, edematous, or firm swellings. They may be mildly erythematous, alopecic, eroded or ulcerated, but are usually neither painful nor pruritic. Lesions can occur anywhere on the body but are most common on the caudal aspect of the thigh (linear granuloma) and chin or lip (swelling). A regional lymphadenomegaly may be present. Oral lesions are characterized by papules, nodules, or well-circumscribed plaques and are found on the tongue or palate. Cats with oral lesions may be dysphagic.

TOP DIFFERENTIALS

Bacterial or fungal granuloma, neoplasia.

DIAGNOSIS

1. Usually based on history, clinical findings, and ruling out other differentials.
2. Cytology (impression smear)—Many eosinophils are seen, but neutrophils and bacteria may predominate if lesion is secondarily infected.
3. Dermatohistopathology—Nodular to diffuse granuloma composed of eosinophils, histiocytes, and multinucleated giant cells with foci of collagen degeneration.
4. Hemogram—Peripheral eosinophilia may be present.

TREATMENT AND PROGNOSIS

1. Identify and manage any underlying allergies.
2. Cutaneous lesions in cats less than 1 year old may resolve spontaneously without treatment.
3. To induce remission give methylprednisolone acetate, 20 mg/cat or 4 mg/kg SC q 2–3 weeks, or give prednisone, 2 mg/kg PO q 12 hours until lesions resolve (approximately 2–8 weeks). Significant improvement should be seen within 2–4 weeks. Once lesions have resolved, oral prednisone therapy should be gradually tapered to the lowest possible alternate-day dosage possible or methylprednisolone acetate given SC q 2–3 months as needed.

4. Alternative glucocorticoids for prednisone or methylprednisolone acetate refractory cases include:

Triamcinolone (induction dose), 0.8 mg/kg PO q 24 hours.

Dexamethasone (induction dose), 0.4 mg/kg PO q 24 hours.

Once lesions have resolved, triamcinolone or dexamethasone therapy should be gradually tapered to the lowest possible dosage q 2–3 days.

5. For steroid-refractory lesions, alternate therapies that may be effective include:

Chlorambucil, 0.2 mg/kg PO q 24–48 hours.

Aurothioglucose, 1 mg/kg IM q 7 days until remission occurs (8–14 weeks), then 1 mg/kg IM q 4 weeks.

6. Treatment with systemic antibiotics for 2–3 weeks may be helpful.
7. Other treatments that may be effective in some cats include surgical excision, laser therapy, and radiation therapy.
8. Prognosis is variable. Cats with underlying allergies that are managed successfully have an excellent prognosis. Cats with recurring lesions for which no underlying cause can be found usually require long-term symptomatic therapy to keep lesions in remission. These cats have a poorer prognosis, as they may become refractory to or develop unacceptable side effects from medical therapy.

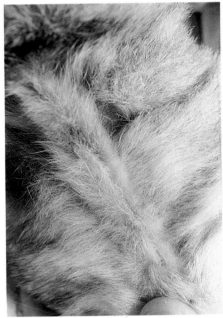

FIGURE 15–9. Feline Eosinophilic Granuloma. Linear region of alopecia and erythema on the caudal rear leg.

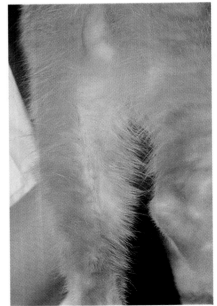

FIGURE 15–8. Feline Eosinophilic Granuloma. A thickened linear region of alopecia and erythema on the caudal rear leg. The inflammation associated with linear eosinophilic granulomas create a distinctive palpable lesion. (Courtesy of D. Angarano)

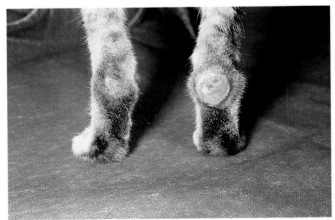

FIGURE 15–10. Feline Eosinophilic Granuloma. A circular eosinophilic granuloma on the rear leg.

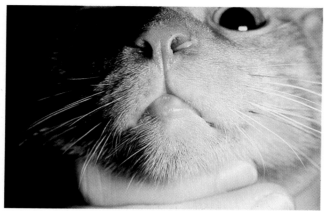

FIGURE 15–11. Feline Eosinophilic Granuloma. Tissue swelling and erythema on the chin and lower lip of a cat. Note the similarity to an indolent ulcer, which usually occurs on the upper lip. (Courtesy of D. Angarano)

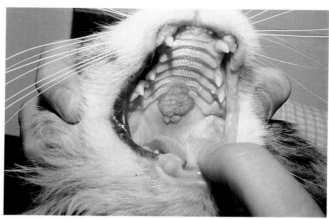

FIGURE 15–13. Feline Eosinophilic Granuloma. Multiple coalescing granulomas on the hard palate of an adult cat. (Courtesy of D. Angarano)

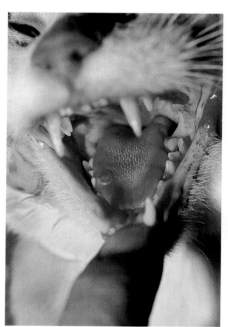

FIGURE 15–12. Feline Eosinophilic Granuloma. A small focal eosinophilic granuloma on the tongue of a young adult cat. (Courtesy of D. Angarano)

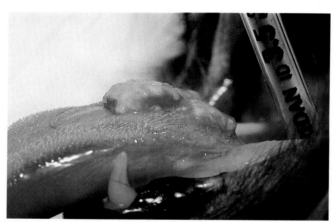

FIGURE 15–14. Feline Eosinophilic Granuloma. These large coalescing granulomas developed on the tongue over several weeks.

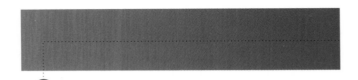

Indolent Ulcer (rodent ulcer, eosinophilic ulcer) (Figs. 15–15 and 15–16)

FEATURES

An ulcerative skin disease that is usually associated with an underlying hypersensitivity (flea bite, food, atopy). Common in cats.

The lesion begins as a small, crater-like ulcer with raised margins that most commonly affects the upper lip. It is usually unilateral but can be bilateral. The ulcer may enlarge progressively and become disfiguring, but it is not painful or pruritic. Regional lymphadenomegaly may be present.

TOP DIFFERENTIALS

Neoplasia.

DIAGNOSIS

1. Usually based on history and clinical findings.
2. Dermatohistopathology—Hyperplastic, ulcerative, superficial perivascular to interstitial dermatitis and fibrosis. Inflammatory cells are primarily neutrophils and mononuclear cells; eosinophils are not typically found.

TREATMENT AND PROGNOSIS

1. Identify and manage any underlying allergies.
2. To induce remission give methylprednisolone acetate, 20 mg/cat or 4 mg/kg SC q 2–3 weeks, or give prednisone, 2 mg/kg PO q 12 hours until lesions resolve (approximately 2–8 weeks). Significant improvement should be seen within 2–4 weeks. Once lesions have resolved, oral prednisone therapy should be tapered gradually to the lowest possible alternate-day dosage or methylprednisolone acetate given SC q 2–3 months as needed.
3. Alternative glucocorticoids for prednisone- or methylprednisolone acetate-refractory cases include:

   Triamcinolone (induction dose), 0.8 mg/kg PO q 24 hours.

   Dexamethasone (induction dose), 0.4 mg/kg PO q 24 hours.

   Once lesions have resolved, triamcinolone or dexamethasome therapy should be tapered gradually to the lowest possible dosage q 2–3 days.

4. For steroid-refractory lesions, alternate therapies that may be effective include:

   Chlorambucil, 0.2 mg/kg PO q 24–48 hours.

   Aurothioglucose, 1 mg/kg IM q 7 days until remission occurs (8–14 weeks), then 1 mg/kg IM q 4 weeks.

5. Treatment with systemic antibiotics for 2–3 weeks may be helpful.
6. Other treatments that may be effective in some cats include laser therapy and radiation therapy.
7. Prognosis is variable, depending on the underlying cause. Cats with underlying allergies that are managed successfully have an excellent prognosis. Cats with recurring lesions for which no underlying cause can be found usually require long-term symptomatic therapy to keep lesions in remission. These cats have a poorer prognosis, as they may become refractory to or develop unacceptable side effects from medical therapy.

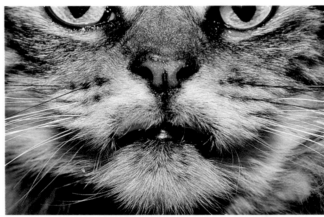

FIGURE 15–15. Indolent Ulcer. Mild swelling and alopecia. The severity of the lesions was not apparent until the lip was examined more closely (see Figure 15–16).

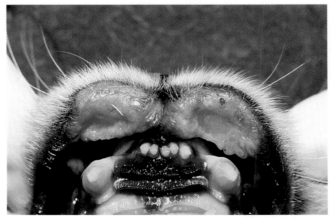

FIGURE 15–16. Indolent Ulcer. Close-up of the cat in Figure 15–15. The tissue swelling and ulceration are characteristic of this disease.

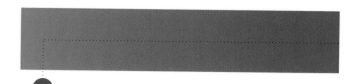

Feline Plasma Cell Pododermatitis (Figs. 15–17 to 15–20)

FEATURES

A plasmacytic inflammatory disease of footpads. Although its exact pathogenesis is unknown, an immune-mediated or allergic etiology is suspected. Rare in cats.

Multiple pads on more than one foot become soft, swollen, and mushy. The metacarpal and metatarsal pads are most commonly affected, but digital pads may also be involved. Affected pads may ulcerate and bleed easily. Cats with ulcerated pads may be painful and lame. Regional lymphadenomegaly may be seen. Occasionally, plasma cell stomatitis, glomerulonephritis, or renal amyloidosis is also present.

TOP DIFFERENTIALS

Eosinophilic, bacterial, or fungal granulomas, neoplasia, autoimmune disorders.

DIAGNOSIS

1. Rule out other differentials.
2. Cytology (aspirate)—Numerous plasma cells. Smaller numbers of lymphocytes and neutrophils may be seen.
3. Dermatohistopathology—Perivascular to diffuse dermal infiltration with plasma cells and Mott cells (plasma cells containing immunoglobulin that stain bright pink). Variable numbers of neutrophils and lymphocytes may also be present.

TREATMENT AND PROGNOSIS

1. Asymptomatic lesions often regress spontaneously without treatment.
2. For painful or ulcerated lesions, treatment with systemic glucocorticoids is usually effective. Give prednisone, 4 mg/kg PO q 24 hours until lesions resolve, then gradually taper off. Improvement should be seen within 2–3 weeks and resolution by 10–14 weeks.
3. Bleeding ulcers may also require surgical intervention.
4. For glucocorticoid-unresponsive or recurring lesions, treatment with aurothioglucose may be effective. Give 1 mg/kg IM q 7 days until lesions resolve (approximately 10–14 weeks). Then give 1 mg/kg IM q 14 days for 2–3 treatments, followed by 1 mg/kg IM q 30 days for maintenance.

5. Alternatively, anecdotal reports suggest that treatment with doxycycline 5 mg/kg PO q 12 hours, may be effective. Improvement should be seen within 1–2 months. Treatment is continued until the footpads have completely healed. In some cats, therapy may need to be continued indefinitely to maintain remission.
6. Prognosis is good for most cats unless concurrent stomatitis or renal disease is present.

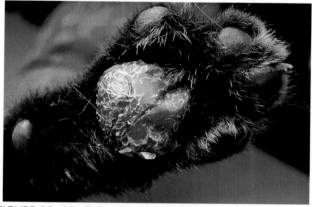

FIGURE 15–17. Feline Plasma Cell Pododermatitis. Swelling with superficial scale and hyperkeratosis of the central footpad. The footpad was soft and spongy on palpation.

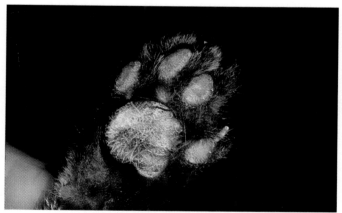

FIGURE 15–18. Feline Plasma Cell Pododermatitis. The hyperkeratotic, scaling footpads were soft and spongy upon palpation.

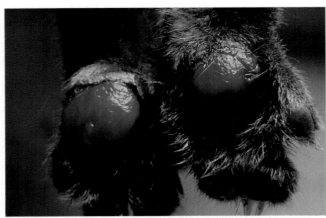

FIGURE 15–19. Feline Plasma Cell Pododermatitis. Ulceration of the central footpads. (Courtesy of Medleau L, Kaswan R, Lovenz M, and Dawe D: Ulcerative Pododermatitis: Immunofluorescent Findings and Response to Chrysotherapy. J Am Anim Hosp Assoc. 18: 449, 1982)

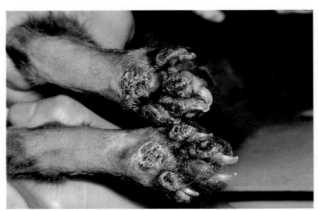

FIGURE 15–20. Feline Plasma Cell Pododermatitis. Same cat as in Figure 15–19. Footpads are begining to heal after surgical debridement of granulation tissue and two weeks of aurothioglucose therapy. (Courtesy of Medleau L, Kaswan R, Lovenz M, and Dawe D: Ulcerative Pododermatitis: Immunofluorescent Findings and Response to Chrysotherapy. J Am Anim Hosp Assoc. 18: 449, 1982)

Feline Idiopathic Ulcerative Dermatosis (Figs. 15–21 and 15–22)

FEATURES

An ulcerative skin disease of unknown etiology. Rare in cats.

The lesion is a heavily crusted, nonhealing ulcer surrounded by a border of thickened skin. It may be painful and occurs most commonly on the dorsal midline of the caudal neck or between the shoulder blades. A peripheral lymphadenomegaly may be present. There are no signs of systemic illness.

TOP DIFFERENTIALS

Injection reaction, foreign body reaction, trauma, burn, bacterial or fungal infection, neoplasia.

DIAGNOSIS

1. Rule out other differentials.
2. Dermatohistopathology—Extensive epidermal ulceration and superficial dermal necrosis with minimal to mild dermal inflammation. Chronic lesions may also have a subepidermal band of dermal fibrosis extending peripherally from the ulcer.

TREATMENT AND PROGNOSIS

1. Wide surgical excision should be attempted but may be unsuccessful.
2. Alternatively, medical therapy with methylprednisolone acetate, 20 mg/cat or 4 mg/kg SC q 2 weeks, until the lesion has resolved may be effective.
3. If the lesion is painful, a restraint device may be needed to prevent the cat from mutilating the affected area.
4. Prognosis is guarded to poor.

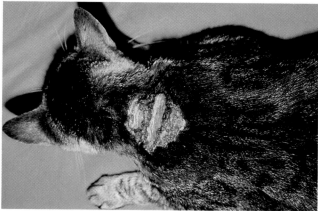

FIGURE 15–21. Feline Idiopathic Ulcerative Dermatosis. A large ulcer on the dorsal cervical region of an adult cat. (Courtesy of D. Angarano)

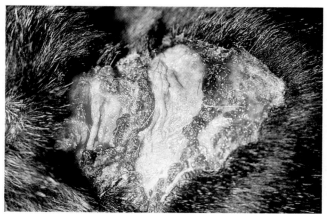

FIGURE 15–22. Feline Idiopathic Ulcerative Dermatosis. Close-up of the cat in Figure 15–21. Deep ulceration. (Courtesy of D. Angarano)

Feline Solar Dermatosis

(Figs. 15–23 to 15–26)

FEATURES

A dermatosis caused by actinic damage to white-haired skin. Initially, the skin becomes sunburned, but with repeated exposure to ultraviolet light, preneoplastic lesions (actinic keratoses, squamous cell carcinoma in situ) and squamous cell carcinoma may develop. Common in older outdoor cats and indoor cats that like to sunbathe.

Initially, there is mild erythema, scaling, and alopecia of the white-haired skin. With continued exposure to sunlight, the skin becomes progressively erythematous and alopecic, crusted, ulcerated, and painful. The ear tips/margins are most commonly affected, but lesions may also occur on white-haired eyelids, nose, or lips.

TOP DIFFERENTIALS

Dermatophytosis, trauma, autoimmune skin disease, vasculitis, squamous cell carcinoma.

DIAGNOSIS

1. Usually based on signalment, history, and clinical findings.
2. Dermatohistopathology—In early lesions, there is epidermal hyperplasia and superficial perivascular dermatitis. Vacuolated epidermal cells, dyskeratotic keratinocytes, and/or basophilic degeneration of elastin (solar elastosis) may be seen. In advanced lesions the epidermis may be dysplastic, without invasion through the basement membrane (actinic keratosis), or the dermis may be invaded by nests of dysplastic epidermal cells (squamous cell carcinoma).

TREATMENT AND PROGNOSIS

1. Keep affected cat indoors and prevent it from sunbathing between 9 A.M. and 4 P.M.
2. If some sun exposure is unavoidable, a waterproof sunscreen with a sun protection factor (SPF) of at least 30 can be applied twice daily to protect ears, but is not recommended for use around the eyes, nose, or mouth in cats.
3. Treatment with beta-carotene, 30 mg/cat PO q 12 hours, may be effective in resolving preneoplastic lesions. It is not effective if squamous cell carcinoma has developed.

4. Retinoids may be effective in the treatment of nonneoplastic actinic lesions. Etretinate, 10 mg/cat PO q 24 hours, has been used; however, this drug is no longer available. Acitretin may possibly be effective when used at ½–1X of the etretinate dosage.

5. Surgical excision, laser therapy, or cryotherapy may be curative.

6. Prognosis is good if further sunlight exposure can be avoided before squamous cell carcinomas develop.

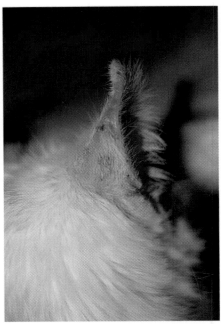

FIGURE 15–25. Feline Solar Dermatosis. Close-up of the cat in Figures 15–23 and 15–24. Alopecia, erythema, erosions, and crusting on the ear pinnae become more apparent as the disease progresses.

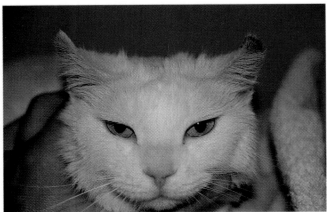

FIGURE 15–23. Feline Solar Dermatosis. Erythema and crust formation on the ear pinnae of an aged cat.

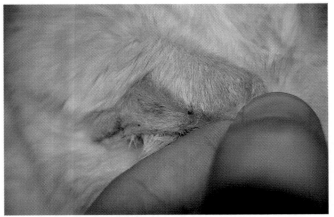

FIGURE 15–24. Feline Solar Dermatosis. Close-up of the cat in Figure 15–23. Erythema and alopecia on the ear margin.

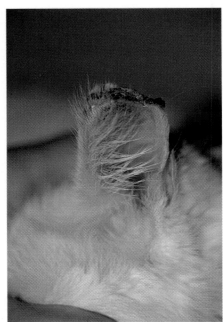

FIGURE 15–26. Feline Solar Dermatosis. Close-up of the cat in Figures 15–23 to 15–25. The lesion on the distal ear margin has progressed to squamous cell carcinoma, destroying the normal ear structure.

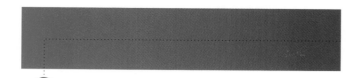

Paraneoplastic Alopecia

(Figs. 15–27 to 15–30)

FEATURES

A unique skin disease in cats that is associated with underlying pancreatic adenocarcinoma or bile duct carcinoma. Rare, with the highest incidence in older cats.

There is a rapidly progressing, bilaterally symmetric alopecia of the ventrum and limbs. Pruritus is usually a feature. The alopecic skin has a shiny and glistening appearance. Focal areas of scaling may be present. Hairs in nonalopecic areas epilate easily. In some cats the footpads are affected and may be painful, dry and fissured, soft and translucent, or erythematous and exudative. Concurrent anorexia, weight loss, and lethargy are usually present.

TOP DIFFERENTIALS

Ectoparasitism (demodicosis, cheyletiellosis, fleas), dermatophytosis, hypersensitivity (flea bite, food, atopy), psychogenic alopecia, hyperadrenocorticism.

DIAGNOSIS

1. Rule out other differentials.
2. Dermatohistopathology—Marked follicular miniaturization, atrophy, and telogenesis.
3. Radiography, ultrasonography, and/or exploratory laparotomy—Pancreatic or biliary tumor.

TREATMENT AND PROGNOSIS

1. The treatment of choice is complete surgical excision of the internal malignancy. If surgery is successful, complete hair regrowth should occur within 10–12 weeks.
2. Prognosis is poor because widespread tumor metastasis has usually occurred by the time of diagnosis.

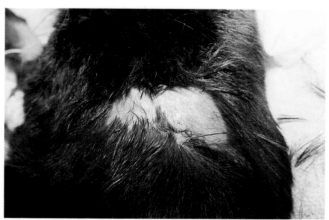

FIGURE 15–28. Paraneoplastic Alopecia. Close-up of the cat in Figure 15–27. This area of alopecia on the dorsum was caused by normal handling during diagnostic procedures.

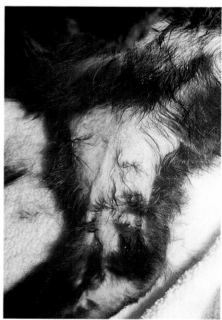

FIGURE 15–27. Paraneoplastic Alopecia. Multifocal alopecia in an adult cat diagnosed with an undifferentiated adenocarcinoma. The hair was epilated easily in large clumps.

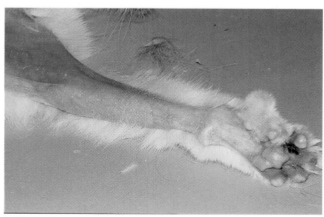

FIGURE 15–29. Paraneoplastic Alopecia. Generalized alopecia of the distal limb of a cat with pancreatic adenocarcinoma. (Courtesy of K. Campbell)

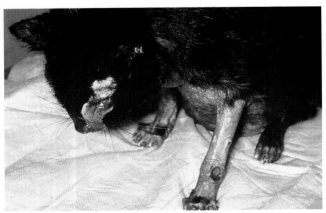

FIGURE 15–30. Paraneoplastic Alopecia. Diffuse alopecia in a cat with pancreatic adenocarcinoma. (Courtesy of K. Campbell)

Suggested Readings

Godfrey D. 1998. A Case of Feline Paraneoplastic Alopecia with Secondary *Malassezia*–Associated Dermatitis. JSAP. 39: 394-396.

Miscellaneous Diseases, pp. 902–955. In Scott DW, Miller WH Jr, and Griffin CE. 1995. Muller & Kirk's Small Animal Dermatology. Ed. 5. W.B. Saunders, Philadelphia, PA.

Overall K. 1997. Pharmacologic Treatments for Behavior Problems. Progr Comp Anim Behav. 27(3): 637–663.

Plumb DC. 1999. Veterinary Drug Handbook. Ed. 3. Iowa State University Press, Ames, IA.

Tasker S, Griffon D, Nuttall T, and Hill P. 1999. Resolution of Paraneoplastic Alopecia Following Surgical Removal of a Pancreatic Carcinoma in a Cat. JSAP. 40(1): 16–19.

16

Diseases of Eyelids, Claws, Anal Sacs, and Ear Canals

- **Blepharitis**

- **Bacterial Claw Infection**

- **Fungal Claw Infection** (onychomycosis)

- **Symmetric Lupoid Onychodystrophy**

- **Squamous Cell Carcinoma**

- **Melanoma**

- **Anal Sac Disease**

- **Perianal Fistulas** (anal furunculosis)

- **Otitis Externa**

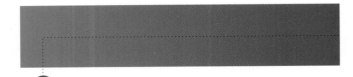

Blepharitis (Figs. 16–1 to 16–6)

FEATURES

Inflammation of the eyelids that may be due to a primary bacterial infection or secondary to an underlying condition such as a parasitic, allergic, or autoimmune skin disease. Eyelid involvement may occur alone or in conjunction with generalized skin disease. Common in dogs. Uncommon in cats.

Bacterial Blepharitis. Affected eyelids are mildly to markedly pruritic. They are often swollen or thickened, erythematous, and alopecic, with pustules, crusts, and sometimes cutaneous fistulae. One or more eyelid glands may be abscessed.

Insect Bite/Sting Hypersensitivity. Acute onset of eyelid erythema, with swelling (angioedema) or raised focal masses.

Contact Hypersensitivity (From Topical Ophthalmic Medication). Acute onset of eyelid alopecia and depigmentation, with marked conjunctival injection.

Allergy. Seasonal (atopy) or nonseasonal (atopy, food hypersensitivity) pruritus (eye rubbing) results in varying degrees of periocular erythema, alopecia, lichenification, and hyperpigmentation. Concurrent conjunctivitis and secondary bacterial blepharitis are common. Other skin involvement is usually present.

Autoimmune Disease. Eyelid erythema, erosions, and crusting, which are not pruritic unless secondary infection is present. Similar lesions involving the dorsum or planum of the nose, lips, ears, footpads, other mucocutaneous junctions, and/or generalized skin lesions are present concurrently.

TOP DIFFERENTIALS

Demodicosis, dermatophytosis, *Malassezia* dermatitis, juvenile cellulitis, viral infections (rhinotracheitis, calicivirus).

DIAGNOSIS

1. Usually based on history, clinical findings, and ruling out other differentials.
2. Cytology (pustule, abscess)—Suppurative inflammation and bacterial cocci if primary or secondary bacterial blepharitis is present.
3. Bacterial culture (pustule, abscess)—*Staphylococcus* is usually isolated if primary or secondary bacterial blepharitis is present.
4. Dermatohistopathology—Findings are variable, depending on the underlying etiology.
5. Allergy workup—Performed if atopy and/or food hypersensitivity are suspected.

TREATMENT AND PROGNOSIS

1. Identify and address any underlying cause.
2. If pruritic, use Elizabethan collar to prevent self-trauma.
3. Apply daily warm water compresses to affected areas to decrease swelling and remove exudate.
4. If bacterial infection is present, apply topical antibiotic-glucocorticoid ophthalmic preparation to affected eye q 8–12 hours for 2–3 weeks. Effective preparations include those containing:

   Bacitracin-neomycin-polymyxin-hydrocortisone.
   Neomycin-prednisone.
   Gentamycin-betamethasone.

5. For bacterial blepharitis, also give appropriate systemic antibiotics for at least 3 weeks.
6. For autoimmune blepharitis, treat with immunosuppressive medications (Chapter 7).
7. Symptomatic treatment with topical ophthalmic preparations containing glucocorticoids or antihistamines may be helpful in cases of allergic blepharitis.
8. Prognosis is good if the underlying cause can be identified and corrected or controlled.

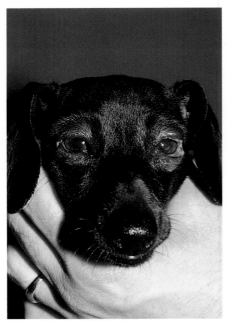

FIGURE 16–1. Blepharitis. The swollen, moist, erythematous dermatitis affecting both eyes was caused by a cutaneous bacterial infection. (Courtesy of S. McLaughlin)

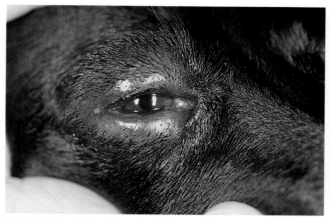

FIGURE 16–2. Blepharitis. Close-up of the dog in Figure 16–1. Alopecia, erythema, and tissue swelling of the periocular skin. (Courtesy of S. McLaughlin)

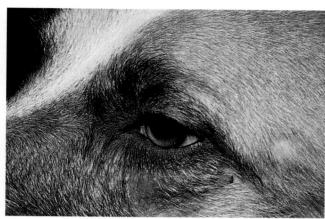

FIGURE 16–5. Blepharitis. The alopecia and hyperpigmentation of the periocular tissue were caused by allergic inflammation and chronic pruritus.

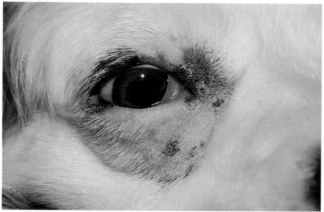

FIGURE 16–3. Blepharitis. Alopecia and erythema affecting the periocular skin associated with a bacterial pyoderma. (Courtesy of E. Willis)

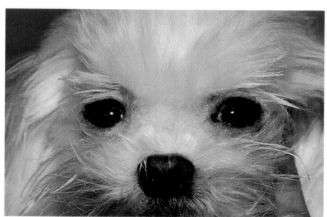

FIGURE 16–6. Blepharitis. Alopecia and erythema associated with atopy.

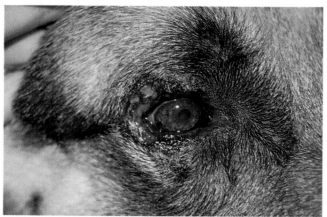

FIGURE 16–4. Blepharitis. The erosive lesions on the eyelids of this adult German shepherd were caused by a bacterial infection.

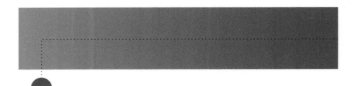

Bacterial Claw Infection

(Figs. 16–7 and 16–8)

FEATURES

Bacterial claw infections are almost always secondary to an underlying cause. When one to a few claws are affected, previous trauma should be suspected. When many claws are infected, underlying conditions to be ruled out include hypothyroidism, hyperadrenocorticism, autoimmune disorders, and symmetric lupoid onychodystrophy.

Affected claw(s) is often fractured and exudative, with associated paronychia, toe swelling, and pain. The nail may slough. Regional lymphadenomegaly may be seen. When multiple claws are involved, fever and depression may be present. Osteomyelitis may develop as a sequela to chronic infection.

TOP DIFFERENTIALS

Trauma, fungal infection, neoplasia, autoimmune skin disorders, symmetric lupoid onychodystrophy.

DIAGNOSIS

1. Usually based on history, clinical findings, and ruling out other differentials.
2. Cytology (exudates from claw or claw fold)—Suppurative to (pyo)granulomatous inflammation with bacteria.
3. Bacterial culture (exudates from claw or claw fold, proximal portion of avulsed claw plate)—*Staphylococcus* is usually isolated. Mixed bacterial infections are common.
4. Radiography (P3)—Evidence of osteomyelitis may be seen.

TREATMENT AND PROGNOSIS

1. Identify and address the underlying cause.
2. Remove any loose claws or fractured portions of traumatized claws. In severe or refractory cases, the affected claw may need to be avulsed under general anesthesia.
3. Give long-term (weeks to months) systemic antibiotics continued at least 2 weeks beyond complete clinical resolution. Antibiotic selection should be based on culture and sensitivity results. Pending these results, antibiotics that may be effective empirically include cephalosporins, clavulanated amoxicillin, potentiated sulfonamides, and fluoroquinolones.
4. Topical foot scrubs with 2–4% chlorhexidine shampoo or foot soaks in 0.025% chlorhexidine solution q 8–12 hours for the first 7–10 days of antibiotic therapy may be helpful.
5. In refractory cases with P3 osteomyelitis, P3 amputation may be necessary.
6. Prognosis for claw regrowth is good (unless P3 has been amputated).

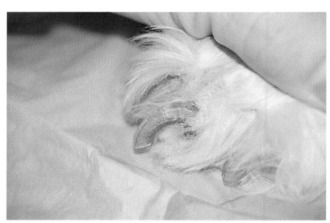

FIGURE 16–7. Bacterial Claw Infection. Flaky dystrophic nails of an adult cocker spaniel with chronic bacterial pododermatitis secondary to food allergy.

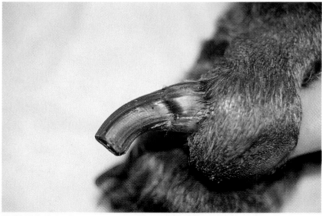

FIGURE 16–8. Bacterial Claw Infection. The base of this nail was split on the midline, and a purulent exudate was exuding from the fractured claw. A mixed bacterial population was cultured from the exudate.

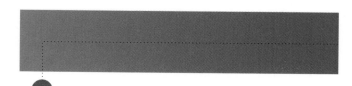

Fungal Claw Infection

(onychomycosis) (Figs. 16–9 to 16–12)

FEATURES

Fungal claw infections are usually caused by dermatophytes, although isolated cases of nail infections from other fungi have been reported. Typically, only one or two claws are affected. Rare in dogs and cats.

Affected claw(s) is often friable and misshapen. Associated paronychia is common. Generalized skin disease may be seen, especially if multiple claws are involved.

TOP DIFFERENTIALS

Trauma, bacterial infection, neoplasia, autoimmune skin disorders, symmetric lupoid onychodystrophy.

DIAGNOSIS

1. Rule out other differentials.
2. Fungal culture (proximal claw shavings)—*Trichophyton* spp. are most commonly isolated, but infections with *Microsporum* spp. and, more rarely, nondermatophytic fungi can occur.
3. Dermatohistopathology (P3 amputation)—Fungal hyphae and arthrospores within keratin.

TREATMENT AND PROGNOSIS

1. Remove any loose or sloughing nails.
2. Give long-term (6 months or longer) systemic antifungal therapy continued at least 1–3 months beyond complete nail regrowth. Perform frequent nail trims to remove infected portion. Submit trimmings for follow-up fungal cultures and continue treatment until culture results are negative.
3. Antifungal drugs that may be effective include:

   Microsize griseofulvin, 50–75 mg/kg PO q 12 hours with high-fat meal.

   Ketoconazole, 5–10 mg/kg PO q 12 hours with food.

   Itraconazole, 5–10 mg/kg PO q 24 hours with food.

4. Concurrent topical therapies that may be helpful include:

   0.025% Chlorhexidine solution as a 5- to 10-minute foot soak q 12 hours.

   0.4% Povidone-iodine solution as a 5- to 10-minute foot soak q 12 hours.

   0.2% Enilconazole solution as a 5- to 10-minute foot soak q 24 hours.

   Thiabendazole (Tresaderm), 1 drop on each claw q 12 hours.

5. Prognosis is guarded to fair. Many dogs have incomplete resolution in spite of aggressive antifungal therapy. In these cases, P3 amputation or long-term, low-dose therapy with ketoconazole or itraconazole may be needed.

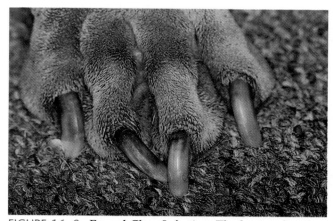

FIGURE 16–9. Fungal Claw Infection. The brown discoloration of this shar pei's nails and nail beds was caused by a secondary *Malassezia* infection associated with allergic dermatitis.

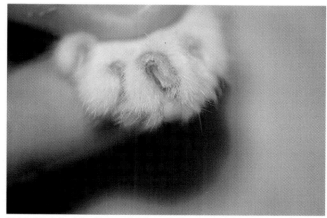

FIGURE 16–10. Fungal Claw Infection. Alopecia and erythema on the nail bed caused by a *Microsporum canis* infection.

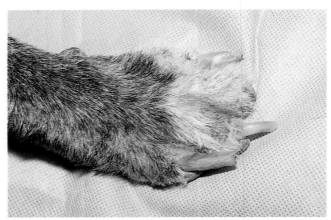

FIGURE 16–11. Fungal Claw Infection. Diffuse alopecia, erythema, and crusting on the foot caused by a *Trichophyton mentagrophytes* infection. The onychomycosis caused dystrophic nails that sloughed. (Courtesy of A. Yu)

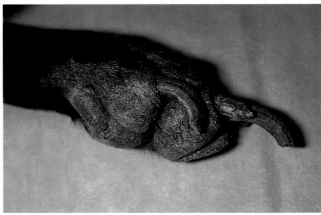

FIGURE 16–12. Fungal Claw Infection. Onychomycosis caused by a *T. mentagrophytes* infection. The nails are dystrophic, and there is an alopecic dermatitis. (Courtesy of D. Angarano)

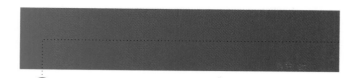

Symmetric Lupoid Onychodystrophy (Figs. 16–13 and 16–14)

FEATURES

A lupus-like disease that causes onychomadesis (claw loss). Uncommon in dogs, with the highest incidence in young adult and middle-aged dogs.

There is usually an acute onset of nail loss. Initially, one or two claws are lost, but over the course of a few weeks to several months, all claws slough. Partial regrowth occurs, but claws are misshapen, soft or brittle, discolored, and friable and often slough again. Affected feet are often painful and/or pruritic. Paronychia is uncommon unless a secondary bacterial infection is present. Affected dogs are otherwise healthy.

TOP DIFFERENTIALS

Fungal and bacterial claw infection, autoimmune skin disorders, drug eruption, vasculitis.

DIAGNOSIS

1. Rule out other differentials.
2. Dermatohistopathology (P3 amputation)—Hydropic and lichenoid interface dermatitis.

TREATMENT AND PROGNOSIS

1. Give appropriate systemic antibiotics to treat secondary bacterial paronychia, if present.
2. Treatment with daily oral fatty acid supplementation given as per label instructions is often effective. Noticeable nail regrowth should be seen within 3 months of initiating therapy.
3. If no improvement is seen with fatty acid supplementation, therapy with vitamin E, 200–400 IU PO q 12 hours, may be effective. Noticeable nail regrowth should be evident within 3 months of initiating therapy.
4. Alternatively, combined tetracycline and niacinamide therapy may be effective. Give 250 mg of each drug (dogs <10 kg) or 500 mg of each drug (dogs >10 kg) PO q 8 hours until noticeable nail regrowth has occurred (approximately 3–6 months). Then give each drug q 12 hours for 2 months, followed by long-term maintenance therapy with each drug given q 24 hours.
5. In severe refractory cases, prednisone therapy may be effective. Give 2–4 mg/kg PO q 24 hours for 2–4 weeks, followed by 1–2 mg/kg PO q 24 hours for 2–4 weeks. Then slowly taper to the lowest possible alternate-day dosage needed to maintain remission.
6. Prognosis for nail regrowth is good, although some nails may remain deformed or friable. In some dogs, therapy can be discontinued after 6 months. In others, long-term maintenance therapy is necessary to maintain remission. In cases refractory to medical therapy, P3 amputation can be considered.

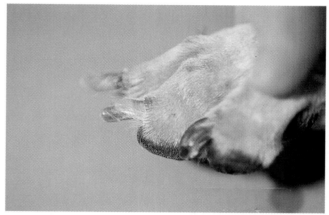

FIGURE 16–13. Symmetric Lupoid Onychodystrophy. Multiple dystrophic nails on multiple feet are characteristic of this disorder. The skin was normal except for iatrogenic changes associated with clipping.

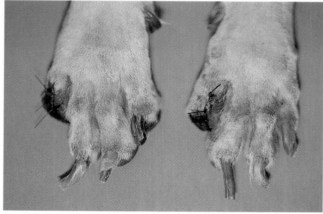

FIGURE 16–14. Symmetric Lupoid Onychodystrophy. Same dog as in Figure 16–13. The dystrophic nails on both front feet are apparent. Two digits were surgically removed for diagnostic evaluation.

Squamous Cell Carcinoma

(Fig. 16–15)

FEATURES

A neoplasm arising from the germinal epithelium of the claw. Uncommon in cats and dogs, with the highest incidence in large breed, black-coated dogs. Black Labrador retrievers and black standard poodles may be predisposed. Usually only one digit is involved, but in Labradors and standard poodles, multiple digits may become affected over a 2- to 4-year period. Claw bed tumors in cats often reflect metastases from other primary sites.

Affected toe is swollen and often painful or pruritic. Paronychia and erosive or ulcerative dermatitis are common. The claw may be misshapen or absent.

TOP DIFFERENTIALS

Other neoplasms, bacterial or fungal infection.

DIAGNOSIS

1. Radiography—Bony lysis of P3 with associated soft tissue swelling.
2. Cytology (often nondiagnostic)—Cells may vary from poorly differentiated, small, round epithelial cells with basophilic cytoplasm to more mature, large, angular, nonkeratinized epithelial cells with abundant cytoplasm, retained nuclei, and perinuclear vacuolation.
3. Dermatohistopathology—Irregular masses of atypical keratinocytes that proliferate downward and invade the dermis. Neoplastic cells are in direct contact with dermis without a basal cell layer.

TREATMENT AND PROGNOSIS

1. Amputate affected digit.
2. Prognosis for cats is poor because digital squamous cell carcinoma is usually an aggressive tumor that metastasizes readily. Prognosis for dogs is good for long-term survival, as digital squamous cell carcinoma is locally invasive but slow-growing and rarely metastasizes. However, if localized metastasis is suspected, regional lymph node excision or limb amputation should be considered.

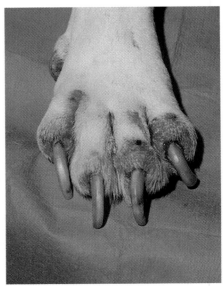

FIGURE 16–15. Squamous Cell Carcinoma. Diffuse swelling and erythema affecting the nail bed and distal toes. Note the similarity to other causes of pododermatitis. (Courtesy of J. MacDonald)

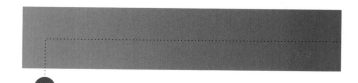

Melanoma (Figs. 16–16 and 16–17)

FEATURES

A benign or malignant proliferation of melanocytes. Most melanomas involving the nailbeds are malignant. Common in older dogs and rare in older cats.

Usually a solitary, well-circumscribed, dome-shaped, firm, brown to black, alopecic, pedunculated or wart-like growth ranging from 0.5 to 10 cm in diameter. Malignant melanomas can be pigmented or nonpigmented (amelanotic), may be ulcerated, and tend to be larger and more rapidly growing than benign melanomas.

TOP DIFFERENTIALS

Other neoplasms, bacterial claw infection/osteomyelitis, fungal infection.

DIAGNOSIS

1. Cytology—Round, oval, stellate, or spindle-shaped cells with a moderate amount of cytoplasm containing granules of brown to green-black pigment. Malignant melanomas may have less pigment and show more pleomorphism, but malignancy cannot be reliably determined cytologically.
2. Dermatohistopathology—Accumulation of neoplastic melanocytes, which may be spindle-shaped, epithelial, or round cell in appearance. Cells may be arranged in clusters, cords, or nerve-like whorls and have variable degrees of pigmentation. Infiltration of pigment-laden macrophages is common. Benign neoplasms are circumscribed and have little nuclear variability and a low mitotic rate. Malignant melanomas may show more invasiveness, cellular pleomorphism, and mitotic figures (including atypical mitotic figures). Mitotic index is the most reliable way to predict biologic behavior; however, 10% of histologically benign melanomas will behave in a malignant manner.
3. Radiography—Soft tissue swelling, bony proliferation, and/or bony lysis of P3 may be seen.
4. Affected animals should be screened for regional lymph node and internal metastasis.

TREATMENT AND PROGNOSIS

1. The treatment of choice is radical surgical excision/P3 amputation because benign melanomas cannot be differentiated clinically from malignant melanomas.
2. Chemotherapy may prolong survival in some cases of malignant disease.
3. Prognosis is good for benign melanomas. Prognosis is poor for malignant melanomas because recurrence following surgery and metastasis are common.

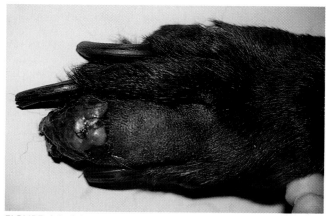

FIGURE 16–16. Melanoma. A large, proliferative tumor of the digit.

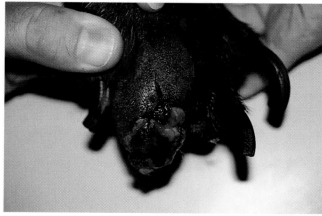

FIGURE 16–17. Melanoma. Same dog as in Figure 16–16. Ulcerated proliferative tumor of the digit.

Anal Sac Disease (Fig. 16–8)

FEATURES

A disease process that results in anal sac impaction, which may be followed by secondary infection (sacculitis) and abscess formation. Recurrent anal sac disease may be often associated with underlying food hypersensitivity or atopy. Common in dogs, with the highest incidence in small-breed dogs. Rare in cats.

Scooting and perineal licking or biting are common symptoms of anal sac impaction and sacculitis. Tenesmus, painful defecation, tail chasing, and perineal pyotraumatic dermatitis may be seen. With abscessation, perianal erythema, swelling, an exudative draining tract (if abscess has ruptured), and fever may be present.

TOP DIFFERENTIALS

Anal sac neoplasia, perianal fistulas, tapeworms.

DIAGNOSIS

1. Digital palpation of distended, obstructed anal sacs.
2. Expression and examination of anal sac contents:

   Normal anal sac—Contains clear or pale yellow-brown fluid.

   Impacted anal sac—Material is thick, brown, and pasty.

   Anal sacculitis—Creamy yellow or thin yellow-green exudates.

   Anal sac abscess—Usually contains a reddish-brown exudate.

TREATMENT AND PROGNOSIS

1. Identify and treat any underlying hypersensitivity.
2. For anal sac impaction, express anal sacs manually.

3. For anal sacculitis, express manually and lavage anal sacs with 0.025% chlorhexidine or 0.4% povidone-iodine solution. Then instill into anal sacs an antibiotic/glucocorticoid ointment (i.e., Panalog, Otomax). Also give appropriate systemic, broad-spectrum antibiotics for 7 days.
4. For anal sac abscess, establish drainage if the anal sac is not already ruptured. Clean and flush anal sac with .025% chlorhexidine or 0.4% povidone-iodine solution and then instill an antibiotic/glucocorticoid ointment (i.e., Panalog, Otomax). Apply warm compresses to affected area or use hydrotherapy q 12–24 hours to ensure drainage and promote healing. Apply topical antibiotic cream or ointment to affected area q 12 hours and give appropriate systemic broad-spectrum antibiotics for 7–10 days.
5. For recurrent impactions, sacculitis, or abscesses, surgical excision of the affected anal sac should be curative. However, temporary or permanent fecal incontinence is a possible postoperative complication, and draining fistulas will develop if the anal sacculectomy is incomplete.
6. Prognosis is variable. Routine manual anal sac expression may be useful to prevent recurrences.

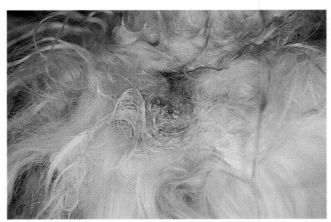

FIGURE 16–18. Anal Sac Disease. Diffuse erythema caused by inflammation and pruritus.

Perianal Fistulas (anal furunculosis) (Figs. 16–19 and 16–20)

FEATURES

A chronic, progressive, debilitating, inflammatory, ulcerative disease of perianal tissues. The cause is unclear, but an immunologic defect is suspected. Food allergy is an incriminated but unproven cause. Uncommon in dogs, with the highest incidence in German shepherds.

Perianal lesions are usually painful, may be mild to severe, and include small draining sinuses, fistulous tracts, erosions, and ulcerations. Associated symptoms may include frequent perianal licking, malodorous mucopurulent anorectal discharge, tenesmus, painful defecations, constipation, low tail carriage, weight loss, and lethargy. Affected dogs may have concurrent inflammatory bowel disease.

TOP DIFFERENTIALS

Perianal adenocarcinomas, ruptured anal sac abscess, pythiosis.

DIAGNOSIS

1. Usually based on history, clinical findings, and ruling out other differentials.

TREATMENT AND PROGNOSIS

1. Identify and treat any underlying food hypersensitivity.
2. Give short-term (10–21 days) systemic antibiotics for secondary bacterial infection.
3. Long-term treatment with prednisone may be effective in some dogs. Give 2 mg/kg PO q 24 hours for 2 weeks, followed by 1 mg/kg PO q 24 hours for 4 weeks and then 1 mg/kg PO q 48 hours for maintenance.
4. Alternatively, long-term (3–5 months) treatment with cyclosporin is effective in many dogs. Give 1.75–5 mg/kg PO q 12 hours continued at least 4 weeks beyond complete resolution. If clinical improvement is not seen after 2 weeks of treatment, the dosage of cyclosporin may need to be increased. If improvement is incomplete, surgical excision of remaining fistulas and anal sacculectomy are often curative. Some dogs may require lifelong therapy with low-dose cyclosporin (i.e., 2.5 mg/kg/day) to maintain remission.
5. Recent anecdotal reports suggest topical cyclosporin or tacrolimus may be effective in some dogs.
6. Surgery to debride ulcers and remove sinuses and fistulas may be effective in some dogs. Surgical procedures include excision, chemical cauterization, cryosurgery, deroofing and fulgaration, and laser excision. However, multiple surgeries may be required, and postsurgical complications (recurrence of fistulas, anal stricture formation, fecal incontinence) are common.
7. Concurrent topical hygiene (clip affected area, cleanse daily with 0.025% chlorhexidine rinses, use tail brace to improve aeration) may be helpful, but by themselves are palliative at best.
8. Prognosis is variable. To date, treatment with cyclosporin and surgical excision of residual lesions (if needed) seems to offer the best prognosis for cure.

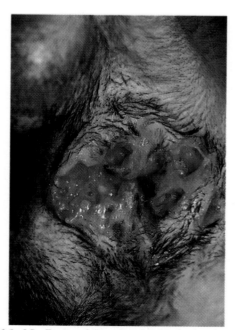

FIGURE 16–19. Perianal Fistulas. Multiple fistulas, severe tissue swelling, and destruction of the perianal tissue.

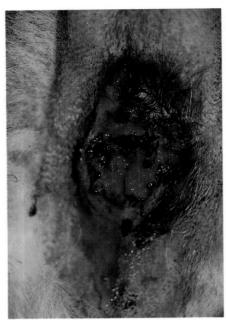

FIGURE 16–20. Perianal Fistulas. Multiple fistulas and severe tissue swelling destroyed the normal anal structure. The purulent exudate is associated with a deep bacterial cellulitis.

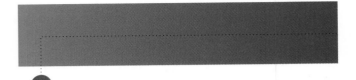

Otitis Externa (Figs. 16–21 to 16–34)

FEATURES

An acute or chronic inflammatory disease of the external ear canal. Its causes are numerous. Predisposing causes of otitis externa make the ear canal susceptible to infection (Table 16–1). Primary factors directly cause otitis externa (Table 16–2). Secondary factors perpetuate otitis externa even if the predisposing and primary causes have been addressed (Table 16–3). Otitis externa is common in dogs and cats.

TABLE 16–1 Predisposing Factors for Otitis Externa

Predisposing Factor	Characteristics	Comments
Conformation	Heavy pendulous ears	May result in decreased air circulation, increased heat, and moisture retention in ear canal. Nidus for infection.
		Especially cocker spaniels, springer spaniels, basset hounds.
	Narrow ear canals	Especially shar-peis, chow chows, English bulldogs.
	Hair in ear canals	Especially poodles.
	Increased glandular tissue	Especially American cocker spaniels, springer spaniels, German shepherds, Labradors.
Maceration (excessive moisture)	Frequent bathing or swimming	May result in ear canal epithelial compromise and loss of stratum corneum barrier function.
	Humid environment	
Iatrogenic irritation	Trauma from cotton swabs	May damage ear canal epithelium.
	Excessive ear cleaning	Chemical irritation and ear canal maceration.

TABLE 16-2 Primary Causes of Otitis Externa

Primary Factor	Characteristics	Comments
Parasites	Otodectes cynotis	Causes approximately 50% of otitis cases in cats and 5–10% of otitis cases in dogs. Dogs and cats can be asymptomatic carriers.
	Demodicosis	Can cause a ceruminous otitis in dogs and cats.
	Sarcoptes scabiei	Typically the ear margin and ventral one-third of outer ear pinna are affected. Otitis externa is not usually a feature of this disease.
	Hard ticks, chiggers	May affect ear pinna and external ear canal.
	Spinous ear ticks	An uncommon cause of otitis externa in dogs and cats.
Foreign bodies		Usually presents as unilateral otitis externa. Look for plant material, dirt, small stones, impacted wax, loose hair, dried medication. Often the inciting foreign body is not identified because it becomes so coated with cerumen that, when removed during ear flushing, it is not recognizable.
Hypersensitivities	Atopy	Otitis externa is seen in 50–80% of atopic dogs. (In 3–5% of these cases, otitis externa is the only symptom.) Usually bilateral otitis.
	Food hypersensitivity	Otitis externa is seen in up to 80% of dogs with food hypersensitives. (In more than 20% of these dogs, otitis externa is the only symptom.)
	Contact dermatitis	Otic medication (i.e., neomycin, propylene glycol) can cause irritant reactions in the ear. Should be suspected any time ear disease worsens significantly while animal is undergoing topical treatment.
Keratinization disorders	Canine primary seborrhea	Bilateral ceruminous otitis. Animals usually have other skin involvement. Cocker spaniels are especially susceptible.
	Facial dermatosis of Persian cats	Bilateral ceruminous otitis externa and seborrheic facial dermatitis. Secondary malasseziasis is common. Uncommon to rare in Persian cats.
	Sebaceous adenitis	May cause dry, scaly ears and mild inflammation. Other skin involvement usually occurs. Rare in dogs, with highest incidence in standard poodles, Akitas, and Samoyeds.
Endocrine	Hypothyroidism	Bilateral ceruminous otitis externa. Most common in middle-aged to older dogs. Usually skin is also involved.
Autoimmune/Immune-mediated diseases		Usually pinna is more involved than ear canals, and other areas of the skin are affected. Lesions may include pustules, vesicles, scales, crusts, erosions, and ulcers.
	Juvenile cellulitis	Acute cellulitis of muzzle and periocular regions, with marked submandibular and prescapular lymphadenomegaly. Exudative otitis externa, fever, and depression may also be present. Uncommon in puppies 3 weeks to 6 months old, with highest incidence in golden retrievers, Labrador retrievers, dachshunds, pointers, and Lhasa apsos.
Inflammatory polyps	Cats	May present as recurrent unilateral otitis externa. Polyps may originate from lining of tympanic cavity, auditory canal, or nasopharynx.
	Dogs	May be sequela to chronic inflammatory or infectious otitis externa.
Neoplasia	Cats	Ceruminous gland adenomas and adenocarcinomas, sebaceous gland adenomas and carcinomas, squamous cell carcinomas, papillomas.
	Dogs	Ceruminous gland adenomas and adenocarcinomas, papillomas, basal cell carcinomas, squamous cell carcinomas.

Otic pruritus or pain is a common symptom of otitis externa. There may be head rubbing, ear scratching, head shaking, aural hematomas, and/or a head tilt, with the affected ear tilted down. An otic discharge that may be malodorous is often present. In acute cases, the inner ear pinna and ear canal are usually erythematous and swollen. The ear canal may also be eroded or ulcerated. Pinnal alopecia, excoriations, and crusts are common. In chronic cases, pinnal hyperkeratosis, hyperpigmentation, and lichenification, as well as ear canal stenosis from fibrosis and/or ossification, are common. Decreased hearing may be noted. Concurrent otitis media should be suspected if otitis externa has been

TABLE 16–3 Secondary Causes of Otitis Externa

Perpetuating Factors	Comments
Bacterial infection	Include *Staphylococcus* spp., *Streptococcus*, *Pseudomonas* spp., *Proteus*, *Escherichia coli*. Recurrent bacterial otitis is often associated with underlying allergies.
Yeast infection	*Malassezia pachydermatis*. Recurrent yeast otitis is often associated with underlying allergies.
Chronic pathologic changes	With chronic inflammation the dermis and subcutis become fibrotic, leading to permanent stenosis of the canal lumen. The auditory cartilage may become calcified. Secretions, desquamated cells, and proliferating microorganisms become trapped. Calcification of ear cartilage is a permanent change that cannot be resolved with medical therapy.
Otitis media	Chronic otitis externa (2 months' duration or longer) often results in extension of the disease into the middle ear. The otitis media can then be a source of recurrent otitis externa.
Overtreatment	The secondary infection has been cleared, but aggressive cleaning and ear medications have been continued too long, leading to a persistent creamy, nonodorous discharge (desquamated cells).
Undertreatment	Client is unwilling or unable to treat the ears appropriately.
Inappropriate treatment	The wrong medication is used and/or the duration of treatment is inadequate, leading to persistent infection or overgrowth of normal microflora.

present for 2 months or longer, even if the tympanic membrane appears to be intact and there are no clinical signs of otitis media (drooping or inability to move the ear or lip, drooling, decreased or absent palpebral reflex, exposure keratitis). Rarely, symptoms of otitis interna (head tilt, nystagmus, ataxia) may be present. Oral examination may reveal pain (severe otitis media), inflammation, or masses (especially polyps in cats). Depending on the underlying cause, concurrent skin disease may be seen.

DIAGNOSIS

1. Based on history and clinical findings.
2. Otoscopic examination—Assess degree of inflammation, stenosis, and proliferative changes, amount and nature of debris and discharge, presence of foreign bodies, ectoparasites, masses, and integrity of tympanic membrane.
3. Microscopy (ear swab)—Look for presence of otodectic and demodectic mites and ova.
4. Cytology (ear swab)—Look for presence of bacteria, yeasts, fungal hyphae, cerumen, leukocytes, and neoplastic cells.
5. Bacterial culture (external and/or middle ear exudate)—Indicated when bacteria are found on cytology in spite of antibiotic therapy or when otitis media is suspected.
6. Radiography (bulla series) or computed tomography (CT) scan—Evidence of bullous involvement (sclerosis, opacifation) is seen in approximately 75% of otitis media cases.
7. Dermatohistopathology (if ear canal mass present)—Indicated when neoplasia is suspected.

TREATMENT AND PROGNOSIS

1. Identify and address the underlying causes of the otitis, if possible.
2. Perform in-hospital ear cleaning and flushing to remove accumulated exudate and debris from the vertical and horizontal ear canals (under sedation or anesthesia if necessary). Repeat procedure q 2–7 days until all debris has been removed. Products that can be used for ear flushing include:

    Water or saline.

    5% Acetic acid (white vinegar) diluted 1:3 in water.

    Povidone-iodine, 0.2–1% solution (may be ototoxic).

    Chlorhexidine, 0.05–0.2% solution (may be ototoxic).

3. Have owner perform at-home ear cleaning q 2–7 days with a ceruminolytic agent (that does not need to be flushed out) to prevent any ear wax and debris from accumulating. Lifelong weekly ear cleaning may be necessary to prevent relapse of otitis. The use of cotton swabs (which may damage the epithelium) is not recommended.
4. Give systemic glucocorticoids if the ear is painful and/or the canal is stenotic from tissue swelling or proliferation. For dogs give prednisone, 0.25–0.5 mg/kg PO q 12 hours for 5–10 days. For cats give prednisone, 0.5–1.0 mg/kg PO q 12 hours for 7–14 days.
5. For ear mites, treat affected and all in-contact dogs and cats. When otic treatments are used, apply a flea spray, powder, or dip q 7 days for 4 weeks or use fipronil spray or spot-on solution twice 2 weeks apart on the body to eliminate any ectopic mites. Effective therapies for ear mites include:

    Otic miticides as per label directions.

    Selamectin, 6–12 mg/kg topically on skin twice 1 month apart (dogs) or once or twice 1 month apart (cats).

Tresaderm or Otomax, 0.125–0.25 ml AU q 12 hours for 2–3 weeks.

Ivermectin, 0.3 mg/kg PO q 7 days for 3–4 treatments or 0.3 mg/kg SC q 10–14 days for two or three treatments.

Fipronil (Frontline Flea Spray), 0.1–0.15 ml AU q 14 days for two or three treatments (based on anecdotal reports).

6. For demodectic otitis, topical treatment with amitraz is usually effective.

Dilute amitraz (1 ml Mitaban or 10 ml Ectodex) in 15 ml mineral oil and instill 2–3 drops AU q 2–3 days, continuing at least 1 week past complete clinical resolution and no evidence of mites on follow-up ear smears.

7. For yeast otitis, antifungal-containing ear preparations should be repackaged into dropper bottle to provide more accurate dosing. Then instill 0.2–0.4 ml (1/4–1/2 dropperful) in the affected ear(s) q 12 hours for at least 2–4 weeks, continued 1–2 weeks beyond complete clinical cure. Effective products include:

Clotrimazole (Otomax, Lotrimin lotion).

Nystatin (Panalog).

Thiabendazole (Tresaderm).

Miconazole (Conofite Lotion).

8. For severe refractory yeast otitis externa and/or otitis media, give systemic antifungal therapy for at least 3–4 weeks, continued 1–2 weeks beyond complete clinical cure. Effective therapies include:

Ketoconazole, 5 mg/kg PO q 12 hours or 10 mg/kg PO q 24 hours with food.

Itraconazole, 5–10 mg/kg PO q 24 hours with food.

9. For bacterial otitis, antibiotic-containing ear preparations should be repackaged into dropper bottle to provide more accurate dosing. Then instill 0.2–0.4 ml (1/4–1/2 dropperful) in the affected ear(s) q 8–12 hours for at least 2–4 weeks, continued 1–2 weeks beyond complete clinical cure. Effective products include:

Gentamycin (Gentocin Otic, Otomax).

Neomycin (Tresaderm, Panalog).

Polymixin B and neomycin (Cortisporin Otic Suspension).

Polymixin E and neomycin) (Coly-Mycin S Otic).

Chloramphenicol (Liquichlor).

Tobramycin (Tobrex Ophthalmic Solution).

Enrofloxacin/silver sulfadiazene (Baytril Otic)

10. For bacterial otitis media use topical and systemic antibiotics, based on culture and sensitivity results, for a minimum of 4 weeks, continued 2 weeks beyond complete clinical cure. Antibiot-

ics that achieve good levels in the ear include:

Ciprofloxacin, 5–15 mg/kg PO q 12 hours.

Enrofloxacin, 10–20 mg/kg PO q 24 hours.

Orbifloxacin, 7.5 mg/kg PO q 24 hours.

Marbofloxacin, 5.5 mg/kg PO q 24 hours.

Ormetoprim-sulfamethoxine, 27.5 mg/kg PO q 24 hours.

Trimethoprim-sulfa, 22 mg/kg PO q 12 hours.

Cephalexin, cephradine, or cefadroxil, 22 mg/kg PO q 8 hours.

Ticarcillin-clavulanic acid, 15–25 mg/kg IV or SC q 6–8 hours.

11. For chronic pseudomonas otitis, use topical and systemic antibiotics for at least 4 weeks, continued 2 weeks beyond complete clinical cure. Select antibiotics based on culture and sensitivity results. Topical agents that may be effective include:

Enrofloxacin (Baytril injectible 22.7 mg/ml), undiluted or diluted 50:50 in water, or propylene glycol, 0.2–0.3 ml instilled q 12 hours.

Amikacin sulfate (Amiglyde V injectable 50 mg/ml), undiluted 0.1–0.2 ml instilled q 12 hours.

Silver sulfadiazine (Silvadene), 0.1% solution (mix 1.5 ml (1/3 tsp) of silvadene cream with 13.5 ml distilled water, or mix 0.1 g silver sulfadiazene powder with 100 ml distilled water) and instill 0.5 ml mixture into ear canal(s) q 12 hours.

Combination 3 ml enrofloxacin (Baytril injectable 22.7 mg/ml) plus 4 mg dexamethasone sodium phosphate plus 12 ml ear cleanser (Epiotic or Dermapet)—instill 0.2–0.4 ml q 12 hours.

Ticarcillin (reconstitute vial as directed, then freeze in TB syringes as 1 ml aliquots. Thaw new syringe each day and keep it refrigerated). Instill 0.2–0.3 ml into affected ear(s) q 8 hours.

Tris EDTA solution (with/without gentamycin, 3 mg/ml, or amikacin, 9 mg/ml), 0.4 ml instilled q 8–12 hours.

12. For swimmer's ear, prevent maceration of ear canals by prophylactically instilling a drying agent after dog gets wet (swimming, bathing) or two or three times per week in very humid climates. Effective products include:

Otic domeboro.

Hydrocortisone/Burows solution (HB 101).

Clear-X Drying Solution.

Ear flushes which contain astringents.

Over-the-counter ear products for human swimmer's ear.

13. For allergic otitis, long-term management in-

cludes controlling the underlying allergies, resolving any secondary bacterial and yeast otitis, and instituting weekly ear cleaning. In animals whose underlying allergies cannot be identified or completely controlled, the judicious use of steroid-containing otic preparations as infrequently as needed may prevent otitis flare-ups. Topical products that may be effective include:

Hydrocortisone/Burows solution (HB 101) instilled q 1–2 days.

Fluocinolone/DMSO (Synotic) instilled q 2–7 days.

Betamethasone (Otomax, Triotic) instilled q 2–7 days.

Dexamethasone (Tresaderm) instilled q 2–7 days.

14. For ceruminous otitis, identify and correct the underlying cause if possible, resolve any secondary bacterial and yeast otitis, and institute weekly ear cleaning. If the underlying cause cannot be identified or corrected, the judicious use of topical otic preparations containing an astringent and/or steroid q 1–7 days, as infrequently as possible, is often helpful in controlling cerumen accumulation.

15. For chronic proliferative otitis, aggressive medical therapy is needed. Institute weekly ear cleaning. For bacterial/yeast otitis externa and media, use long-term (minimum 4 weeks) systemic and topical antibiotics and/or antifungal medications continued 2 weeks beyond complete clinical resolution of the infection. To reduce tissue proliferation give prednisone, 0.5 mg/kg PO q 12 hours for 2 weeks, then give 0.5 mg/kg PO q 24 hours for 2 weeks, followed by 0.5 mg/kg PO q 48 hours for 2 weeks. These ears rarely return to complete normalcy, so long-term maintenance therapy with steroid-containing otic preparations, as described for allergic otitis, is almost always necessary.

16. Indications for surgery include:

Surgical excision of resectable otic polyps or masses.

Lateral ear canal resection aids in ventilation and drainage, and allows easier application of medication, but rarely results in cure because a large amount of diseased tissue is still present.

Vertical ear canal ablation if proliferative changes are present in the vertical canal but the horizontal canal is not affected.

Total ear canal ablation and bulla osteotomy is indicated when there is otitis media and severe, irreversible proliferation and/or calcification of the horizontal and vertical auricular cartilages.

17. Prognosis is variable, depending on whether the underlying cause can be identified and corrected, and on the chronicity and severity of the otitis externa.

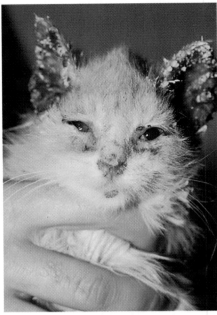

FIGURE 16–21. Otitis Externa. Severe erosive, crusting lesions on the ear pinnae of a young kitten with food allergy. The ocular and nasal erosions were associated with a rhinotracheitis viral infection.

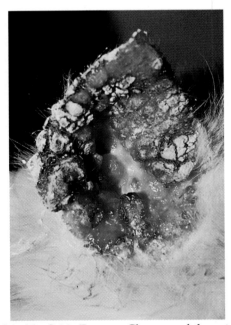

FIGURE 16–22. Otitis Externa. Close-up of the cat in Figure 16–21. Cutaneous crusts, erosions, and tissue swelling completely occluded the ear canal. The gray clumps within the crusts were medicinal clay that had been packed into the ear by the owner.

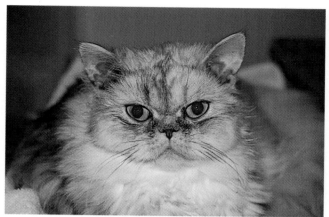

FIGURE 16–23. Otitis Externa. Bilateral otitis with a brown, waxy exudate in a food-allergic Persian cat.

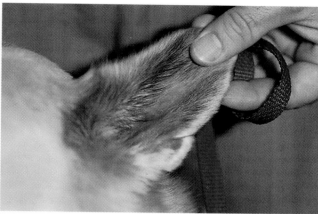

FIGURE 16–25. Otitis Externa. Erythema of the ear pinnae caused by an acute allergic reaction.

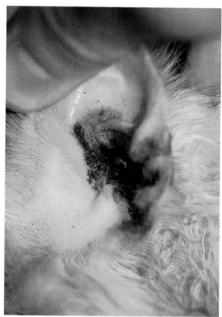

FIGURE 16–24. Otitis Externa. Close-up of the cat in Figure 16–23. The brown, waxy exudate was caused by a secondary yeast infection.

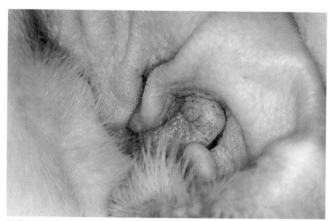

FIGURE 16–26. Otitis Externa. The erythema and cobblestone texture of the ear pinnae are characteristic of chronic allergic otitis. Note that there is no active secondary infection.

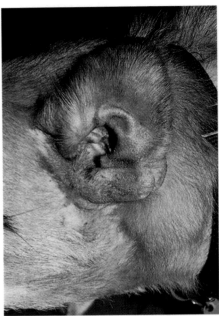

FIGURE 16–27. Otitis Externa. The hyperpigmentation and lichenification of the ear base and pinnae were caused by chronic allergy. There is no active secondary infection.

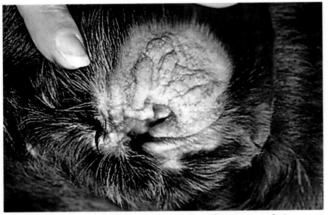

FIGURE 16–28. Otitis Externa. Lichenification and tissue proliferation caused by a secondary *Malassezia* infection associated with allergic otitis.

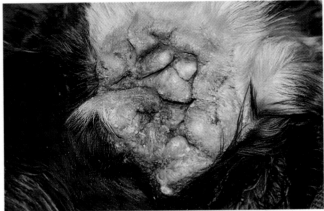

FIGURE 16–29. Otitis Externa. Severe tissue proliferation and calcification of the ear canal in an adult cocker spaniel.

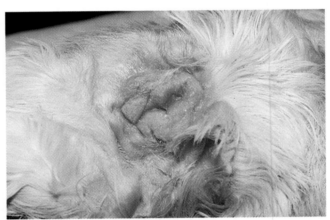

FIGURE 16–30. Otitis Externa. Severe inflammation and tissue proliferation at the site of a previous total ear canal ablation. The secondary infection and underlying allergy had not been identified and controlled.

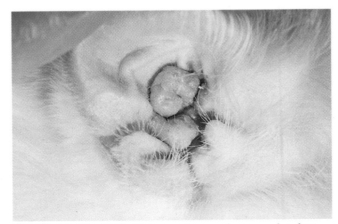

FIGURE 16–31. Otitis Externa. A nasopharyngeal polyp protruding from the ear canal of a cat. (Courtesy of S. Sanderson)

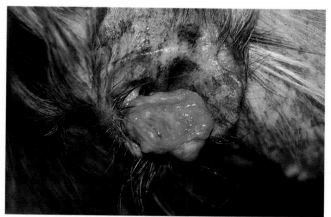

FIGURE 16-32. Otitis Externa. This squamous cell carcinoma was the cause of a chronic recurrent bacterial otitis. Once the tumor was removed and the secondary infections were treated, the otitis resolved.

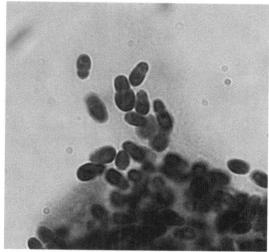

FIGURE 16-34. Otitis Externa. Cytology demonstrating *Malassezia*.

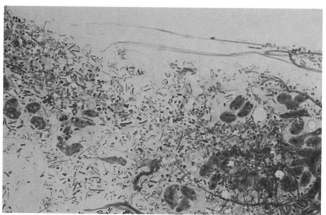

FIGURE 16-33. Otitis Externa. Otic cytology demonstrating the mixed bacterial population and inflammatory cells.

Suggested Readings

Bedford PGC. 1999. Diseases and Surgery of the Canine Eyelid, pp. 559–561. In Gelatt KN (ed). Veterinary Ophthalmology. Lippencott Williams and Wilkins, Philadelphia, PA.

Diseases of Eyelids, Claws, Anal Sacs, and Ear Canals, pp. 956–989. In Scott DW, Miller WH Jr, and Griffin CE. 1995. Muller & Kirk's Small Animal Dermatology. Ed. 5. W.B. Saunders, Philadelphia, PA.

Ellisonn GW. 1995. Treatment of Perianal Fistulas in Dogs. J Am Vet Med Assoc. 206: 1680–1682.

Foster A, DeBoer D. 1998. The Role of *Pseudomonas* in Canine Ear Disease. Compen Cont Edu Pract Vet. 20(8): 909–918.

Griffin C. 2000. *Pseudomonas* Otitis Therapy. In Bonagura JD (ed). Kirk's Current Veterinary Therapy, XII, Small Animal Practice. W.B. Saunders, Philadelphia, PA.

Griffiths LG, Sullivan M, and Borland WW. 1999. Cyclosporin as the Sole Treatment for Anal Furunculosis: Preliminary Results. J Small Anim Pract. 40: 569–572.

Mathews KA, Ayres SA, Tano CA, Riley SM, Sukhiani HR, and Adams C. 1997. Cyclosporin Treatment of Perianal Fistulas in Dogs. Can Vet J. 38: 39–41.

Mathews KA and Sukhiani HR. 1997. Randomized Controlled Trial of Cyclosporine for Treatment of Perianal Fistulas. J Am Vet Med Assoc. 211: 1249–1253.

McKeever PJ. 1996. Otitis Externa. Compend Cont Edu Pract Vet. 18: 759–773.

McKeever PJ and Globus H. 1995. Canine Otitis Externa, pp 647–658. In Bonagura JD (ed). Kirk's Current Veterinary Therapy, XII, Small Animal Practice. W.B. Saunders, Philadelphia, PA.

Merchant SR. 1997. Medically Managing Chronic Otitis Externa and Media. Vet Med. 518–534.

Mueller RS, Friend S, Shipstone MA, and Burton G. 2000. Diagnosis of Canine Claw Disease—a Prospective Study of 24 Dogs. Vet Dermatol. 11: 133–142.

Nutall T. 1998. Use of Ticarcillin in the Management of Canine Otitis Externa Complicated by *Pseudomonas aeruginosa*. J Small Anim. Pract. 39: 165–168.

Plumb DC. 1999. Veterinary Drug Handbook. Ed. 3. Iowa State University Press, Ames, IA.

Rosychuk RAW. 1995. Diseases of the Claw and Claw Fold, pp 641–646. In Bonagura JD (ed). Kirk's Current Veterinary Therapy, XII, Small Animal Practice. W.B. Saunders, Philadelphia, PA.

Scott D and Miller WH Jr. 1992. Disorders of the Claw and Clawbed in Dogs. Compend Cont Edu Pract Vet. 14: 1448–1459.

17

Neoplastic and Non-neoplastic Tumors

KIMBERLY LOWER

- **Intracutaneous Cornifying Epithelioma** (keratoacanthoma, infundibular keratinizing acanthoma)

- **Squamous Cell Carcinoma**

- **Basal Cell Tumors**

- **Hair Follicle Tumors**

- **Sebaceous Gland Tumors**

- **Perianal Gland Tumors**

- **Apocrine Gland Tumors**

- **Fibropruritic Nodule**

- **Fibroma**

- **Fibrosarcoma**

- **Nodular Dermatofibrosis**

- **Hemangioma**

- **Hemangiosarcoma**

- **Hemangiopericytoma**
- **Lipoma**
- **Mast Cell Tumor**
- **Nonepitheliotropic Lymphoma** (lymphosarcoma)
- **Epitheliotropic Lymphoma** (mycosis fungoides)
- **Plasmacytoma**
- **Histiocytoma**
- **Cutaneous Histiocytosis**
- **Systemic Histiocytosis**
- **Malignant Histiocytosis**
- **Melanoma**
- **Transmissible Veneral Tumor**
- **Collagenous Nevus**
- **Follicular Cyst—Epidermal Inclusion Cyst** (infundibular cyst)
- **Cutaneous Horn**
- **Skin Tag** (fibrovascular papilloma)
- **Calcinosis Circumscripta**

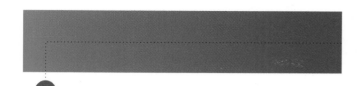

Intracutaneous Cornifying Epithelioma (keratoacanthoma, infundibular keratinizing acanthoma)
(Figs. 17–1 and 17–2)

FEATURES

A benign neoplasm of hair follicle origin. Uncommon in dogs, with the highest incidence in Norwegian elkhounds.

Single to multiple (as many as 40–50) firm to fluctuant, well-circumscribed dermal or subcutaneous nodules ranging from 0.5 to 4 cm in diameter. The nodules may be partially alopecic. Most have variably sized, dilated central pores that open directly to the skin surface from which gray-brown keratinaceous material can be expressed. Large pores may contain a hard, horn-like keratin plug (cutaneous horn). Deep dermal and subcutaneous tumors usually do not have pores. Lesions can be anywhere on the body but are most common on the dorsal neck, back, and tail.

DIAGNOSIS

1. Cytology (usually nondiagnostic)—Amorphous cellular debris and mature cornified squamous epithelial cells with cholesterol crystals.
2. Dermatohistopathology—Lamellated, keratin-filled cavity (which may contain a pore to the skin surface) lined with stratified epithelial cells. Focal rupture may release keratin into the dermis, inciting a pyogranulomatous reaction in surrounding tissue.

TREATMENT AND PROGNOSIS

1. Surgically excise the tumor(s) if one to few in number.
2. For multiple lesions, treatment with etretinate, 1 mg/kg PO q 24 hours, may be effective in some dogs but is no longer available. A new retinoid, Acitretin, may also be effective (0.5–1 mg/kg PO q 24 hours). A good response should be seen after 3 months of treatment. Animals that respond usually require lifelong therapy to maintain remission.
3. Following surgical removal, prognosis for cure is good for dogs with one lesion, but dogs with more than one tumor are likely to develop new tumors at other sites. Prognosis for resolving multiple lesions with medical treatment is fair to good. These tumors are benign and do not metastasize.

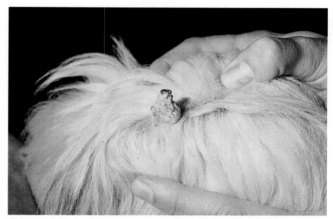

FIGURE 17–1. Intracutaneous Cornifying Epithelioma. This cutaneous horn developed over several weeks from an underlying intracutaneous cornifying epithelioma. (Courtesy of D. Angarano)

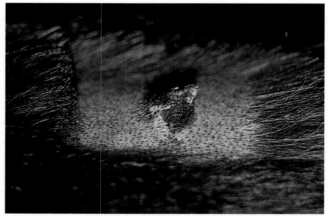

FIGURE 17–2. Intracutaneous Cornifying Epithelioma. An intracutaneous cornifying epithelioma and cutaneous horn on the lateral thorax of a young adult German shepherd.

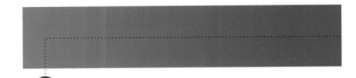

Squamous Cell Carcinoma
(Figs. 17–3 to 17–8)

FEATURES

A malignant neoplasm of keratinocytes. It occurs most often in thinly haired, nonpigmented, sun-damaged skin and may be preceded by solar dermatosis. The incidence of solar-induced squamous cell carcinoma is highest in geographic areas with intense sunlight. Common in dogs, with the highest incidence in older dogs. Common in cats, with the highest incidence in older, white cats.

Dogs. Usually a single proliferative and/or ulcerative lesion. Proliferative tumors often have a cauliflower-like appearance, vary in size, and may ulcerate and bleed easily. Crater-like ulcerative lesions begin as crusted-over, shallow erosions that deepen. Tumors occur most commonly on the trunk, limb, digit, scrotum, nose, and/or lip. Nail bed tumors usually involve one digit but can be multiple, especially in large black-coated dogs. Affected digits are typically swollen and painful and have a misshapen or absent nail.

Cats. Proliferative, crusting, and/or ulcerative lesion(s) that may bleed easily. The tumors most commonly involve white-haired skin on the ear pinnae, nose, and/or eyelids.

DIAGNOSIS

1. Cytology (often nondiagnostic)—Cells may vary from poorly differentiated small, round epithelial cells with basophilic cytoplasm to more mature, large, angular, nonkeratinized epithelial cells with abundant cytoplasm, retained nuclei, and perinuclear vacuolation.
2. Dermatohistopathology—Irregular masses of atypical keratinocytes that proliferate downward and invade the dermis. Neoplastic cells are in direct contact with dermis without a basal cell layer.

TREATMENT AND PROGNOSIS

1. The treatment of choice is complete surgical excision.
2. For lesions that cannot be excised, radiotherapy or electron beam radiation therapy may be effective.
3. Alternatively, intralesional chemotherapy (cisplatin, 5-fluorouracil), hyperthermia, or photodynamic therapy may be effective in some cases.

4. To prevent new solar-induced lesions from developing, avoid future ultraviolet light exposure.
5. Prognosis for dogs is variable, depending on the degree of differentiation and the site of the lesion. Most tumors are locally invasive and slow to metastasize, although squamous cell carcinoma of the nail bed tends to be more aggressive and may metastasize more readily. Prognosis in cats depends on the degree of differentiation, with well-differentiated tumors having a better prognosis than poorly differentiated ones.

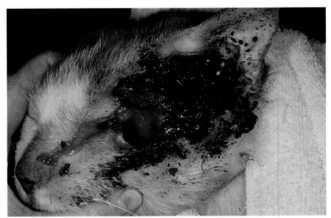

FIGURE 17–3. Squamous Cell Carcinoma. Severe tissue destruction and tumor proliferation on the face and periocular tissue of a cat. (Courtesy of S. McLaughlin)

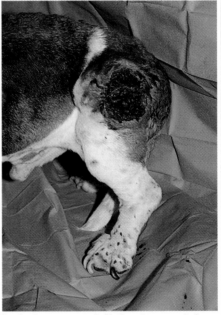

FIGURE 17–4. Squamous Cell Carcinoma. A large, ulcerated tumor on the hip of an aged basset hound.

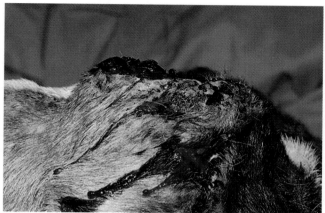

FIGURE 17–5. Squamous Cell Carcinoma. Close-up of the dog in Figure 17–4. This raised tumor has a deep ulcer with tissue destruction forming a central crater.

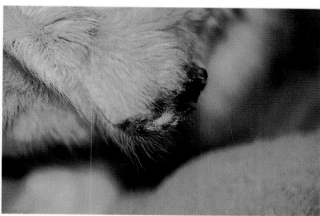

FIGURE 17–7. Squamous Cell Carcinoma. Necrosis and crusting of the distal ear margin of an adult white cat.

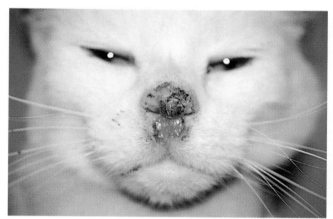

FIGURE 17–6. Squamous Cell Carcinoma. Erythema, ulceration, and crusting on the nose of an adult white cat. The initial lesions were typical of solar dermatosis.

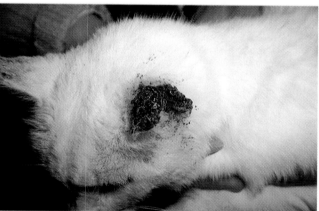

FIGURE 17–8. Squamous Cell Carcinoma. This tumor was allowed to progress, causing the eventual destruction of the entire ear pinnae.

Basal Cell Tumors (Figs. 17–9 and 17–10)

FEATURES

A neoplasm of epidermal or adnexal epithelial basal cells that may be benign (basal cell tumor) or malignant (basal cell carcinoma). Basal cell tumors are uncommon in cats, with Siamese, Himalayan, and Persian cats possibly predisposed. Basal cell carcinomas are common in cats and uncommon in dogs, with the highest incidence in older animals.

A benign basal cell tumor (cats) is usually a solitary, well-circumscribed, 1–2 cm in diameter, raised, round, firm nodule that may be pigmented, alopecic, and/or ulcerated. The tumor is most commonly found on the head, neck, or dorsum of the back.

A basal cell carcinoma (dogs and cats) is usually a solitary well-circumscribed, firm to fluctuant, round, raised, 0.5–10 cm in diameter tumor that is often alopecic, pigmented, and ulcerated. It tends to occur on the head, neck, or thorax.

DIAGNOSIS

1. Cytology—Basal cell tumors contain small, fairly uniform, round to cuboidal epithelial cells with scant basophilic cytoplasm, which may be arranged in groups or ribbons. Basal cell carcinomas may show standard criteria for malignancy, but can be difficult to differentiate cytologically from a benign tumor.
2. Dermatohistopathology

Basal Cell Tumor. Well-circumscribed, nonencapsulated, often multilobulated intradermal mass composed of cords or nests of hyperchromatic cells with scant cytoplasm which resemble basal cells. The tumor may be melanotic or cystic.

Basal Cell Carcinoma. In cats, the tumor appears as irregular dermal masses of multiple epithelial cell aggregates of varying size and shape embedded in a fibrous stroma which may infiltrate subcutis and muscle. The tumor may have cystic or adnexal differentiation and may be melanotic. In dogs, the tumor tends to have angular dermal islands of atypical epithelial cells, which contain central areas of squamous differentiation.

TREATMENT AND PROGNOSIS

1. Surgical excision of the tumor is curative.
2. If surgery is otherwise contraindicated, observation without treatment is reasonable because these tumors tend to be benign.
3. Prognosis is good. Basal cell tumors are benign, and basal cell carcinomas are of low-grade malignancy and very rarely metastasize.

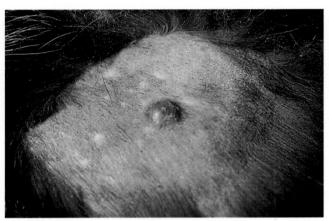

FIGURE 17–9. Basal Cell Tumors. This pigmented nodule on the trunk of an adult cat is typical of this tumor.

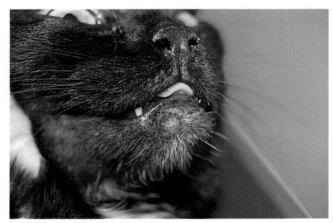

FIGURE 17–10. Basal Cell Tumors. A pigmented nodule on the chin of an adult cat.

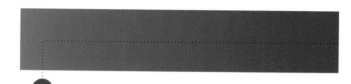

Hair Follicle Tumors (Figs. 17–11 to 17–14)

FEATURES

Common, usually benign neoplasms of germinal hair follicle cells that are classified on the basis of the direction of adnexal differentiation.

Trichoblastoma • Usually a benign neoplasm of cells originating from primitive hair germ epithelium. Common in dogs and cats, with the highest incidence in middle-aged to older animals. In dogs, poodles and cocker spaniels may be predisposed. The tumor is a 1–2 cm solitary, firm, dome-shaped, alopecic nodule that occurs most commonly on the head or neck in dogs. In cats, the tumor most frequently is found on the cranial half of the trunk.

Trichoepithelioma • Usually a benign tumor of cells which differentiate toward hair follicle and shaft structures. Uncommon in dogs and cats, with the highest incidence in middle-aged to older animals. Bassett and coon hounds, golden retrievers, setters, spaniels, and Persians cats may be predisposed. The tumor is usually a solitary (but often multiple in bassett hounds), alopecic, firm, white to gray, multilobulated mass which may be ulcerated. The tumor may range in size from 1 mm to 2 cm in diameter. It is often located on the trunk or limb in dogs and on the tail or limb in cats.

Tricholemmoma • A benign tumor of cells which differentiate toward the outer root sheath of hair follicles. Rare in dogs and cats, with the highest incidence in middle-aged to older animals. In dogs, Afghans may be predisposed. The tumor is a 1–7 cm diameter, firm, circumscribed nodule that is often found on the head or neck.

Trichofolliculoma • A benign hair follicle tumor, which may actually be a follicular and/or pilosebaceous hamartoma rather than a true neoplasm. Rare in dogs and cats. The tumor is a solitary, dome-shaped nodule which may have a central depression or opening containing hair or sebaceous material.

Dilated pore of Winer • A benign hair follicle tumor or cyst. Uncommon in older cats. The tumor is a solitary, firm mass or cyst (<1 cm) that has a keratin-filled central opening. The keratin may form a cutaneous horn. The lesion is most commonly found on the head or neck.

Pilomatrixoma • A benign neoplasm arising from cells of hair bulb/matrix. Uncommon in dogs and very rare in cats, with the highest incidence in middle-aged to older animals. In dogs, Kerry blue terriers, poodles, Bedlington terriers, schnauzers, and Old English sheepdogs may be predisposed. The tumor is a solitary, firm, plaque-like to dome-shaped dermal or subcutaneous mass. The nodule is well circumscribed, often alopecic, and may be calcified. It ranges in size from 1 to 10 cm in diameter and occurs most commonly on the trunk.

DIAGNOSIS

1. Cytology (often nondiagnostic)—Hair follicle tumors are characterized by mature cornified squamous epithelial cells and amorphous cellular debris. Small, uniform, basal-type epithelial cells can occasionally be seen.
2. Dermatohistopathology

Trichoblastoma • Tumor appearance can vary from winding and branching ribbons of small basophilic basaloid cells in a fibrous stroma to well-circumscribed nodules of lobular groups of basaloid cells with peripheral palisading. There is no epidermal contiguity.

Trichoepithelioma • Multiple well-circumscribed, nonencapsulated nodules of basal cells (which resemble primitive follicular bulbs) with central cystic areas of keratinization. Cysts are lined with basal to squamous epithelial cells.

Tricholemmoma • Well-circumscribed dermal nodules made up of small polyhedral cells with clear cytoplasm due to increased glycogen content, similar to outer root sheath cells of the hair bulb. There may be small central foci of keratinization. Tumor follicles are surrounded by thick, homogeneous basement membrane.

Trichofolliculoma • Well-circumscribed, unencapsulated dermal nodule comprised of a cystic, dilated primary follicular structure surrounded by a tree-like pattern of secondary follicles and sebaceous glands in various stages of maturation.

Dilated pore of Winer • Markedly dilated, cup-shaped follicle lined with hyperplastic squamous epithelium and filled with laminated keratin, which protrudes through the central pore.

Pilomatrixoma • Well-circumscribed dermal/subcutaneous tumor composed of multiple cystic structures lined by basaloid cells which resemble hair matrix cells. Cysts contain masses of eosinophilic keratinized ghost or shadow cells, which are often calcified.

TREATMENT AND PROGNOSIS

1. Observation without treatment is reasonable because these tumors are benign.
2. Surgical excision of the tumor is curative.
3. Prognosis is good. Hair follicle tumors are not locally invasive, do not metastasize, and rarely recur following surgical removal.

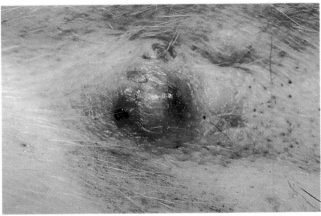

FIGURE 17–13. Hair Follicle Tumors. Close-up of the dog in Figure 17–12. The pigmentation and ulceration of this nodule are typical of trichoepitheliomas.

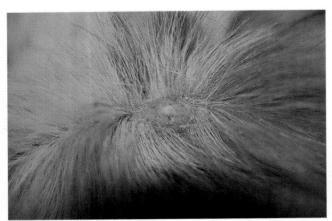

FIGURE 17–11. Hair Follicle Tumors. This small, nonpigmented nodule is typical of follicular tumors.

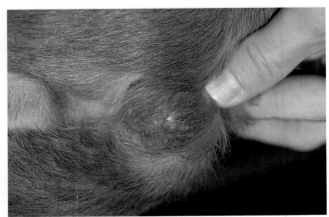

FIGURE 17–14. Hair Follicle Tumors. This large cyst on the ventral thorax of an aged hound mix was associated with a follicular tumor.

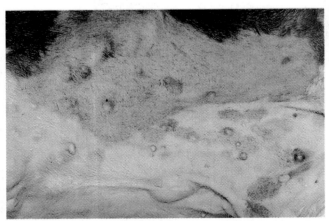

FIGURE 17–12. Hair Follicle Tumors. Multiple trichoepitheliomas on the flank of an aged basset hound.

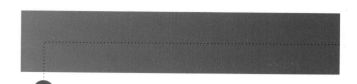

Sebaceous Gland Tumors (Figs. 17–15 to 17–18)

FEATURES

Nodular sebaceous hyperplasia, sebaceous epitheliomas, and sebaceous adenomas are benign tumors of sebocytes. They are common in older dogs, with the highest incidence in poodles, cocker spaniels, miniature schnauzers, and terriers. Benign sebaceous gland tumors are uncommon in older cats, with Persian cats possibly predisposed. Sebaceous gland carcinomas are malignant tumors of sebocytes. They are rare in older dogs and cats. In dogs, cocker spaniels are predisposed.

Benign sebaceous gland tumors are usually firm, elevated, wart- or cauliflower-like growths ranging from a few millimeters to several centimeters in diameter. They may be yellowish or pigmented, alopecic, oily, or ulcerated. Sebaceous epitheliomas and sebaceous adenomas usually occur as a solitary tumor, whereas sebaceous hyperplastic nodules can be multiple. A sebaceous carcinoma tends to be a solitary, <4 cm diameter, intradermal nodule. The tumor may be alopecic, erythematous, and/or ulcerated. It may invade into the subcutis. Sebaceous gland tumors occur most commonly on the trunk, legs, head, and eyelids.

DIAGNOSIS

1. Cytology

   Nodular sebaceous hyperplasia and adenomas • Cells exfoliate in groups and appear similar to normal sebaceous cells, with foamy pale blue cytoplasm and small, dark nuclei.

   Sebaceous epithelioma • Small, fairly uniform, sometimes melanotic epithelial cells with small numbers of sebaceous cells.

   Sebaceous carcinoma • Extremely basophilic basal-type cells with nuclear and cellular pleomorphism.

2. Dermatohistopathology

   Nodular sebaceous hyperplasia • Multiple enlarged, mature sebaceous lobules with a single peripheral layer of basaloid germinal cells and a central duct. No mitotic figures are seen.

   Sebaceous adenoma • Similar to sebaceous hyperplasia, but with increased numbers of basaloid germinal cells and immature sebocytes. There is

low mitotic activity and loss of organization around the central duct. Cystic degeneration (acellular eosinophilic material) is frequently present in center of lobules.

Sebaceous epithelioma • Multiple lobules of basaloid epithelial cells interspersed with reactive collagenous tissue and secondary inflammation. Fairly high mitotic activity. There may be scattered areas of sebaceous differentiation, squamous metaplasia, or melanization.

Sebaceous carcinoma • Poorly defined lobules of large epithelial cells with varying degrees of sebaceous differentiation and cytoplasmic vacuolation. Nuclei are large, and mitotic activity is moderately high. Lobules are divided by connective tissue trabeculae.

TREATMENT AND PROGNOSIS

1. For benign sebaceous gland tumors, observation without treatment is reasonable.
2. Surgical excision of benign sebaceous tumors is usually curative.
3. For dogs with cosmetically unacceptable multiple benign sebaceous tumors that are too numerous to excise, treatment with isotretinoin, 1–2 mg/kg PO q 24 hours, may induce lesion regression. Response is gradual, but benefit should be seen within 45 days. Etretinate, 1 mg/kg PO q 24 hours, may be effective in some dogs but is no longer available. A new retinoid, Acitretin, may also be effective (0.5–1 mg/kg PO q 24 hours).
4. For sebaceous adenocarcinomas, the tumor should be completely excised surgically.
5. Prognosis is good. Benign sebaceous gland tumors are not locally invasive, do not metastasize, and rarely recur following surgical removal. Sebaceous gland carcinomas are locally infiltrative and occasionally involve regional lymph nodes, but distant metastases are uncommon.

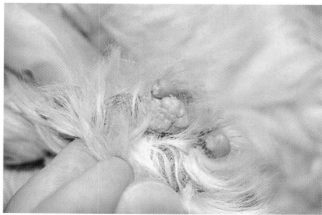

FIGURE 17–15. Sebaceous Gland Tumors. This sebaceous adenoma on the toe of an aged cocker spaniel demonstrates the characteristic cauliflower appearance.

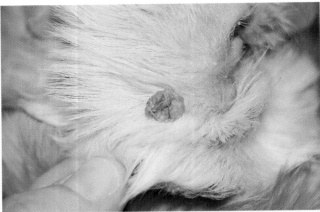

FIGURE 17–16. Sebaceous Gland Tumors. The sebaceous adenoma on the ear pinnae of this aged cocker spaniel had persisted for several years, with little progression.

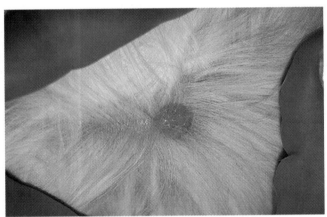

FIGURE 17–17. Sebaceous Gland Tumors. This small, alopecic plaque with a cobblestone texture is typical of sebaceous hyperplasia.

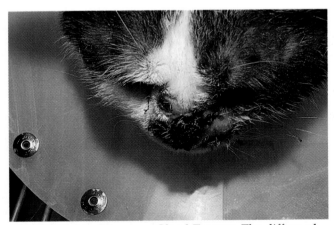

FIGURE 17–18. Sebaceous Gland Tumors. The diffuse ulceration and tissue destruction on the nose of this aged cat were caused by a sebaceous adenocarcinoma.

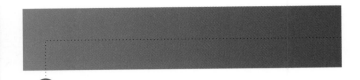

Perianal Gland Tumors

(Figs. 17–19 and 17–20)

FEATURES

Benign or malignant neoplasm arising from the circumanal (hepatoid) gland cells, possibly secondary to androgenic stimulation. Perianal adenomas are common in older intact male dogs and uncommon in female and neutered male dogs. Perianal gland adenocarcinomas are uncommon in older dogs and occur with equal frequency in intact and neutered male and female dogs.

Adenomas are solitary or multiple slow-growing, firm, round to lobular dermal nodules of variable size which may ulcerate. The tumors usually occur adjacent to the anus but may also occur on the tail, tail head, perineum, or prepuce. They can also appear as a diffuse bulging ring of tissue around the anus. Perianal adenocarcinomas appear similar to adenomas but tend to grow rapidly and ulcerate.

DIAGNOSIS

1. Cytology—Clumps of large, round to polyhedral hepatoid epithelial cells containing abundant pale blue cytoplasm, round to oval nuclei, and one or two nucleoli. A second population of smaller epithelial "reserve cells" is also commonly present. Adenocarcinomas cannot be reliably differentiated cytologically from adenomas.
2. Dermatohistopathology—Lobules of polygonal cells resembling hepatocytes, with abundant, finely vacuolated eosinophilic cytoplasm and central round nuclei. A rim of basal reserve cells surrounds each lobule. Squamous metaplasia may occur. Mitotic figures are rarely seen in adenomas. Adenocarcinomas appear similar to adenomas but have increased anisocytosis/anisokaryosis and frequent mitotic figures.

TREATMENT AND PROGNOSIS

1. For perianal adenomas in intact male dogs, castration is the treatment of choice.
2. Surgical excision is also indicated for recurrent or ulcerative adenomas in male dogs and for adenomas occurring in female or neutered male dogs.
3. For perianal adenocarcinomas, complete surgical excision is the treatment of choice. Radiation therapy or chemotherapy may slow the progression of incompletely excised tumors.

4. Prognosis for perianal adenomas is good, as tumors are benign and do not usually recur after castration. Prognosis for perianal adenocarcinomas is fair to guarded, as recurrence with local invasion following surgery or metastasis may occur.

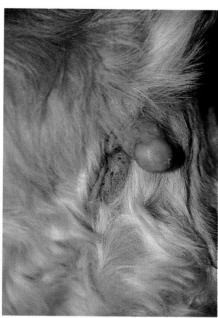

FIGURE 17–19. Perianal Gland Tumors. An elongated, pedunculated tumor on the perianal tissue of an aged cocker spaniel.

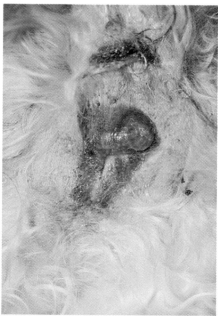

FIGURE 17–20. Perianal Gland Tumors. An ulcerated nodule on the perianal tissue of an aged cocker spaniel.

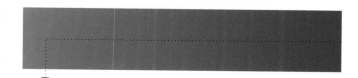

Apocrine Gland Tumors

(Figs. 17–21 and 17–22)

FEATURES

Apocrine gland adenomas and carcinomas can arise from apocrine gland or apocrine duct cells. Uncommon in older dogs and cats, with Siamese cats possibly predisposed to carcinomas.

Dogs. An apocrine gland adenoma is usually a solitary, raised, alopecic, circumscribed dermal or subcutaneous tumor. It may have a bluish tint and may be firm, cystic, or ulcerated. The tumor ranges in size from 0.5 to 4 cm in diameter. An apocrine gland carcinoma is usually a solitary growth that may appear clinically similar to an adenoma or may be a poorly circumscribed, rapidly enlarging, infiltrative plaque or erosive mass. Apocrine gland tumors are most common on the head, neck, legs, and axillary or inguinal areas.

Cats. Apocrine adenomas and carcinomas are clinically indistinguishable from each other. Both are usually solitary, well-circumscribed, raised, firm or cystic tumors ranging from a few millimeters to a few centimeters in diameter. The tumor may have a bluish tinge, may be ulcerated, and is most common on the head, neck, abdomen, and leg.

DIAGNOSIS

1. Cytology (often nondiagnostic)

Apocrine adenoma • Few medium, round, or oval cells with eccentric nuclei and large intracytoplasmic droplets of secretory product.

Apocrine carcinoma • Groups of small basophilic epithelial cells with scant blue cytoplasm. Most cells may appear fairly uniform, with a subpopulation of larger, more pleomorphic cells.

2. Dermatohistopathology

Apocrine adenoma • Circumscribed dermal nodule comprised of multiple cysts lined by columnar epithelium and containing clear or eosinophilic fluid. Proliferation of epithelium may result in intraluminal papillary growths. Mitotic activity is low.

Apocrine carcinoma • Architecturally similar to adenoma. However, nuclear pleomorphism and increased mitotic activity are present, and neoplastic cells may be locally invasive and incite a marked scirrhous reaction.

TREATMENT AND PROGNOSIS

1. The treatment of choice is complete surgical excision.
2. Prognosis for apocrine adenomas is good, as surgical removal is curative. Prognosis for apocrine carcinomas is variable. Carcinomas may be locally invasive and recur following surgery, with up to 20% of them having lymphatic involvement and/or distant metastasis.

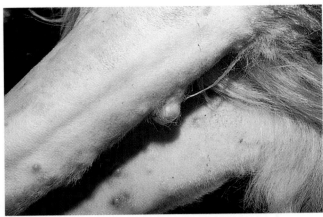

FIGURE 17–22. Apocrine Gland Tumor. An apocrine gland cyst on the leg of an adult dog.

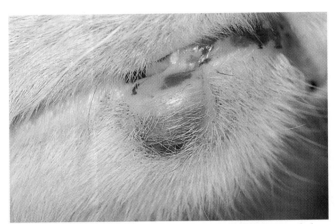

FIGURE 17–21. Apocrine Gland Tumor. The blue nodule on the lower lip of this adult cat is typical of apocrine tumors.

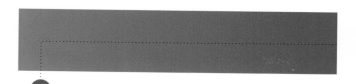

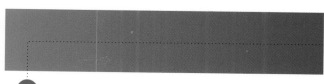

Fibropruritic Nodule (Fig. 17–23)

FEATURES

Although the pathogenesis is unknown, fibropruritic nodules occur only in dogs with chronic flea bite hypersensitivity. Uncommon in dogs, with the highest incidence in older dogs, especially pure-breed and mixed-breed German shepherds.

Multiple alopecic, firm, 0.5–2 cm diameter sessile or pedunculated nodules develop that may be erythematous or hyperpigmented. Lesions may be smooth or hyperkeratotic and occasionally ulcerate. They are found along the dorsal lumbosacral area in dogs with chronic flea bite hypersensitivity.

DIAGNOSIS

1. Usually based on history and clinical findings.
2. Dermatohistopathology—Severely hyperplastic, sometimes ulcerated epidermis overlying dermal fibrosis and inflammation which may obscure adnexal structures.

TREATMENT AND PROGNOSIS

1. Treat the underlying flea bite hypersensitivity.
2. Cosmetically unacceptable lesions can be surgically excised.
3. Prognosis is good. Although fibropruritic nodules rarely resolve spontaneously, they are benign lesions that do not affect the dog's quality of life. Flea control should prevent further lesions from developing.

Fibroma (Fig. 17–24)

FEATURES

A benign neoplasm of dermal or subcutaneous fibroblasts. Uncommon in middle-aged to older cats and dogs, with the highest incidence in boxers, golden retrievers, and Doberman pinschers.

The tumor is usually a solitary, well-circumscribed, firm dermal or subcutaneous mass. It may be dome-shaped or pedunculated and range from 1 to 5 cm in diameter. The overlying epidermis may be alopecic and atrophic. The tumor can occur anywhere on the body but is most common on the limb or flank.

DIAGNOSIS

1. Cytology (often nondiagnostic)—Few uniform spindle cells with round or oval dark nuclei containing one or two small nucleoli.
2. Dermatohistopathology—Well-circumscribed dermal or subcutaneous nodule of mature fibroblasts with abundant collagen production, which displaces normal dermal adnexal structures. Mitotic figures are very rare.

TREATMENT AND PROGNOSIS

1. Observation without treatment is reasonable because these tumors are benign.
2. Cosmetically unacceptable lesions can be surgically excised.
3. Prognosis is good. Fibromas are benign, noninvasive, and nonmetastatic.

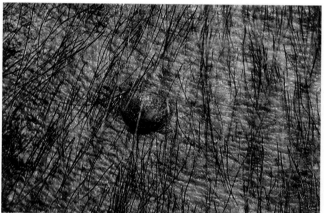

FIGURE 17–23. Fibropruritic Nodule. This small, pigmented nodule developed on the lumbar region of an adult schnauzer with severe flea allergy dermatitis.

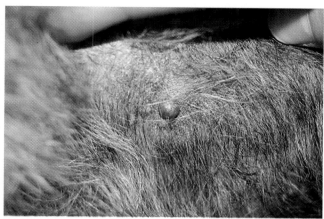

FIGURE 17–24. Fibroma. A small, nonpigmented nodule on the lateral thorax of an aged schnauzer.

Fibrosarcoma (Figs. 17–25 to 17–28)

FEATURES

A malignant neoplasm arising from dermal or subcutaneous fibroblasts. In dogs it occurs spontaneously. In cats, it may arise spontaneously, be induced by feline sarcoma virus (FeSV), or be vaccine-induced. Uncommon in dogs, with the highest incidence in older animals, especially golden retrievers and Doberman pinschers. Common in cats, with the highest incidence in animals <5 years old for FeSV-induced lesions and in older cats for tumors not associated with FeSV.

Dogs. Usually a solitary, firm subcutaneous or dermal mass that is poorly circumscribed, nodular to irregular in shape, and ranges from 1 to 15 cm in diameter. Its surface may be alopecic and ulcerated. The tumor often arises on the head or proximal limb and may be fixed to the underlying tissue.

Cats. Rapidly infiltrating dermal or subcutaneous mass(es) that are firm, poorly circumscribed, nodular to irregular in shape, and range from 0.5 to 15 cm in diameter. The tumors may be alopecic and ulcerated. FeSV-associated fibrosarcomas are usually multicentric, whereas those not caused by FeSV are usually solitary. Tumors most commonly involve the trunk, distal limbs, and ear pinnae. Vaccination-induced fibrosarcomas arise at previous vaccination sites.

DIAGNOSIS

1. Feline leukemia test—Positive for cats with FeSV-induced tumors.
2. Cytology (often nondiagnostic)—Cells may be fusiform, oval, or stellate and may contain multiple nuclei. Cellular pleomorphism, nuclear size, and cytoplasmic basophilia vary with degree of tumor differentiation.
3. Dermatohistopathology—Haphazardly interlacing bundles of plump spindle cells, which are infiltrative and nonencapsulated. Mitotic activity, numbers of multinucleated cells, and collagen production are variable. In vaccination-induced lesions, there is also peripheral lymphoid and granulomatous inflammation with epithelioid macrophages and multinucleated histiocytic giant cells, which contain an intracytoplasmic, amorphous basophilic material (presumed to be adjuvant).

TREATMENT AND PROGNOSIS

1. Treatment of choice for solitary tumors is wide surgical excision or amputation of the affected limb.
2. Radiation therapy is often used pre- or postoperatively in cases where complete excision is difficult.
3. Prognosis for solitary tumors is variable. Factors influencing prognosis include tumor size, histologic grade, location, and depth of invasion. Small, superficial low-grade tumors or tumors on extremities treated with amputation have a better prognosis, whereas large, deep, truncal, vaccine-induced or high-grade tumors have a poor prognosis and usually recur locally after surgery. Distant metastasis is uncommon.
4. Prognosis for multiple FeSV-induced tumors is poor. Surgery is ineffective for cats with tumors induced by FeSV due to multicentric nature of disease.

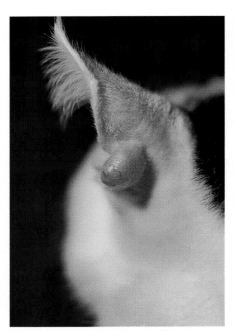

FIGURE 17–25. Fibrosarcoma. A small fibrosarcoma on the ear pinnae of an adult cat.

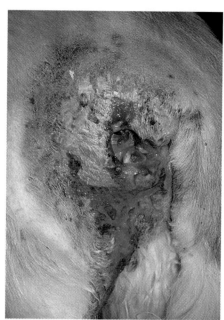

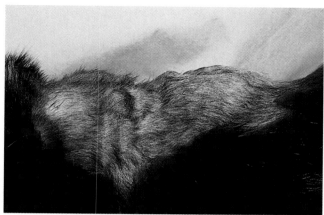

FIGURE 17–28. Fibrosarcoma. The multiple tumors on the back of this cat developed following surgical removal of the original primary tumor. Wide surgical margins were not achieved, and the aggressive, invasive nature of this tumor caused its recurrence.

FIGURE 17–26. Fibrosarcoma. This large area of ulceration with draining tracts on the lateral hip of this aged golden retriever was caused by an invasive fibrosarcoma.

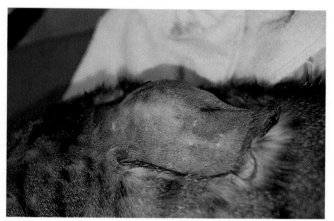

FIGURE 17–27. Fibrosarcoma. A large vaccine-induced tumor on the dorsal thorax of an adult cat.

Nodular Dermatofibrosis

(Figs. 17–29 and 17–30)

FEATURES

A syndrome in which the appearance of dermal fibrotic nodules is associated with concurrent renal cystic disease. Though its exact pathogenesis is unknown, an autosomal dominant mode of inheritance has been postulated in affected German shepherd dogs. Rare in dogs, with the highest incidence in middle-aged to older German shepherds.

The disease is characterized by the sudden appearance of multiple cutaneous nodules. Nodules are firm, well circumscribed, dermal to subcutaneous, and range from several millimeters to 4 cm in diameter. The skin overlying the nodules may be thickened, hyperpigmented, alopecic, or ulcerated. The lesions are most commonly found on the limbs, head, and ears. Concurrent unilateral or bilateral renal epithelial cysts, cystadenomas, or cystadenocarcinomas are present.

DIAGNOSIS

1. Dermatohistopathology—Circumscribed dermal or subcutaneous mass composed of structurally normal collagenous bundles.
2. Radiography, ultrasonagraphy, or exploratory laparotomy—Renal cystic disease.

TREATMENT AND PROGNOSIS

1. The treatment of choice is nephrectomy if only one kidney is involved. Unfortunately, the renal disease is usually bilateral.
2. The prognosis is poor, as the underlying renal cystic disease is invariably fatal. Affected dogs should not be bred.

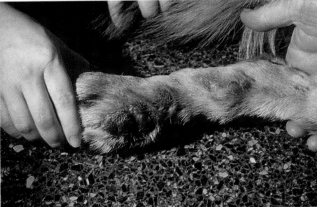

FIGURE 17–29. Nodular Dermatofibrosis. Multiple alopecic, hyperpigmented nodules on the distal limbs of an adult German shepherd. (Courtesy of D. Angarano)

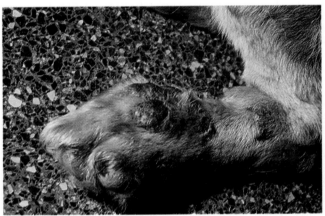

FIGURE 17–30. Nodular Dermatofibrosis. Close-up of the dog in Figure 17–29. Multiple alopecic, hyperpigmented nodules. (Courtesy of D. Angarano)

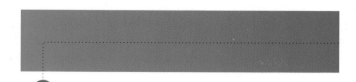

Hemangioma

FEATURES

A benign tumor of blood vessel endothelial cells. Uncommon in dogs, with the highest incidence in older dogs, especially those with lightly pigmented and sparsely haired ventrums, suggesting ultraviolet light exposure as a causal factor. Rare in cats, with the highest incidence in older, male cats.

Usually a solitary, rounded, well-circumscribed, firm to fluctuant, raised, bluish to reddish-black dermal or subcutaneous growth ranging from 0.5 to 4 cm in diameter. Hemangiomas of the glabrous skin can appear as clusters or plaque-like aggregates of blood vessels. Tumors are more common on the trunk and limbs (dogs) and on the head and limbs (cats).

DIAGNOSIS

1. Cytology (often nondiagnostic)—Mostly blood with a few normal-appearing endothelial cells, which may be oval, stellate, or spindle cells with moderate blue cytoplasm and a medium-sized, round nucleus with one or two small nucleoli.
2. Dermatohistopathology—Well-circumscribed dermal or subcutaneous nodule formed by dilated blood-filled spaces lined by relatively normal-appearing, flattened endothelial cells. No mitotic figures are seen.

TREATMENT AND PROGNOSIS

1. Observation without treatment is reasonable, as these tumors are benign.
2. Surgical excision is curative.
3. To prevent new solar-induced lesions from developing, avoid future ultraviolet light exposure.
4. Prognosis is good. Hemangiomas are benign, not invasive, and do not recur following surgical excision. However, malignant transformation of solar-induced lesions may occasionally occur.

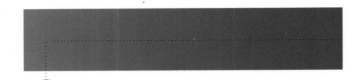

Hemangiosarcoma (Fig. 17–31)

FEATURES

A malignant neoplasm of blood vessel endothelial cells which can involve the skin as a primary or metastatic site. Tumors of ventral glabrous skin may be solar-induced in short-coated, lightly pigmented dogs. Uncommon in older dogs and cats.

The tumors can occur in the dermis (especially of the ventral glabrous skin) or subcutaneous tissue. They may appear clinically similar to hemangiomas (bluish to reddish-black plaques or nodules <4 cm in diameter) or can present as poorly defined subcutaneous spongy dark red to black masses up to 10 cm in diameter. Alopecia, bleeding, and ulceration are common. Hemostatic abnormalities such as thrombocytopenia and disseminated intravascular coagulation may occur. The tumors occur most commonly on the limbs and trunk in dogs and on the head, ears, and limbs in cats.

DIAGNOSIS

1. Cytology (may be nondiagnostic)—Mostly blood with neoplastic endothelial cells, which vary in appearance from normal to large, pleomorphic cells with basophilic cytoplasm and prominent nucleoli.
2. Dermatohistopathology—Dermal or subcutaneous infiltrative mass of atypical pleomorphic, hyperchromatic spindle cells with a tendency to form vascular channels. Mitotic rate is variable.
3. Affected animals should be screened for internal neoplasia and metastasis (radiography/ultrasound).

TREATMENT AND PROGNOSIS

1. Radical surgical excision is usually adequate for dermal tumors.
2. Adjunctive chemotherapy may be indicated for tumors that involve structures deeper than the dermis.
3. Prognosis for strictly dermal tumors is good, while prognosis for subcutaneous tumors is poor. Local recurrence or metastasis of primary skin hemangiosarcoma may occur.

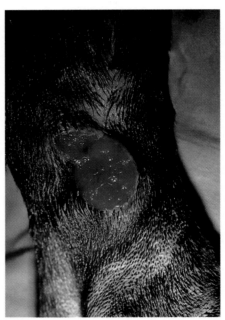

FIGURE 17–31. Hemangiosarcoma. An ulcerated proliferative tumor on the distal limb of a dog. (Courtesy of L. Schmeitzel)

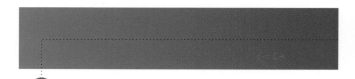

Hemangiopericytoma (Figs. 17–32 and 17–33)

FEATURES

A neoplasm arising from vascular pericytes. Common in older dogs, with the highest incidence in large breeds. Rare in cats.

Usually a solitary, well-circumscribed, firm to fatty, multinodular dermal to subcutaneous tumor ranging from 2–25 cm in diameter. The tumor may be fixed to the underlying tissue, and its surface may be hyperpigmented, alopecic, and/or ulcerated. It is most commonly found on the stifle, elbow, thorax, and flank.

DIAGNOSIS

1. Cytology (may be nondiagnostic)—Tumor cell morphology varies from spindle-shaped to stellate, with wispy light to medium blue cytoplasm and a round or oval nucleus with uniformly stippled chromatin and one or two prominent nucleoli.
2. Dermatohistopathology—Multilobular unencapsulated subcutaneous or dermal mass consisting of small spindle and polygonal cells with few mitotic figures arranged in sheets and concentric whorls around a central vascular lumen.

TREATMENT AND PROGNOSIS

1. The treatment of choice is radical surgical excision of the tumor or amputation of the affected limb if complete excision is not possible.
2. Adjunctive radiation therapy may prolong the disease-free interval for animals with incompletely resected tumors.
3. Prognosis is variable. Tumors may recur locally after surgery, but metastasis is rare.

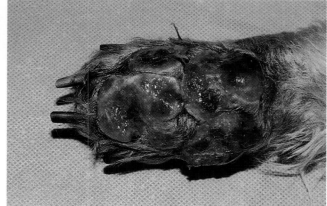

FIGURE 17–32. Hemangiopericytoma. This alopecic, ulcerated tumor on the dorsal surface of the paw is typical of hemangiopericytomas.

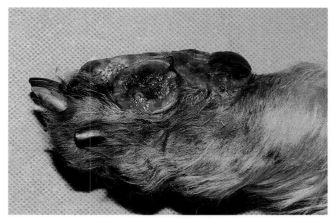

FIGURE 17–33. Hemangiopericytoma. Close-up of the dog in Figure 17–32. The ulcerated proliferative tumor extends above the foot.

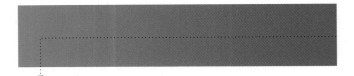

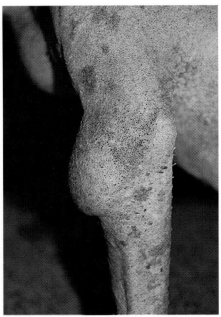

Lipoma (Figs. 17–34 to 17–37)

FEATURES

A benign neoplasm of subcutaneous (occasionally dermal) lipocytes. Common in middle-aged to older dogs. Uncommon in older cats, with Siamese cats possibly predisposed.

Tumors are single to multiple movable, well-circumscribed, dome-shaped to multilobulated, soft to firm subcutaneous masses ranging from 1 to 30 cm in diameter. Less commonly, the tumors are large, soft, poorly circumscribed masses which infiltrate the underlying muscle, tendons, and fascia (infiltrative lipoma). Lipomas most often occur on the thorax, abdomen, and limbs.

FIGURE 17–34. Lipoma. This soft tumor developed over several years on the front leg of this aged dog.

DIAGNOSIS

1. Cytology—Aspirates are grossly oily and often dissolve in alcohol-containing stains, leaving behind clear areas with variable numbers of lipocytes containing pyknotic nuclei, which are compressed to the cell membrane by intracellular fat globules.
2. Dermatohistopathology—Lipomas are well-circumscribed nodules composed of solid sheets of mature lipocytes which may have a capsule of mature fibrous tissue. Mitotic figures are not present. Infiltrative lipomas are composed of sheets of mature lipocytes, which spread along fascial planes into muscle bundles and connective tissue.

TREATMENT AND PROGNOSIS

1. For small, well-circumscribed tumors, observation without treatment is reasonable.
2. Surgical excision is the treatment of choice for cosmetically unacceptable or rapidly enlarging lipomas.
3. For infiltrative lipomas the treatment of choice is early aggressive surgery, which can be followed by radiation therapy or chemotherapy if excision is incomplete.
4. Although the intralesional injection of 10% calcium chloride solution will result in tumor regression, it is not recommended because it causes tissue necrosis.
5. Prognosis is good for well-encapsulated lipomas. Prognosis is guarded for infiltrative lipomas, which often recur after surgery. Infiltrative lipomas frequently cause muscle and connective tissue destruction, but they are not metastatic.

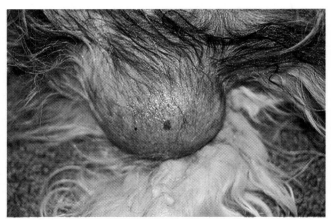

FIGURE 17–35. Lipoma. A large lipoma on the ventral chest of an aged schnauzer.

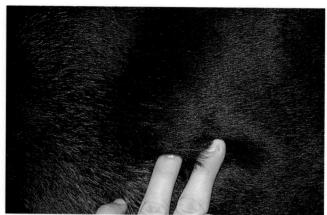

FIGURE 17–36. Lipoma. The lipoma on the lateral thorax of this aged mixed-breed Labrador was difficult to visualize but was easily palpated.

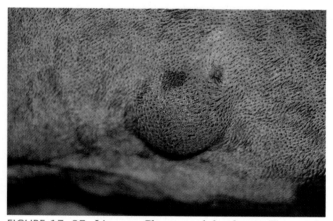

FIGURE 17–37. Lipoma. Close-up of the dog in Figure 17–36. The clipped fur coat allows the tumor to be visualized more easily.

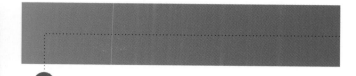

Mast Cell Tumor (Figs. 17–38 to 17–43)

FEATURES

A malignant tumor arising from mast cells. Common in dogs and cats, with the highest incidence in older animals. Boxers, pugs, Boston terriers, and Siamese cats are predisposed.

Dogs. Tumors are usually solitary but may be multiple. Their appearance is variable and may include dermal or subcutaneous edema, papules, nodules, or pedunculated masses ranging from a few millimeters to several centimeters in diameter. The tumors may be poorly or well circumscribed and soft or firm. They may be alopecic, ulcerated, erythematous, hyperpigmented, and/or flesh-colored. They are most commonly found on the perineum, trunk, hind legs, and genitalia. Concurrent gastric or duodenal ulcers and/or coagulopathy may be seen secondary to release of mast cell granules containing histamine and heparin.

Cats. Usually a solitary intradermal nodules which may be erythematous, alopecic, or ulcerated and ranges in size from 0.2 to 3 cm. The tumor may be diffusely swollen and infiltrative. In young adult Siamese cats, multiple clusters of subcutaneous nodules ranging in size from 0.5 to 1 cm have been described (histiocytic mast cell tumors). Mast cell tumors are most commonly found on the head and neck. Concurrent systemic abnormalities are rarely seen.

DIAGNOSIS

1. Cytology—Many round cells with round nuclei and basophilic intracytoplasmic granules which stain variably, depending on degree of tumor differentiation. Eosinophils may also be seen in association with tumor cells.
2. Dermatohistopathology—Nonencapsulated, infiltrative sheets or densely packed cords of round cells with central nuclei and abundant cytoplasm with variably basophilic granules. Eosinophils may be numerous. Histiocytic mast cell tumors of young Siamese cats are poorly granulated and contain lymphoid aggregates.
3. Affected animals should be screened for internal metastasis (radiography, ultrasound, +/− liver, spleen, and/or bone marrow aspirate).

TREATMENT AND PROGNOSIS

1. For solitary tumors, wide surgical excision (minimum 3 cm margins) is the treatment of choice.
2. Radiation therapy can prolong the disease-free interval of animals with incompletely excised tumors.
3. Intralesional triamcinolone and deionized water have been used to treat selected animals with incompletely resected or nonresectable tumors, with variable results.
4. For disseminated lesions in dogs, treatment with prednisone, 2 mg/kg/day PO for 2 weeks, then 1 mg/kg/day for 2 weeks, then 1 mg/kg every other day indefinitely, may induce temporary remission.
5. Additional palliative therapy for metastatic disease includes use of H2 blockers (cimetidine, famotidine, ranitidine) to decrease gastrointestinal (GI) effects from hyperhistaminemia.
6. Chemotherapy is generally of limited value in disseminated disease; however CCNU (lomustine), vinblastine, and vincristine may be partially effective.
7. Prognosis in dogs is variable. The most important prognostic factor is the histologic grade of tumor; complete excision of grade I (well-differentiated) tumor is usually curative, whereas dogs with grade III tumors (poorly differentiated) often succumb to local recurrence or metastasis within months. Tumor location is also prognostically important: tumors in the inguinal and perineal regions, on the muzzle, and in the oral or nasal cavity frequently metastasize, whereas appendicular tumors have a better prognosis. Primary cutaneous mast cell tumors in cats are usually benign, and excision is curative. Histiocytic mast cell tumors in young Siamese cats may regress spontaneously.

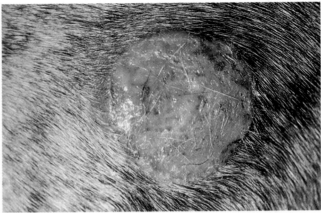

FIGURE 17–39. Mast Cell Tumor. A circumscribed, ulcerated tumor on the trunk of a dog. (Courtesy of D. Angarano)

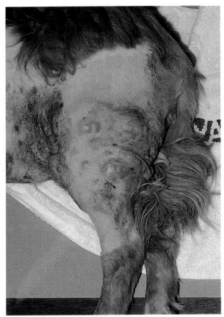

FIGURE 17–40. Mast Cell Tumor. Multiple tumors on the distal limb of an aged golden retriever. The purple appearance was caused by bruising of the tissue.

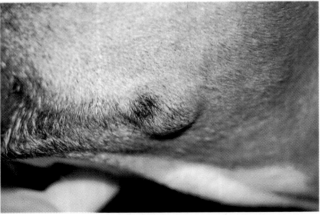

FIGURE 17–38. Mast Cell Tumor. A large nodule on the ventral mandible of an adult boxer.

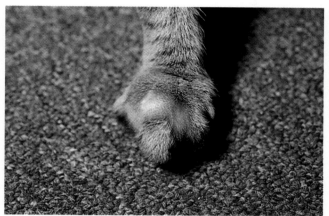

FIGURE 17–41. Mast Cell Tumor. The diffuse swelling of this cat's foot was caused by a mast cell tumor. Previous attempts to remove the tumor surgically failed.

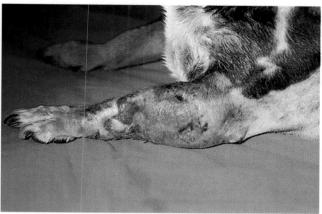

FIGURE 17–43. Mast Cell Tumor. Close-up of the dog in Figure 17–42. The forelimb has swollen due to angioedema caused by the released histamine. (Courtesy of D. Angarano)

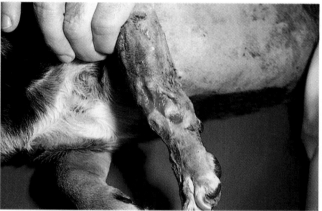

FIGURE 17–42. Mast Cell Tumor. Multiple nodules and ulcerations on the distal limb. Just after this picture was taken, the limb began to swell due to histamine release during diagnostic palpation of the tumor (see Figure 17–43). (Courtesy of D. Angarano)

Nonepitheliotropic Lymphoma

(lymphosarcoma) (Figs. 17–44 to 17–47)

FEATURES

A malignant neoplasm that may arise from B or T lymphocytes. Uncommon in dogs and cats, with the highest incidence in older animals.

Usually there are multiple firm dermal to subcutaneous nodules that may be alopecic and ulcerated. The tumors occur most frequently on the trunk, head, and extremities. Oral mucosal involvement is rare. Concurrent signs of systemic involvement are common.

DIAGNOSIS

1. Cytology—Numerous neoplastic lymphocytes.
2. Dermatohistopathology—Nodular to diffuse infiltration of dermis and/or subcutis by sheets of homogeneous neoplastic lymphocytes, which do not involve glands or hair follicles.
3. Affected animals should be screened for internal metastasis.

TREATMENT AND PROGNOSIS

1. For solitary lesions, surgical excision or radiation therapy is the treatment of choice.
2. For disseminated disease, combination chemotherapy may induce temporary remission.
3. Treatment with isotretinoin, 3–4 mg/kg/day PO for dogs or 10 mg/cat q 24 hours, may result in partial improvement.
4. Prognosis is poor. Tumors are highly malignant and metastasize readily.

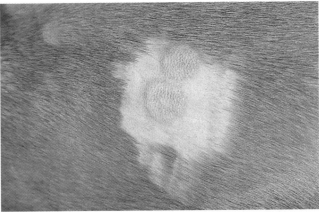

FIGURE 17–45. Nonepitheliotropic Lymphoma. Close-up of the dog in Figure 17–44. The area has been clipped to provide better visualization of the tumors. (Courtesy of J. MacDonald)

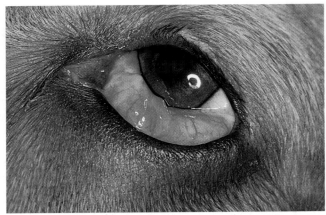

FIGURE 17–46. Nonepitheliotropic Lymphoma. The conjunctival tissue was infiltrated with neoplastic lymphocytes. (Courtesy of J. MacDonald)

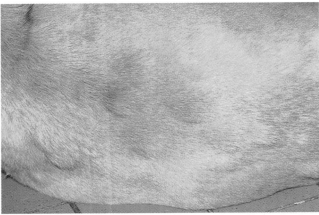

FIGURE 17–44. Nonepitheliotropic Lymphoma. Multiple nodules on the dorsum of an aged Labrador. (Courtesy of J. MacDonald)

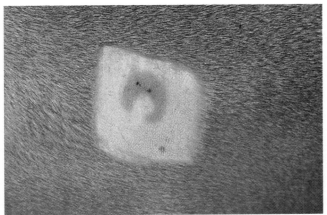

FIGURE 17–47. Nonepitheliotropic Lymphoma. A C-Shaped tumor on the trunk of an aged dog. (Courtesy of D. Angarano)

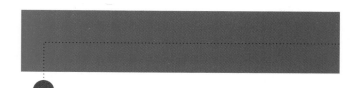

Epitheliotropic Lymphoma
(mycosis fungoides) (Figs. 17–48 to 17–53)

FEATURES

A malignant neoplasm which arises from T lymphocytes. Uncommon in dogs and cats, with the highest incidence in older animals.

Dogs. The lesions may include single to multiple plaques and/or nodules, which range from a few millimeters to several centimeters in diameter. There may be generalized erythema, alopecia, scaling, and pruritus. Mucocutaneous depigmentation and ulceration, and/or ulcerative stomatitis, may be present. The disease is usually slowly progressive, and in chronic cases peripheral lymphadenomegaly and signs of systemic involvement may be seen.

Cats. There may be pruritic and exfoliative erythroderma with alopecia and crusting. Erythematous plaques or nodules may occur, especially on the head and neck. Oral and mucocutaneous involvement is less common than in the dog.

DIAGNOSIS

1. Cytology—Abundant round neoplastic lymphoid cells which are often histiocytic, with basophilic cytoplasm and pleomorphic, indented to lobular nuclei.
2. Dermatohistopathology—Lichenoid band of pleomorphic neoplastic lymphocytes which infiltrate the superficial dermis and surface follicular and sweat gland epithelia. Neoplastic cells may occur within small intraepidermal vesicles (Pautrier's microabcesses).
3. Affected animals should be screened for internal metastasis.

TREATMENT AND PROGNOSIS

1. For solitary lesions, surgical excision or radiation therapy (especially electron beam therapy) is the treatment of choice.
2. Topical nitrogen mustard is helpful in some cases, but there is a high incidence of allergic/irritant contact dermatitis in humans exposed to the drug. Nitrogen mustard should not be used in cats due to common side effects of bone marrow suppression and GI upset.
3. Treatment with combination chemotherapy (prednisone and cytotoxic drugs) is only minimally effective. Anecdotally, L-asparaginase or CCNU (Lomustine) may be more effective than other drugs.
4. Treatment with isotretinoin, 3–4 mg/kg/day PO for dogs or 10 mg/cat q 24 hours, may improve clinical signs in some animals.
5. Supplementation with safflower oil (which contains high levels of linoleic acid), 3 ml/kg PO mixed with food twice weekly, may improve clinical signs in some animals.
6. Regardless of the treatment, the prognosis is poor, with most animals surviving for less than 1 year after diagnosis.

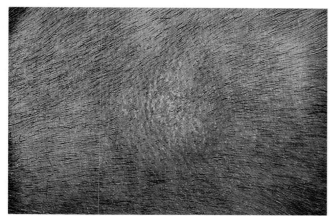

FIGURE 17–48. Epitheliotropic Lymphoma. This erythematous, scaling plaque is typical of mild tumor lesions.

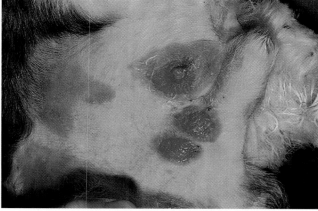

FIGURE 17–49. Epitheliotropic Lymphoma. Close-up of the dog in Figure 17–48. More severe erythematous, ulcerated lesions.

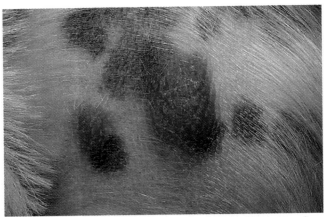

FIGURE 17–50. Epitheliotropic Lymphoma. Close-up of the dog in Figures 17–48 and 17–49. Erythematous nodules on the trunk.

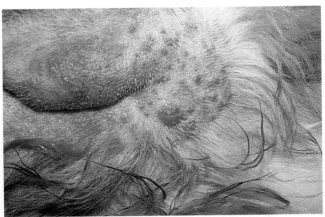

FIGURE 17–52. Epitheliotropic Lymphoma. Multiple erythematous papules and nodules. Note the similarity to lesions typical of folliculitis.

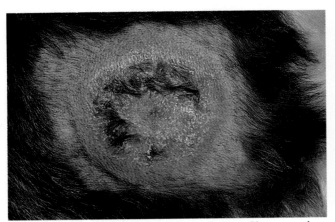

FIGURE 17–51. Epitheliotropic Lymphoma. Close-up of the dog in Figures 17–48 to 17–50. This large, erythematous, alopecic tumor has a central crater-like depression.

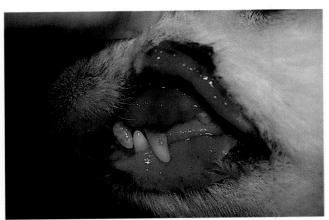

FIGURE 17–53. Epitheliotropic Lymphoma. The mucosal ulceration and tissue proliferation are typical of epitheliotropic lymphoma. Note the similarity to autoimmune skin disease.

Plasmacytoma (Figs. 17–54 to 17–57)

FEATURES

A neoplasm of plasma cell origin. Uncommon in dogs, with the highest incidence in older animals. Cocker spaniels may be predisposed. Very rare in cats.

The lesion is usually a solitary, well-circumscribed, soft or firm, occasionally pedunculated dermal nodule. The tumor may be ulcerated and erythematous and is usually 1–2 cm in diameter. The tumor is most often found in the external ear canal, on the lip, and on the digit. Digital lesions may be ulcerated and bleed easily. Concurrent multiple myeloma is rare in dogs but may be more common in cats.

DIAGNOSIS

1. Cytology—many round cells which may appear like typical plasma cells, with perinuclear halos, or may be less plasmacytoid, with a moderate amount of dark blue cytoplasm and round, eccentric nuclei with stippled chromatin. Binucleate and multinucleate cells are common.
2. Dermatohistopathology—Well-circumscribed round cell tumor with cells arranged in small, solid lobules by a delicate stroma. Marked cellular pleomorphism, occasional binucleate cells, and a moderate to marked mitotic index are present. Recognizable plasma cells with perinuclear halos are visible mostly on the periphery.

TREATMENT AND PROGNOSIS

1. The treatment of choice is surgical excision.
2. Prognosis is good in dogs. Local recurrence and metastasis are rare. In cats, prognosis is guarded. Although few cases have been described in cats, systemic disease or metastasis to regional lymph nodes was reported in two of three cases.

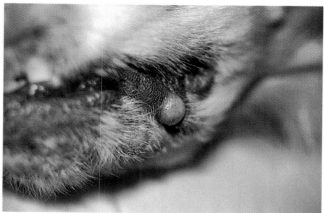

FIGURE 17–54. Plasmacytoma. Small, alopecic nodule on the lower lip of a mixed-breed adult dog.

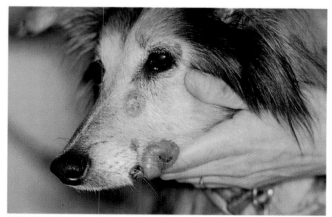

FIGURE 17–55. Plasmacytoma. Multiple alopecic, erythematous tumors on the face of an aged Shetland sheepdog.

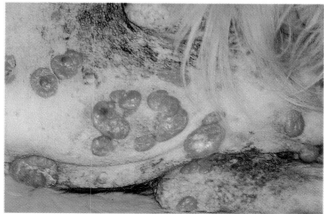

FIGURE 17–56. Plasmacytoma. Close-up of the dog in Figure 17–55. Multiple alopecic, erythematous, cauliflower-shaped tumors on the trunk.

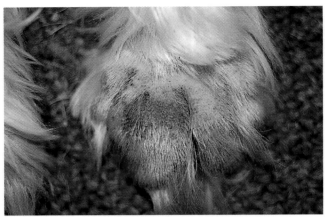

FIGURE 17–57. Plasmacytoma. Diffuse swelling on the toe of an adult dog caused by the infiltration of neoplastic plasma cells.

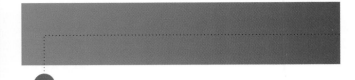

Histiocytoma (Figs. 17–58 to 17–61)

FEATURES

A benign neoplasm of mononuclear cells derived from epidermal Langerhans cells. Common in dogs, with the highest incidence in young dogs <4 years old. Rare in cats.

Usually a solitary, rapidly growing, firm, well-circumscribed, raised dermal nodule. The tumor is erythematous, may be ulcerated, and is up to 3 cm in diameter. It occurs most commonly on the head, ear pinna, and limb.

DIAGNOSIS

1. Cytology—Large round cells with a moderate amount of pale blue, finely granular cytoplasm and round or kidney bean-shaped nuclei with lacey chromatin, multiple indistinct nucleoli, and occasional mitotic figures. Aspirates from regressing lesions will also contain lymphocytes.
2. Dermatohistopathology—Circumscribed, dense dermal infiltrative sheets of homogeneous histiocytes. Mitotic figures may be seen, and lymphocytic infiltration is common. Older lesions often contain multifocal areas of necrosis.

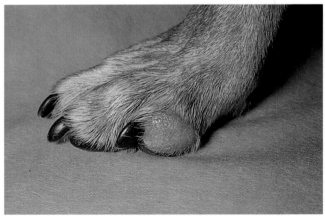

FIGURE 17–58. Histiocytoma. The alopecic, erythematous tumor on the foot of this young dog is typical of cutaneous histiocytomas. (Courtesy of D. Angarano)

TREATMENT AND PROGNOSIS

1. Observation without treatment is reasonable because most lesions regress spontaneously within 3 months.
2. Surgical excision is curative for lesions which do not regress spontaneously.
3. Prognosis is good.

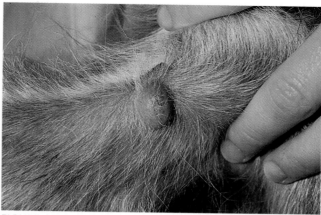

FIGURE 17–61. Histiocytoma. The alopecic, erythematous tumor on the distal limb of this young dog is typical of this neoplasia. (Courtesy of D. Angarano)

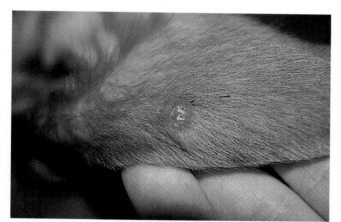

FIGURE 17–59. Histiocytoma. A small, alopecic, erythematous nodule on the ear pinnae of a young adult dog.

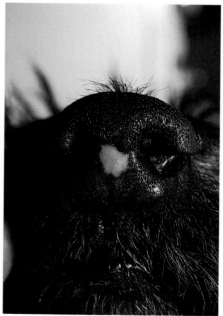

FIGURE 17–60. Histiocytoma. A depigmented, erythematous macule on the nose of an adult Scottish terrier.

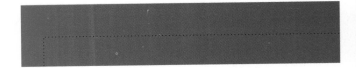

Cutaneous Histiocytosis

(Figs. 17–62 and 17–63)

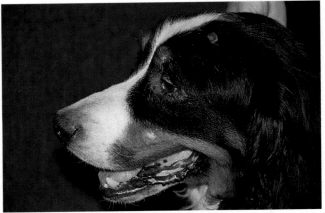

FIGURE 17–62. Cutaneous Histiocytosis. Multiple alopecic nodules on the head of an adult Bernese mountain dog.

FEATURES

A rare benign histiocytic proliferative disorder in dogs which involves cutaneous structures only. Affected dogs range in age from 2 to 13 years. Shelties and collies may be predisposed.

Multiple (a few to over 50) dermal (rarely subcutaneous), erythematous nodules or plaques. The tumors are nonpainful and nonpruritic, may be alopecic or ulcerated, and range in size from 1 to 5 cm. They tend to wax and wane or regress and appear at new sites. Tumors occur most frequently on the head, neck, perineum, scrotum, and extremities. Nasal mucosal involvement may occur.

DIAGNOSIS

1. Dermatohistopathology—Diffuse, often periadnexal or perivascular accumulations of a mixture of large histiocytes with large vesicular and often indented nuclei, as well as lymphocytes, plasma cells, and neutrophils. Mitotic figures are numerous, and vascular involvement or thrombosis may occur. Special stains are required to rule out infectious causes of histiocytic inflammation.

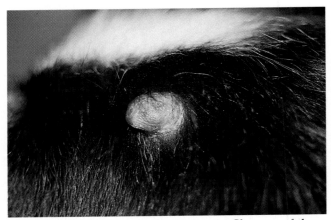

FIGURE 17–63. Cutaneous Histiocytosis. Close-up of the dog in Figure 17–62. Alopecic nodule on the head.

TREATMENT AND PROGNOSIS

1. Approximately 50% of cases respond to immunosuppressive doses of glucocorticoids. The addition of cytotoxic drugs may improve the response.
2. Cyclosporin A and leflunomide are useful in cases that respond poorly to glucocorticoid therapy.
3. Surgical excision is successful in a minority of cases.
4. Prognosis is guarded. Although systemic involvement is not present, most cases are episodic or continually progressive and need long-term immunosuppressive therapy for control.

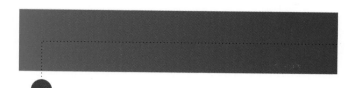

Systemic Histiocytosis

FEATURES

A proliferative disorder of histiocytes which involves skin and internal organs. Rare in dogs, with the highest incidence in young adult to middle-aged male Bernese mountain dogs.

There are multifocal haired or alopecic papules, plaques, and nodules which may be ulcerated. Nodules are up to 4 cm in diameter, may extend into the subcutis, and are not painful or pruritic. The tumors affect the eyelids, muzzle, planum nasale, extremities, and scrotum most severely. Generalized lymphadenomegaly may occur. Lesions may also develop in the lung, spleen, liver, bone marrow, and nasal cavity, causing noncutaneous signs of anorexia, weight loss, and respiratory stertor. In some dogs the disease is rapidly progressive. In others the course is more prolonged, with alternating episodes of exacerbation and remission.

DIAGNOSIS

1. Histopathology of skin/affected internal organs—Diffuse, often periadnexal or perivascular accumulations of a mixture of large histiocytes with large vesicular and often indented nuclei, as well as lymphocytes, plasma cells, and neutrophils. Mitotic figures are numerous, and vascular involvement or thrombosis is common. Special stains are required to rule out infectious causes of histiocytic inflammation.

TREATMENT AND PROGNOSIS

1. Immunosuppressive doses of glucocorticoids are usually ineffective.
2. Treatments with cyclosporin A or leflunomide have been used successfully in some cases. After cessation of therapy, some dogs may remain asymptomatic for an indefinite period, while others need continuous therapy to maintain remission.
3. Prognosis is guarded to poor. Most cases are episodic or continually progressive and need long-term immunosuppressive therapy for control.

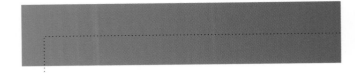

Malignant Histiocytosis

(Figs. 17–64 and 17–65)

FEATURES

A malignant neoplasm of histiocytes. Rare in dogs, with the highest incidence in older animals, especially Bernese mountain dogs.

Cutaneous lesions are uncommon but, if present, are characterized by multiple firm dermal to subcutaneous nodules that may be alopecic or ulcerated. The tumors may be anywhere on the body. Spleen, lymph nodes, lung, and bone marrow are the organ systems primarily affected. Dogs with widespread disease may also have lesions in the liver, central nervous system (CNS), and kidney. Common clinical symptoms include lethargy, weight loss, lymphadenomegaly, hepatosplenomegaly, pancytopenia, respiratory signs, and CNS disease.

DIAGNOSIS

1. Cytology (may be nondiagnostic)—Large pleomorphic, atypical histiocytes with abundant, finely granulated or vacuolated cytoplasm and single or multiple oval to reniform nuclei. Phagocytosis of erythrocytes and leukocytes by multinucleated tumor cells is commonly seen.
2. Histopathology (skin or affected internal organs)—Nonencapsulated, poorly demarcated proliferation of pleomorphic anaplastic histiocytes, which may be round or spindle-shaped. Multinucleate giant cells, cells with abnormal nuclei, and bizarre mitotic figures are common. Special stains are required to rule out infectious causes of histiocytic inflammation.

TREATMENT AND PROGNOSIS

1. Chemotherapy may prolong survival in some cases.
2. Prognosis is poor. Malignant histiocytosis is a highly malignant, rapidly progressive, fatal disease.

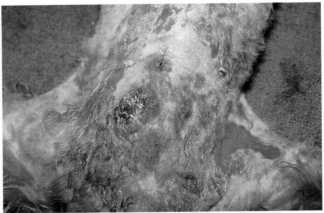

FIGURE 17–64. Malignant Histiocytosis. Generalized areas of alopecia, erythema, erosions, and crusting. (Courtesy of D. Angarano)

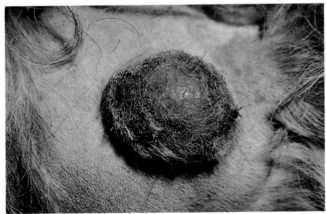

FIGURE 17–65. Malignant Histiocytosis. Close-up of the dog in Figure 17–64. Alopecia, erythema, and erosions on the scrotum. (Courtesy of D. Angarano)

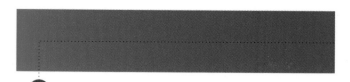

Melanoma (Figs. 17–66 to 17–69)

FEATURES

A benign or malignant proliferation of melanocytes. Most (85%) well-differentiated cutaneous melanomas are benign. Common in older dogs and rare in older cats. In dogs, predisposed breeds may include Scottish terriers, Airedales, Doberman pincers, cocker spaniels, and schnauzers.

Benign and malignant melanomas are usually solitary, well-circumscribed, dome-shaped, firm, brown to black, alopecic, pedunculated, or wart-like growths ranging from 0.5 to 10 cm in diameter. Plaque-like tumors can also occur. Malignant melanomas can be pigmented or nonpigmented (amelanotic), may be ulcerated, and tend to be larger and more rapidly growing than benign melanomas. Melanomas can be anywhere on the body but in dogs occur most commonly on the head, trunk, and digits. In cats, tumors are found most commonly on the head, neck, and digits.

DIAGNOSIS

1. Cytology—Round, oval, stellate, or spindle-shaped cells with a moderate amount of cytoplasm containing granules of brown to green-black pigment. Malignant melanomas may have less pigment and show more pleomorphism, but malignancy cannot be reliably determined cytologically.
2. Dermatohistopathology—Accumulation of neoplastic melanocytes, which may be spindle-shaped, epithelial, or round cell in appearance. Cells may be arranged in clusters, cords, or nerve-like whorls and have variable degrees of pigmentation. Infiltration of pigment-laden macrophages is common. Benign neoplasms are circumscribed and have low nuclear variability and a low mitotic rate. Malignant melanomas may show more invasiveness, cellular pleomorphism, and mitotic figures (including atypical mitotic figures). Mitotic index is the most reliable way to predict biologic behavior; however, 10% of histologically benign melanomas behave in a malignant manner.
3. Affected animals should be screened for regional lymph node and internal metastasis.

TREATMENT AND PROGNOSIS

1. The treatment of choice is radical surgical excision because benign melanomas cannot be differentiated clinically from malignant melanomas.
2. Chemotherapy may prolong survival in some cases of malignant disease.
3. Prognosis is good for benign melanomas. Prognosis is poor for malignant melanomas, especially if the tumor is large. Recurrence following surgery and metastasis are common. Tumor location is prognostic: most oral and mucocutaneous melanomas (except those of the eyelid) and one-third of the melanomas involving the nail beds are malignant.

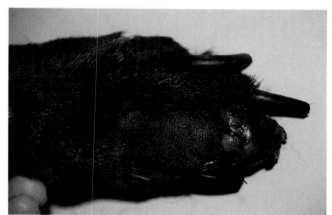

FIGURE 17–66. Melanoma. A large, ulcerative, proliferative melanoma of the digit.

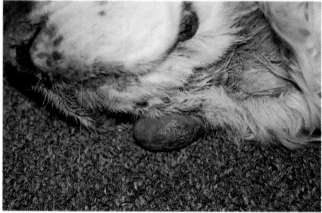

FIGURE 17–67. Melanoma. An ulcerated, amelanotic melanoma on the ventral neck of an aged cocker spaniel.

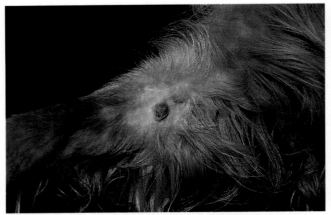

FIGURE 17–68. Melanoma. A small, pigmented nodule on the distal limb of an adult golden retriever.

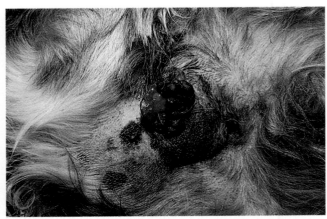

FIGURE 17–69. Melanoma. Tissue proliferation, hyperpigmentation, and ulceration caused by an aggressive melanoma on the scrotum of an adult dog.

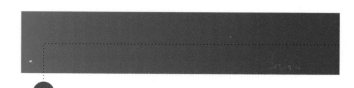

Transmissible Venereal Tumor (Figs. 17–70 and 17–71)

FEATURES

A benign to malignant neoplasm of unknown cell origin which may be virus-induced. Viable neoplastic cells are most often transplanted during coitus but can be inoculated into multiple sites by licking, sniffing, or scratching. Uncommon in dogs, with the highest incidence in sexually active female dogs in the tropics and subtropics.

Single to multiple, firm to friable, dermal or subcutaneous nodular or wart-like masses ranging from 1 to 20 cm in diameter. Tumors most commonly involve the external genitalia but may also be found elsewhere on the body, especially on the face and limbs. Ulceration and secondary bacterial infection may be present. Metastasis is rare but can occur, especially in immunosuppressed dogs and in puppies.

DIAGNOSIS

1. Cytology—Large, pleomorphic round cells with a moderate amount of medium blue, distinctly vacuolated cytoplasm and round nuclei with coarse chromatin and one or two large nucleoli. Mitotic figures and small numbers of lymphocytes, plasma cells, and histiocytes may be seen.
2. Dermatohistopathology—Sheets of uniform round cells interspersed with a delicate collagenous stroma. Nuclei are large and hyperchromatic, and cells contain abundant light blue vacuolated cytoplasm. Mitotic index is high. Necrosis or lymphocytic infiltration may be present.

TREATMENT AND PROGNOSIS

1. The treatment of choice is vincristine. Give 0.025 mg/kg IV q 7 days until complete clinical remission occurs (approximately 4–6 weeks).
2. Alternatively, treatment with doxorubicin may be effective.
3. Prognosis is generally good. Although tumors can regress spontaneously, treatment is recommended to prevent metastasis.

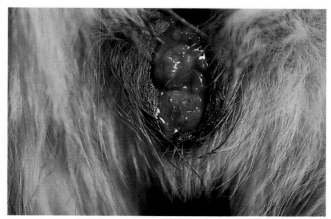

FIGURE 17–70. Transmissible Venereal Tumor. A multilobulated tumor on the vaginal mucosa of an adult dog. The cauliflower-shaped mass is typical of transmissible venereal tumors.

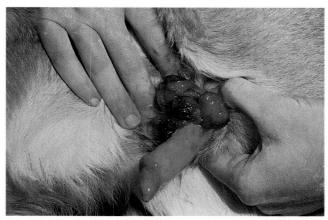

FIGURE 17–71. Transmissible Venereal Tumor. A large, multilobulated mass on the base of the penis of an adult dog. The hemorrhage was caused by the prepuce traumatizing the tumor. (Courtesy of C. Calvert)

Collagenous Nevus (Figs. 17–72 and 17–73)

FEATURES

A developmental defect of the skin, which may or may not be congenital, that is characterized by collagenous hyperplasia. Uncommon in dogs.

Usually a solitary, firm, well-circumscribed, flat to dome-shaped dermal nodule. The nodule may have a pitted surface, may be alopecic and hyperpigmented, and is usually <1 cm in diameter. It can occur anywhere on the body but is most commonly found on the head, neck, and limb.

DIAGNOSIS

1. Dermatohistopathology—Poorly cellular mass of mature collagen which does not usually displace adnexal structures.

TREATMENT AND PROGNOSIS

1. Observation without treatment is reasonable because these are benign lesions.
2. Cosmetically unacceptable lesions can be excised surgically.
3. Prognosis is good, as tumors are not neoplastic.

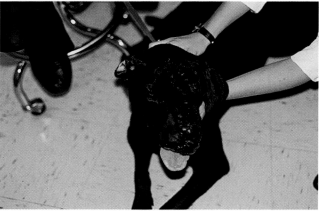

FIGURE 17–72. Collagenous Nevi. Multiple nodules and tumors on the head of an adult Labrador. (Courtesy of the University of Florida: case material)

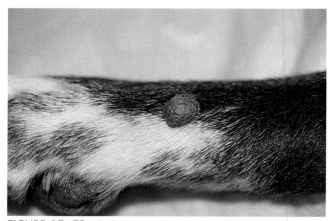

FIGURE 17–73. Collagenous Nevus. This solitary alopecic, hyperpigmented nodule is typical of this tumor.

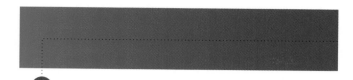

Follicular Cyst—Epidermal Inclusion Cyst (infundibular cyst)
(Figs. 17–74 to 17–77)

FEATURES

A nonneoplastic cystic structure which contains an epithelial lining. Common in dogs and uncommon in cats, with the highest incidence in middle-aged animals. In dogs, predisposed breeds may include boxers, shih tzus, schnauzers, and bassett hounds.

Usually a solitary, well-circumscribed, firm to fluctuant intradermal swelling. It may be alopecic and is usually <2 cm in diameter. The cyst may become inflamed, secondarily infected, painful, and pruritic, and may rupture, discharging thick gray to yellow-brown caseous material. The lesion is most commonly found on the head, trunk, or proximal limb in dogs and on the head, neck, and trunk in cats.

DIAGNOSIS

1. Cytology (may be nondiagnostic)—Amorphous cellular debris and mature, keratinized epithelial cells with cholesterol crystals.
2. Dermatohistopathology—A cystic structure filled with lamellated keratin and lined by normal stratified squamous epithelium. Rupture of cyst contents may incite a surrounding pyogranulomatous inflammatory response.

TREATMENT AND PROGNOSIS

1. Observation without treatment is reasonable because lesions are benign.
2. Surgical excision is curative.
3. The cyst contents should not be expressed manually because if the cyst wall ruptures through the dermis, a foreign body reaction and infection may develop.
4. Prognosis is good, as tumors are not neoplastic.

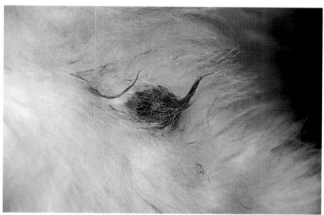

FIGURE 17–75. Follicular Cysts. Close-up of the dog in Figure 17–74. The follicular cyst ruptured upon palpation.

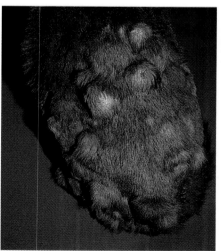

FIGURE 17–74. Follicular Cysts. This alopecic, erythematous nodule is typical of small follicular cysts. When the cyst was palpated, it ruptured (see Figure 17–75).

FIGURE 17–76. Follicular Cysts. Multiple follicular cysts on the trunk of an adult cat. (Courtesy of D. Angarano)

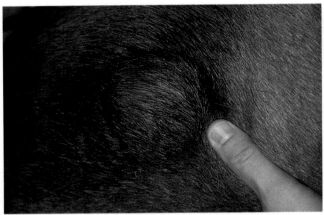

FIGURE 17–77. Follicular Cyst. This large follicular cyst was on the dorsum of a dog.

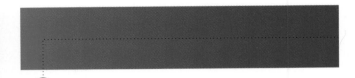

Cutaneous Horn (Figs. 17–78 and 17–79)

FEATURES

A circumscribed conical or cylindrical mass of keratin which may originate from an underlying solar dermatosis, squamous cell carcinoma, papilloma, dilated pore, or intracutaneous cornifying epithelioma. It is also seen as a unique entity on the footpads of cats infected with feline leukemia virus. Uncommon in dogs and cats.

Single or multiple conical to cylindrical horn-like masses of firm keratin, which are several millimeters in diameter and up to 2 cm in length.

DIAGNOSIS

1. Dermatohistopathology—A well-demarcated area of papillomatous epidermal hyperplasia from which a compact column of keratin (with orthokeratotic to parakeratotic cells) protrudes, resembling a claw. The epidermis of feline leukemia-associated cutaneous horns may show dyskeratotic or multinucleate keratinocytes.
2. Cats with footpad lesions should be screened for feline leukemia virus infection.

TREATMENT AND PROGNOSIS

1. The treatment of choice is complete surgical excision.
2. While cutaneous horns themselves are benign, prognosis is variable, depending on the underlying cause.

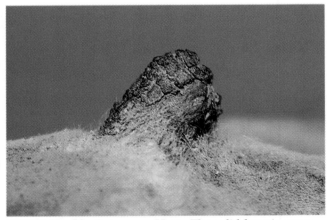

FIGURE 17–78. Cutaneous Horn. The solid keratin structure of this cutaneous horn is apparent.

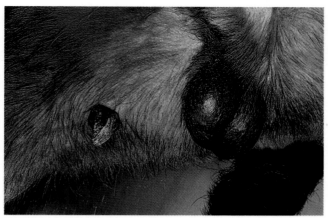

FIGURE 17–79. Cutaneous Horn. A cutaneous horn on the caudal thigh of an adult mixed-breed dog.

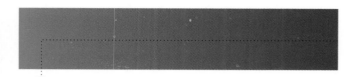

Skin Tag (fibrovascular papilloma)
(Figs. 17–80 to 17–82)

FEATURES

A benign growth of fibrovascular origin, which may be a hyperplastic skin response to repetitive trauma. Uncommon in dogs, with the highest incidence in middle-aged to older large and giant breeds. Rare in cats.

Firm, pedunculated growths 1–2 cm long and a few millimeters in diameter. Larger lesions may become ulcerated. Skin tags are most common on the sternum, bony prominences, and trunk.

DIAGNOSIS

1. Dermatohistopathology—Hyperplastic epidermis overlying a core of vascularized collagenous connective tissue. Adnexa are absent.

TREATMENT AND PROGNOSIS

1. Observation without treatment is reasonable because these lesions are benign.
2. Surgical excision is curative.
3. Prognosis is good, as growths are not neoplastic.

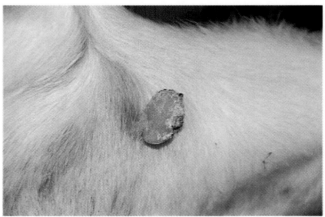

FIGURE 17–80. Skin Tag. The large, pedunculated tumor developed on the lateral forearm of this aged Saint Bernard over several years.

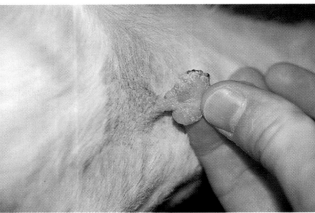

FIGURE 17–81. Skin Tag. Close-up of the dog in Figure 17–80. The small pedicle that attaches the skin tag to the body is visible.

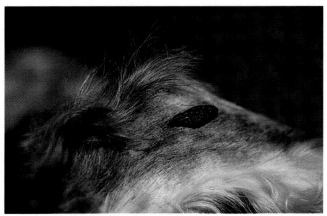

FIGURE 17–82. Skin Tag. A pigmented skin tag on the trunk of an adult schnauzer.

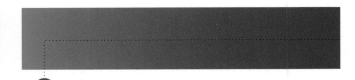

Calcinosis Circumscripta

(Fig. 17–83)

FEATURES

A focal area of dystrophic calcification that occurs at sites of repetitive or previous trauma.

Multiple nodules have also been described in association with hypertrophic osteodystrophy (HOD) and polyarthritis. Uncommon in dogs, with the highest incidence in young large-breeds dogs, especially German shepherds. Rare in cats.

Usually a solitary, firm, haired or alopecic, dome-shaped subcutaneous or deep dermal mass which may ulcerate and discharge a white, gritty substance. The mass may range from 0.5 to 7 cm in diameter. Lesions are most frequently seen over bony prominences such as the elbow but can also occur on the footpads, at ear cropping sites, and at sites of injection or injury.

DIAGNOSIS

1. Cytology (may be nondiagnostic)—Amorphous gritty white material, which becomes basophilic when stained.
2. Dermatohistopathology—Multifocal accumulations of finely or coarsely granular, amorphous basophilic debris in the deep dermal or subcutaneous tissue surrounded by granulomatous inflammation.

TREATMENT AND PROGNOSIS

1. Complete surgical excision is curative.
2. Multiple or symmetrical lesions associated with HOD or polyarthritis may resolve spontaneously with resolution of the associated disease.
3. Prognosis is good, as growths are not neoplastic.

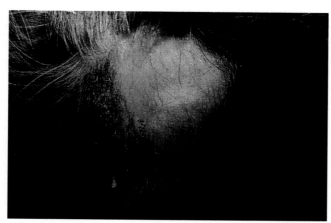

FIGURE 17–83. Calcinosis Circumscripta. The alopecia allows visualization of the calcified material within the skin. (Courtesy of M. Austel)

Suggested Readings

Affolter V and Moore P. 2000. Canine Cutaneous Histiocytic Diseases, pp. 588–591. In Kirk's Current Veterinary Therapy, XIII, Small Animal Practice. W.B. Saunders, Philadelphia, PA.

Bergman PJ, Withrow SJ, Straw RC, and Powers BE. 1994. Infiltrative Lipoma in Dogs: 16 Cases (1981–1992). JAVMA. 205: 322–324.

Cowell R, Tyler R, and Meinkoth J. 1999. Diagnostic Cytology and Hematology of the Dog and Cat. Ed. 2. ed. Mosby, St. Louis, MO.

Goldschmidt M and Shofer F. 1992. Skin Tumors of the Dog and Cat. Pergamon Press, Oxford.

Gomes LAM, Ferreira AMR, Ferrreira de Almeida LE, and Paes de Almeida E. 2000. Squamous Cell Carcinoma Associated with Actinic Dermatitis in Seven White Cats. Feline Practice. 28: 14–17.

Gross T, Ihrke P, and Walder E. 1992. Veterinary Dermatopathology. Mosby, St. Louis, MO.

Jubb K, Kennedy P, and Palmer N. Pathology of Domestic Animals. Ed. 4. Academic Press, San Diego, CA.

Lana S, Ogilivie G, Withrow S, Straw R, and Rogers K. 1997. Feline Cutaneous Squamous Cell Carcinoma of the Nasal Planum and the Pinnae: 61 Cases. JAAHA. 33: 329–332.

Morrison W. 1998. Cancer in Dogs and Cats: Medical and Surgical Management. Williams & Wilkins, Baltimore, MD.

Moulton J (ed.). 1978. Tumors in Domestic Animals. University of California Press, Berkeley, CA.

Neoplastic and Non-Neoplastic Tumors, pp. 990–1126. In Scott DW, Miller WH Jr, and Griffin CE. 1995. Muller & Kirk's Small Animal Dermatology. Ed. 5. W.B. Saunders, Philadelphia, PA.

Ogilve G and Moore A. 1995. Managing the Veterinary Cancer Patient. Veterinary Learning Systems, Trenton, NJ.

Paterson S, Boydell P, and Pike R. 1995. Systemic Histiocytosis in the Bernese Mountain Dog. JSAP. 36: 233–236.

Peterson A, Wood S, and Rosser E. 1999. The Use of Safflower Oil for the Treatment of Mycosis Fungoides in Two Dogs. Proceedings of the 15th AAVD/ACVD Meeting, pp. 49–50.

Plumb DC. 1999. Veterinary Drug Handbook. Ed. 3. Iowa State University Press, Ames, IA.

Power H and Ihrke P. 1995. The Use of Synthetic Retinoids in Veterinary Medicine, pp. 585–590. In Bonagura J (ed). Kirk's Current Veterinary Therapy, XII, Small Animal Practice. W.B. Saunders, Philadelphia, PA.

Ramsey I, McKay J, Rudorf H, and Dobson J. 1996. Malignant Histiocytosis in Three Bernese Mountain Dogs. Vet Rec. 138: 440–444.

Ruslander D, Kaser-Hortz B, and Sardinas J. 1997. Cutaneous Squamous Cell Carcinoma in Cats. Compend Cont Edu Pract Vet. 19(10): 1119–1130.

Walder EJ. 1995. Fibropruritic Nodules in the Dog, p. 635. In Bonagura JD (ed). Kirk's Current Veterinary Therapy, XII, Small Animal Practice. W.B. Saunders, Philadelphia, PA.

Weigand C and Brewer W. 1996. Vaccination-Site Sarcomas in Cats. Compend Cont Edu Pract Vet. 18(8): 869–875.

White SD, Rosychuk RA, Scott KV, Trettien AL, Jonas L, and Denerolle P. 1993. Use of Isotretinoin and Etretinate for the Treatment of Benign Cutaneous Neoplasia and Cutaneous Lymphoma in Dogs. JAVMA. 202: 387–390.

Withrow S and MacEwan EG. 1996. Small Animal Clinical Oncology. Ed. 2. W.B. Saunders, Philadelphia, PA.

Yager J and Wilcoct B. 1994. Color Atlas and Text of Surgical Pathology of the Dog and Cat. Wolfe, London.

Antimicrobial, Antiseborrheic, and Antipruritic Shampoos and Conditioners

Ingredient	Therapeutic Effect	Usage	Disadvantages
Chlorhexidine	Antibacterial Antifungal Antiviral	A mild topical ingredient with excellent antimicrobial activity.	
Benzoyl peroxide	Antibacterial Follicular flushing Degreasing Keratolytic	A potent degreasing, follicular flushing topical ingredient with excellent antibacterial effects. Mildly antiseborrheic. Good for crusting and oily seborrheic disorders.	Drying Skin irritation May bleach fabrics
Triclosan	Antibacterial	A moderately effective antibacterial ingredient added to topicals.	
Ethyl lactate	Antibacterial Decreases skin pH Degreasing Comedolytic	A mild degreasing, antiseborrheic shampoo with good antibacterial activity. Good for dry, scaling seborrhea.	
Povidone-iodine	Antibacterial Antifungal Antiviral	A mild topical ingredient with excellent antimicrobial activity but limited duration of effect.	Short duration of effect Staining Skin irritation Thyroid dysfunction Metabolic acidosis
Ketoconazole	Antifungal	A mild topical ingredient with good antifungal activity.	Expensive
Miconazole	Antifungal	A mild topical ingredient with good antifungal activity.	Expensive
Sulfur/salicylic acid	Keratolytic Keratoplastic	A moderately well tolerated shampoo with good antiseborrheic activity. Good for crusting or dry, seborrheic disorders.	
Tar	Keratolytic Keratoplastic Degreasing Antipruritic Vasoactive	A potent degreasing and antiseborrheic shampoo. Good for severe oily, seborrheic disorders.	Toxic to cats Drying Skin irritation Staining Photosensitization Superficial migratory necrolytic dermatitis
Selenium sulfide	Keratolytic Keratoplastic Degreasing	A potent degreasing shampoo with good antiseborrheic activity. Good for oily, seborrheic disorders. Moderate activity against yeast.	Drying Skin irritation

Appendix A continued on following page

Ingredient	Therapeutic Effect	Usage	Disadvantages
Oatmeal	Decreases prosta-glandins Antipruritic Soothing	A mild topical ingredient with moderate antipruritic activity.	
Diphenhydramine	Antipruritic	A mild topical ingredient with good antipruritic activity.	Contact sensitivity
Pramoxine	Antipruritic	A mild topical ingredient with good antipruritic activity.	
Hydrocortisone	Anti-inflammatory Antipruritic	A mild topical ingredient with good antipruritic activity.	Immunosuppression Cutaneous atrophy

A p p e n d i x   B

Topical Therapeutic Drugs

Drug Name	Brand Name	How Supplied
Aluminum acetate 5% solution	Otic Domeboro Solution: Bayer; West Haven, CT	2% acetic acid in aqueous aluminum, 2 fl oz dropper bottles
Amitraz solution	Mitaban: Pharmacia & Upjohn; Kalamazoo, MI	19.9% amitraz in 10.6 ml bottles
	Taktic EC: Hoechst Russell Vet; Warren, NJ	12.5% amitraz in 760 ml containers
	Ectodex: Hoechst Roussel Vet (not available in United States)	5% amitraz in 50 ml bottles
Amitraz collars	Preventic Collar: Allerderm/Virbac; Ft. Worth, TX	9% amitraz 25 in. plastic collar
Amphotericin B 3% lotion, cream, and ointment	Fungizone: Apothecon; Princeton, NJ	Lotion: 30 ml bottles Cream: 20 g tubes Ointment: 20 g tubes
Benzoyl peroxide 5% Gel	Cytoxl-AQ gel: Vetgenix; Coral Gables, FL	Benzoyl peroxide in 170 g bottle with dispensing tip
	Pyoben Gel: Allerderm/Virbac; Ft. Worth, TX	Benzoyl peroxide in 30 g plastic tubes
	Oxydex Gel: DVM; Miami, FL	Benzoyl peroxide in 30 g tubes
Burow's solution/hydrocortisone	Bur-O-Cort 2:1: QA Labs; Kansas City, MO	In 10 oz and 16 oz bottles
	Burow's H Solution: Vetus; Farmer's Branch, TX	In 1 oz squeeze bottles, 2 oz spray bottles, and 16 oz bottle
	Cort/Astrin Solution: Vedco; St. Joseph, MO	In 1 oz dropper bottles and 16 oz bottles
	Corti-Derm Solution: First Priority; Elgin, IL	In 16 oz bottles
	Hydro-Plus: Phoenix; St. Joseph, MO	In 1 oz and pint bottles
	Many other generics	
Clindamycin 1% gel, lotion, and solution	Clindamycin Phosphate: Geneva; Broomfield, CO	Gel: 30 g tubes Lotion: 60 ml bottles Solution: 30 ml and 60 ml bottles
	Cleocin T: Upjohn; Exton, PA	Gel: 7.5 g and 30 g tubes Lotion: 60 ml bottles Solution: 30 ml and 60 ml bottles
	Clinda-derm: Paddock; Minneapolis, MN	Solution: 60 ml bottles
	C/T/S: Hoescht Marion Russell; Kansas City, MO	Solution: 30 ml and 60 ml containers

Appendix B continued on following page

Drug Name	Brand Name	How Supplied
Chlorhexadine ointment	Chlorhexadine Ointment: Davis Veterinary Products; Scottdale, GA	2% Chlorhexadine Ointment in 4 oz containers
	Nolvasan Antiseptic Ointment: Fort Dodge; Fort Dodge, IA	1% Chlorhexadine Ointment in 1 oz, 7 oz, and 16 oz tubes
	Many other generics	
Chlorhexadine 2% solution	Nolvason Solution: Fort Dodge; Fort Dodge, IA	1 gal containers
	Hexasol: Vetus, Farmer's Branch, TX	1 gal containers
	Many other generics	
Clotrimazole 1% cream, lotion, and solution	Clotrimazole: Taro; Hawthorne, NY	Cream: 15 g, 30 g, and 45 g tubes Solution: 30 ml bottles
	Fungoid: Pedinol; Farmingdale, NY	Cream: 30 g tubes Solution: 30 ml bottles
	Lotrimin: Schering-Plough; Kenilworth, NJ	Lotion: 30 ml containers Solution: 10 ml and 30 ml containers
	Lotrimin AF: Schering-Plough; Kenilworth, NJ (OTC)	Lotion: 20 ml bottles Solution: 10 ml bottles
Dimethyl sulfoxide 20% Gel	Domoso: Fort Dodge; Ft. Dodge, IA	In 2.1 oz and 4.2 oz tubes and 15 oz containers
Econazole 1% cream	Spectazole: Ortho Pharmaceutical Corporation; Raritan, NJ	In 15 g, 30 g, and 85 g tubes
Enilconazole 1% solution	Imaverol: Janssen Pharmaceutical (not available in United States)	In 100 ml and 1L containers
Erythromycin solution	Staticin: Westwood Squibb; Buffalo, NY	1.5% erythromycin in 60 ml bottles with applicator
	Erythromycin Topical: Bausch & Lomb; Claremont, CA	2% erythromycin in 60 ml bottles
	Many other generics	
Fipronil spray and solution	Frontline Spray and Top Spot: Merial; Iselin, NJ	29% spray: 3.4 oz and 8.5 oz containers 9.7% solution: 0.5 ml, 0.67 ml, 1.34 ml, 2.68 ml, and 4.02 ml pipettes
Fipronil/(s)-methoprene solution	Frontline-Plus: Merial; Iselin, NJ	9.8% fipronil and 8.8% (s)-methoprene (dogs) or 11.8% methoprene (cats): 0.5 ml, 0.67 ml, 1.34 ml, 2.68 ml, and 4.02 ml pipettes
Gentamicin-betamethasone valerate spray	Genta-Spray: Vetus; Farmer's Branch, TX	In 60 ml, 120 ml, and 240 ml bottles
	Gentaved Topical Spray: Vedco; St. Joseph, MO	
	Gentocin Topical Spray: Schering-Plough; Union, NJ	
Icthamol 20% ointment	Icthamol: Butler; Dublin, OH, and Phoenix; St. Joseph, MO	In 1 lb jars
	Icthamol Ointment: First Priority; Elgin, OH	In 4 oz and 1 lb jars

Drug Name	Brand Name	How Supplied
	Icthamol Ointment: Aspen; Kansas City, MO	In 1 lb jars
	Many other generics	
Imidacloprid solution	Advantage: Bayer Corp.; Shawnee Mission, KS	9.1% solution: in 0.4 ml, 0.8 ml, 1.0 ml, 2.5 ml, and 4.0 ml tubes
Ketoconazole 2% cream	Nizoral 2% Cream: Janssen Pharmaceutical, Inc.; Titusville, NJ	In 15 g, 30 g, and 60 g tubes
Lidocaine spray and gel	Allerspray: Evsco; Buena, NJ	2.5% lidocaine HCl in 4 oz and 12 oz containers
	Dermacool with lidocaine HCl: Allerderm/Virbac; Ft. Worth, TX	Hamamelis extract and lidocaine HCl (no concentration given) in 4 oz bottles
	Vetmark Anti-itch gel and spray: Bioderm; Longview, TX	Gel: 2.46% lidocaine HCl in 2 oz bottles Spray: 2.46% lidocaine HCl in 4 oz containers
Lime-sulfur solution	Lymdyp: DVM, Miami, FL	In 12 oz and 1 gal containers
Metronidazole 0.75% gel	Metro Gel: Galderma; Ft. Worth, TX	In 28.4 g tubes
Miconazole 1% spray, lotion, and cream	Micaved: Vedco; St. Joseph, MO Micazole: Vetus; Carrollton, TX Miconosol: Med-Pharmex; Pomona, CA	Spray: 120 ml and 240 ml containers Lotion: 60 ml bottles
	Conofite: Schering-Plough; Union, NJ	Cream: 15 g tubes Spray: 60 ml bottle Lotion: 30 ml containers
Mupirocin 2% ointment	Bactoderm: Pfizer Animal Health; Exton, PA	In 15 g tubes
Mupirocin 2% cream	Bactoban: SmithKline Beecham; Exton, PA	In 15 g and 30 g tubes
Neomycin ointment and powder	Forte Topical: Pharmacia & Upjohn; Exton, PA	Neomycin sulfate/procaine penicilin G/ polymyxin B sulfate/hydrocortisone acetate/hydrocortisone sodium succinate in 10 ml tubes
	Neo-Predef: Pharmacia & Upjohn; Exton, PA	Neomycin sulfate/isoflupredone acetate/tetracaine HCl topical powder in 15 g bottles
	Triple Antibiotic Ointment: Legere; Scottsdale, AZ	Neomycin sulfate/polymyxin B sulfate/ bacitracin in 1/2 oz tubes
	Tritop: Pharmacia & Upjohn; Exton, PA	Neomycin sulfate/isoflupredone acetate/tetracaine HCl in 10 g tubes
	Many other generics	
Nystatin-neomycin-thiostrepton-triamcinolone acetonide	Animax: Pharmaderm; Melville, NY	Ointment: 7.5 ml, 15 ml, 30 ml tubes and 240 ml bottles
	Panalog: Solvay; Mendota Heights, MN	Ointment: 7.5 ml, 15 ml, 30 ml, and 240 ml
	Many other generics	Cream: 7.5 g and 15 g tubes
Povidine-iodine 10% solution	Betadine: Perdue-Frederick;	15 ml, 120 ml, 237 ml, 1 pt, 1 qt, and 1 gal containers
	Povidem Solution: Vetus; Farmer's Branch, TX	1 gal containers
	Many other generics	

Appendix B continued on following page

Drug Name	Brand Name	How Supplied
Pramoxine HCl 1% solution	Heska Pramoxine Spray: Heska; Ft. Collins, TX	In 12 oz bottles
	Relief Spray: DVM; Miami, FL	In 6 oz containers
	Corium-Tx: VRx; Harbor City, CA	In 2 oz bottles
Salicylic acid-sodium lactate-urea gel	Kerasolv: DVM; Miami, FL	In 1 oz tubes
Selamectin solution	Revolution: Pfizer; Exton, PA	6–12% solution in 0.25 ml, 0.75 ml, 0.5 ml, 1 ml, and 2 ml tubes
Silver sulfadiazine 1% cream	SSD cream: Boots [Knoll]; Mt. Olive, NJ	In 25 g, 50 g, 85 g, 400 g, and 1000 g tubes
	Silvadene: Hoescht Marion Russell; Kansas City, MO	In 20 g, 50 g, 85 g, 400 g, and 1000 g tubes
	Thermazene: Sherwood [Kendall]: Mansfield, MA	In 50 g, 400 g, and 1000 g tubes
Tetracycline solution and ointment	Topicycline: Roberts; Eatontown, NJ	2.2 mg/ml solution when reconstituted; supplied as powder with diluent for 70 ml
	Achromycin: Lederle; Pearl River, NY	3% ointment in 14.2 g and 30 g tubes
Tretinoin gel and cream	Retin-A: Ortho; Raritan, NJ	Gel: 0.01% in 15 g and 45 g tubes 0.025% in 15 g and 45 g tubes 0.1% in 20 g and 45 g tubes Cream: 0.01% in 20 g and 45 g tubes 0.025% in 20 g and 45 g tubes 0.1% in 20 g and 45 g tubes
Triamcinolone cream	Vetalog Cream: Fort Dodge; Ft. Dodge, IA	In 15 g tubes

Appendix C

Otic Therapeutic Drugs

Drug Name	Brand Name	How Supplied
Acetic acid-hydrocortisone	Clearx Ear Drying Solution: DVM; Miami, FL	25% acetic acid; 2% colloidal sulfur; 1% hydrocortisone in 30 ml containers
	Bur-Otic Ear Treatment: Allerderm/ Virbac; Fort Worth, TX Many other generics	1% hydrocortisone; also contains Burow's solution, acetic acid, and benzalkonium chloride in 30 ml containers
Chloramphenicol/prednisolone (otic)	Chlora-Otic: Vetus; Farmer's Branch, TX Liqui-Chlor: Evsco; Buena, NJ	In 10 ml tubes and 12 oz bottles
Clotrimazole 1% (otic)	Otibiotic Ointment: Vetus; Farmer's Branch, TX Tri-Otic: Med-Pharmex; Pomona, CA Otomax: Schering-Plough; Union, NJ	Gentamicin sulfate/betamethasone valerate/clotrimazole ointment in 7.5 ml, 15 ml, 30 ml, and 240 ml tubes
Enrofloxacin/silver sulfadiazene	Baytril Otic: Bayer; Shawnee Mission, KS	0.5% enrofloxacin and 1.0% silver sulfadiazene in 15 and 30 ml bottles
Fluocinolone-dimethyl sulfoxide (otic)	Syn-Otic Solution: Fort Dodge; Fort Dodge, IA	0.01% fluocinolone acetonide, 0.01 dimethyl sulfoxide in 8 ml and 60 ml dropper vials
Gentamicin-betamethasone valerate	Genta-Spray: Vetus; Farmer's Branch, TX Gentaved Topical Spray: Vedco; St. Joseph, MO Gentocin Topical Spray: Schering-Plough; Union, NJ	In 60 ml, 120 ml, and 240 ml bottles
Gentamicin	Gen-Otic: Vetus; Farmer's Branch, TX Gentaved Otic: Vedco; St. Joseph, MO Gentocin Otic: Schering-Plough; Union, NJ	Gentomicin sulfate/betamethasone valerate in 7.5 ml, 15 ml, and 240 ml squeeze bottles
	Otibiotic: Vetus; Farmer's Branch, TX Otomax: Schering-Plough; Union, NJ Tri-Otic: Med-Pharmex; Pomona, CA	Gentomicin sulfate/betamethasone valerate/clotimazole in 7.5 ml, 15 ml, and 240 ml squeeze bottles

Appendix C continued on following page

333

Drug Name	Brand Name	How Supplied
Nystatin-neomycin-thio-streptone-triamcino-lone acetonide, cream and ointment	Animax: Pharmaderm; Melville, NY	Ointment: 7.5 ml, 15 ml, and 30 ml tubes and 240 ml bottles
	Panaolg: Solvay; Mendota Heights, MN	Ointment: 7.5 ml, 15 ml, 30 ml, and 240 ml Cream: 7.5 g and 15 g tubes
	Many other generics	
Otic miticides	Acarexx: IDEXX; Blue Ridge Pharmaceuticals; Greensboro, NC	0.01% ivermectin in 0.5 ml ampules
	Aurimite: Schering-Plough; Union, NJ	Pyrethrin/piperonyl butoxide in 10 oz and 16 oz bottles
	Cerumite: Evsco; Buena, NJ	Pyrethrin/piperonyl butoxide in 15 ml bottles
	Ear Miticide: Vedco; St. Joseph, MO	Rotenone/cube resins in 2 oz and 4 oz containers
	Ear Mite Lotion: Duravet; Blue Springs, MO	Same as above in 4 oz containers
	Mita-Clear: Pfizer Animal Health; Exton, PA	N-octyl bicycloheptene dicarboximide/di-n-propyl isocinchomeronate in 12 ml bottles
	Mitaplex-R: Tomlyn; Buena, NJ	Rotenone in 2 oz and 4 oz bottles
	Otomite Plus Ear Mite Treatment: Allerderm/Virbac; Ft. Worth, TX	Pyrerthrin/piperonyl butoxide/N-octyl bicycloheptene dicarboxide/di-n-propyl isocinchomeronate in ½ oz bottles
	Many others	
Silver sulfadiazine	Silvadene: Hoescht Marion Russell; Kansas City, MO	1% cream in 20 g, 50 g, 85 g, 400 g, and 1000 g tubes
	Silver Sulfadiazine, Micronized: Spectrum Laboratory Products; Gardena, CA	Powder in 10 g, 25 g, 100 g, and 1 kg containers
Thiabendazole-dexamethasone-neomycin solution	Tresaderm: Merck Ag Vet; Rahway, NJ	In 7.5 ml and 15 ml dropper bottles
Tobramycin 0.3% solution	Tobramycin: Bausch & Lomb; Tampa, FL	In 5 ml bottles
	AKTob: Akorn; Buffalo Grove, IL	
	Tobradex Alcon Laboratories; Fort Worth, TX	
	Many other generics	

Systemic Therapeutic Drugs

Drug Name	Brand Name	How Supplied
Acitretin	Soriatane: Roche; Nutley, NJ	Capsules: 10 mg and 25 mg
Allopurinol	Allopurinol: Boots [Knoll]; Mt. Olive, NJ Geneva; Broomfield, CO Major; Livonia, MI Mylan; Morgantown, WV Parmed; Niagara Falls, NY Vangard; Glasgow, KY	Tablets: 100 mg and 200 mg
	Zyloprim: GlaxoWellcome; Research Triangle Park, NC	Tablets (scored): 100 mg and 200 mg
Amikacin sulfate	Amiglyde-V Injection: Fort Dodge; Ft. Dodge, IA Amiject-D: Vetus; Farmer's Branch, TX Amikacin C: Phoenix; St. Joseph, MO Amikacin sulfate Injection: Vet Tek; Blue Springs, MO	Injectable solution: 50 mg/ml in 50 ml vials
Amino acid 10% infusion (Crystalline)	Aminosyn 10%; Abbott; Abbott Park, IL	Injectable solution: 500 ml and 1000 ml containers
Amitriptyline HCl	Elavil: AstraZeneca; Westboro, MA Amitriptyline HCl: Geneva; Broomfield, CO Many other generics	Tablets: 10 mg, 25 mg, 50 mg, 75 mg, 100 mg, and 150 mg
Amoxicillin (clavulanated)	Clavamox: Pfizer Animal Animal Health, manufactured by SmithKline Beecham; Exton, PA	Oral suspension: 62.5 mg/ml (12.5 mg clav. acid, 50 mg amox.) 15 ml bottles Tablets: 62.5 mg (50 mg amox./12.5 mg clav. acid) 125 mg (100 mg amox./25 mg clav. acid) 250 mg (200 mg amox./50 mg clav. acid 375 mg (300 mg amox./75 mg clav. acid)
Amphotericin B injection	Amphotericin B: Pharm-Tek; Huntington, NY	Powder for injection: 50 mg vials

Appendix D continued on following page

Drug Name	Brand Name	How Supplied
Amphotericin B injection (cont.)	Fungizone IV: Bristol Myers Squibb; Princeton, NJ	Powder for injection: 50 mg vials
	Amphotec: Sequus Pharmaceuticals; Menlo Park, CA	Powder for injection: 50 mg and 100 mg vials
	Ambisome: Fujisawa; Deerfield, IL	Powder for injection: 50 mg in 20 ml vials and 100 mg in 50 ml vials
	Abelcet: Liposome Co.; Princeton, NJ	Powder for injection (liposomal complex): 50 mg vials
		Suspension for injection (lipid complex): 100 mg vials
Asparginase	Elspar: Merck; West Point, PA	Powder for injection: 10,000 units in 10 ml vials
Aurothioglucose	Solganal: Schering; Liberty Corner, NJ	Injection suspension: 50 mg/ml in 10 ml vials
Azathioprine	Imuran: GlaxoWellcome; Research Triangle Park, NC	Tablets (scored): 50 mg
Betamethasone	Betasone: Schering-Plough; Union, NJ	Injection suspension: betamethasone dipropionate (2 mg/ml) and betamethasone sodium phosphate (2 mg/ml) in 5 ml vials
Brompheniramine maleate	Dimetane-Dx: A.H. Robins Co; Richmond, VA	Oral syrup: 0.4 mg/ml in pint bottles
Calcitrol	Rocaltrol: Roche; Nutley, NJ	Capsules: 0.25 μg and 0.5 μg Oral solution: 1 μg/ml in 15 ml bottles
Cefadroxil	Cefa-Tabs, Cefa-drops: Fort Dodge; Fort Dodge, IA	Tablets: 50 mg, 100 mg, and 200 mg Tablets (scored): 1 g Oral suspension: 50 mg/ml in 15 ml and 50 ml dropper bottles
Cephalexin	Keflex: Dista; Indianapolis, IN	Oral suspension: 25 mg/ml and 50 mg/ml in 100 ml and 200 ml bottles
	Cephalexin: Novopharm; Schaumberg, IL	Capsules: 250 mg and 500 mg
Cephradine	Velosef: Bristol-Myers Squibb; Princeton, NJ	Powder for injection: 250 mg, 500 mg, and 1 g vials
	Cephradine: Geneva Pharmaceuticals, Inc.; Broomfield, CO	Oral suspension: 25 mg/ml in 100 ml and 200 ml bottles Capsules: 250 mg and 500 mg
	Many other generics	
Cetirizine HCl	Zyrtec: Pfizer; New York, NY	Oral syrup: 1 g/ml in 120 ml and pint bottles Tablets: 5 mg and 10 mg
Chlorambucil	Leukeran: GlaxoWellcome; Research Triangle Park, NC	Tablets: 2 mg
Chloramphenicol	Chloramphenicol Capsules: V.P.C.; Pomona, NY	Capsules: 100 mg, 250 mg, and 500 mg

Drug Name	Brand Name	How Supplied
	Duricol Chloramphenicol Capsules U.S.P.: Nylos; Pomona, NY	Capsules: 50 mg, 100 mg, 250 mg, and 500 mg
Chlorpheniramine maleate	Chlor-Trimeton Allergy: Schering-Plough; Union, NJ	Tablets: 4 mg, 8 mg, and 12 mg Oral syrup: 0.4 mg/ml in 118 ml bottles
	Chlorpheniramine Maleate: Geneva Pharmaceuticals, Inc.; Broomfield, CO	Tablets: 4 mg
Cimetidine	Tagamet: SmithKline Beecham; Philadelphia, PA	Tablets: 100 mg, 200 mg, 300 mg, 400 mg, and 800 mg Oral liquid: 60 mg/ml
	Many other generics	
Ciprofloxacin	Cipro: Bayer Corporation; Shawnee Mission, MS	Tablets: 100 mg, 250 mg, 500 mg, and 750 mg Injectable solution: 2 mg/ml in 100 ml and 200 ml bottles and 10 mg/ml in 20 ml and 40 ml vials
Clarithromycin	Biaxin: Abbott Laboratories; North Chicago, IL	Tablets: 250 mg and 500 mg Oral suspension: 25 mg/ml and 50 mg/ml in 50 ml and 100 ml bottles
Clemastine	Tavist: Novartis; East Hanover, NJ	Tablets (scored): 2.68 mg Oral syrup: 0.134 mg/ml syrup in 118 ml bottles
	Clemastine Fumarate: various manufacturers	Tablets: 1.34 mg
	Antihist-1: Rugby (Watson); Corona, CA	Tablets: 1.34 mg
	Clemastine Fumarate: various manufacturers	Tablets: 2.68 mg
Clindamycin HCl	Antirobe: Pharmacia & Upjohn; Kalamazoo, MI	Capsules: 25 mg, 75 mg, and 150 mg Oral solution: 25 mg/ml in 30 ml bottles
	Clindrops: Vetus; Farmer's Branch, TX	Oral solution: 25 mg/ml in 30 ml bottles
	Many other generics	
Clofazimine	Lamprene: Geigy[Novartis]; East Hanover, NJ	Capsules: 50 mg
Clomipramine HCl	Clomicalm: Novartis; East Hanover, NJ	Tablets: 20 mg, 40 mg, 80 mg, and 160 mg
	Clomipramine HCl: Teva; Montgomeryville, PA	Capsules: 25 mg, 50 mg, and 75 mg
	Anafranil: Novartis; East Hanover, NJ	Capsules: 25 mg, 50 mg, and 75 mg
Cyclophosphamide	Cytoxan: Mead Johnson Oncology (Bristol Myers Oncology), Princeton, NJ	Tablets: 25 mg and 50 mg Powder for injection: 100 mg, 200 mg, and 500 mg vials and 1 g and 2 g vials

Appendix D continued on following page

Drug Name	Brand Name	How Supplied
Cyclophosphamide (cont.)	Neosar: Pharmacia & Upjohn; Peapack, NJ	Powder for injection: 100 mg, 200 mg, 500 mg, and 1 g and 2 g vials
Cyclosporin	Neoral: Sandoz; East Hanover, NJ	Gelatin capsules: 25 mg and 100 mg Oral solution: 100 mg/ml in 50 ml vials
	(Neoral) generic: Elan Labs; Lavelton, NY	Gelatin capsules: 25 mg and 100 mg Oral solution: 100 mg/ml in 50 ml vials
Cyproheptadine HCL	Periactin: Merck; West Point, PA	Tablets (scored): 4 mg Oral solution: 0.4 mg/ml
	Cyproheptadine HCL: Moore Medical Corp; New Britain, CT	Tablets: 4 mg
	Cyproheptadine HCL: Geneva; Broomfield, CO	Syrup: 0.4 mg/ml in 118 ml, 1 pt, and 1 gal containers
	Many other generics	
Dapsone	Dapsone: Jacobus; Princeton, NJ	Tablets (scored): 25 mg and 100 mg
Dexamethasone	Pet-Derm III Chewable Tablets, King Pharmaceutical; Bristol, TN	Tablets (scored): 0.25 mg
	Dexamethasone: Rugby Pharmaceuticals; Livonia, MI	Tablets: 0.25 mg and 0.50 mg
	Azium Solution, Schering-Plough; Union, NJ	Injectable solution: 2 mg/ml IV/IM in 100 ml vials
	Aspen: Kansas City, MO Butler, Dublin, OH Phoenix, St. Joseph, MO	Injectable solution: 2 mg/ml in 100 ml vials
	Dexaject, Vetus; Farmer's Branch, TX	
Diazepam	Valium: Roche Products; Manati, Puerto Rico	Tablets (scored): 2 mg, 5 mg, and 10 mg Injectable solution: 5 mg/ml in 10 ml vials
	Many other generics	
Diphenhydramine HCl	Benadryl: Warner-Lambert; Morris Plains, NJ	Capsules (OTC): 25 mg Tablets (OTC): 12.5 mg and 25 mg Oral solution (OTC): 2.5 mg/ml Injectable solution: 50 mg/ml in 1 ml and 10 ml vials
	Diphenhydramine HCL: Geneva Pharmaceutials, Inc.; Broomfield, CO	Capsules: 25 mg and 50 mg
	Diphenhydramine HCL: Rugby Labs, Inc.; Corona, CA	Syrup: 2.5 mg/ml
	Many other generics	
Doramectin	Dectomax Injectable Solution; Pfizer Animal Health; Exton, PA	Injectable solution: 10 mg/ml in 100 ml, 250 ml, and 500 ml vials
Doxepin HCl	Sinequan: Roering-Pfizer; New York, NY	Capsules: 10 mg, 25 mg, 50 mg, 75 mg, 100 mg, and 150 mg

Drug Name	Brand Name	How Supplied
	Doxepin HCl: UDL; Loves Park, IL	Capsules: 10 mg, 25 mg, 50 mg, 75 mg, 100 mg, and 150 mg Oral concentrate: 10 mg/ml in 120 ml bottles
Doxycycline	Vibramycin: Pfizer; New York, NY	Tablets: 100 mg Oral suspension: 5 mg/ml in 60 ml bottles Oral syrup: 10 mg/ml in 60 ml bottles
	Doxycycline: Lederle; Pearl River, NY	Capsules: 50 mg
	Periostat: CollaGenex; Newton, PA	Capsules: 20 mg
Enrofloxacin	Baytril: Bayer Corporation; Shawnee Mission, MS	Tablets (double scored): 22.7 mg, 68 mg, and 136 mg Injectable solution: 22.7 mg/ml in 20 ml vials
Epinephrine	Many manufacturers	Injectable solution: 1 mg/ml
Erythromycin	Erythromycin: Abbott; North Chicago, IL Many other generics	Tablets: 250 mg, 500 mg
Estrogen	Premarin: Wyeth-Ayerst; Philadelphia, PA	Tablets: 0.3 mg, 0.625 mg, 0.9 mg, 1.25 mg, and 2.5 mg
Ethambutol HCl	Myambutol: Lederle; Pearl River, NY	Tablets: 100 mg Tablets (scored): 400 mg
Fenbendazole	Panacur: Hoecst Russell Vet [Global]; Warren, NJ	Granules: 22 mg/g in 1 g, 2 g, and 4 g packages and 454 g jars
Fluconazole	Diflucan: Roering; New York, NY	Tablets: 50 mg, 100 mg, 150 mg, and 200 mg Oral suspension: 10 mg/ml in 30 ml bottles and 40 mg/ml 35 ml bottles Injectable solution: 2 mg/ml in 100 ml and 200 ml bottles
Flucytosine	Ancoban: Roche; Nutley, NJ	Capsules: 250 mg and 500 mg
Fluoxetine HCl	Prozac: Dista; Indianapolis, IN	Tablets (scored): 10 mg Capsules: 10 mg and 20 mg Oral solution: 4 mg/ml in 120 ml bottles
Gentamycin	Gentaject: Vetus; Farmer's Branch, TX Gentocin injection: Schering-Plough; Union, NJ Gentaved 50: Vedco; St. Joseph, MO	Injectable solution: 50 mg/ml in 50 ml vials
Goserelin acetate	Zoladex: AstraZeneca; Wayne, PA	Implants: 3.6 mg and 10.8 mg
Griseofulvin, micro-size	Fulvicin U/F: Schering-Plough; Liberty Corner, NJ	Tablets (scored): 250 mg and 500 mg

Appendix D continued on following page

Drug Name	Brand Name	How Supplied
Griseofulvin, micro-size (cont.)	Grifulvin V: Ortho Derm; Raritan, NJ	Tablets (scored): 250 mg and 500 mg Oral suspension: 125 mg/ml in 120 ml bottles
	Grisactin: Wyeth-Ayerst, Philadelphia, PA	Capsules: 250 mg
Griseofulvin, ultra-microsize	Fulvicin P/G: Schering-Plough, Liberty Corner, NJ	Tablets (scored): 125 mg, 165 mg, and 250 mg
	Grisactin Ultra: Wyeth-Ayerst, Philadelphia, PA	Tablets (scored): 125 mg, 250 mg, and 330 mg
Hydrocodone	Hycodan: DuPont; Wilmington, DE	Tablets (scored): 5 mg Oral syrup: 1 mg/ml in 473 ml bottles
	Hydrocodone Compound Syrup: various manufacturers	
Hydroxyzine	Atarax: Pfizer; New York, NY	Tablets: 10 mg, 25 mg, 50 mg, and 100 mg Oral syrup: 2 mg/ml in pint bottles
	Vistaril: Pfizer; New York, NY	Capsules: 25 mg, 50 mg, and 100 mg Oral suspension: 5 mg/ml in 120 ml and 473 ml bottles
	Many other generics	
Imipramine HCl	Tofranil: Novartis; Summit, NJ	Tablets: 10 mg, 25 mg, and 50 mg
	Imipramine HCl: various manufacturers	
Interferon-alpha 2B	Intron A: Schering; Liberty Corner, NJ	Powder for injection: 3 million units, 5 million units, 10 million units, 18 million units, 25 million units and 50 million units in vials
		Injectable solution: 3 million units, 5 million units, 10 million units, 18 million units and 25 million units in vials
Isoniazid (isonicotinic acid hydrazide)	Isoniazid: Schein; Florham Park, NJ	Tablets: 50 mg
	Laniazid: Lannett; Philadelphia, PA	Tablets (scored): 50 mg Oral syrup: 10 mg/ml in 480 ml bottles
	Isoniazid: Carolina Medical; Farmville, NC	Tablets: 100 mg Tablets: 300 mg
	Many other generics	
Isotrentinoin	Accutane: Roche; Nutley, NJ	Capsules: 10 mg, 20 mg, and 40 mg
Itraconazole	Sporanox: Janssen pharmaceutical; Titusville, NJ	Capsules: 100 mg Oral solution: 10 mg/ml in 150 ml containers

Drug Name	Brand Name	How Supplied
Ivermectin	Ivomec: Merial; Iselin, NJ	Injectable solution: 2.7 mg/ml in 200 ml collapsible soft packs 10 mg/ml in 50 ml bottles and 200 ml, 500 ml, and 1000 ml collapsible soft packs Injectable solution: 10 mg/ml in 50 ml bottles and 200 ml and 500 ml collapsible soft packs
	Double Impact: Agrilabs; St. Joseph, MO	Oral suspension: 10 mg/ml in 100 ml bottles
	Equvalen: Merial; Iselin, NJ	
Ketoconazole	Nizoral: Janssen Pharmaceutical; Titus-ville, NJ	Tablets (scored): 200 mg
	Ketoconazole: Novopharm USA, Inc.; Schaumburg, IL	Tablets: 200 mg
Ketophen fumarate	Zaditor: CibaVision; Duluth, GA	0.025% solution in 5 ml, 7.5 ml for ophthalmic use
Leuprolide acetate	Lupron: TAP Pharma; Deerfield, IL	Injectable solution: 5 mg/ml in 2.8 ml vials Injection depot: 3.75 mg, 7.5 mg, 11.25 mg, 22.5 mg, and 30 mg
Levamisole	Levasole Sheep Wormer: Schering-Plough; Union, NJ	Boluses: 184 mg
Levothyroxine	Soloxine: Daniels; St. Louis, MO	Tablets: 0.1 mg, 0.2 mg, 0.3 mg, 0.4 mg, 0.5 mg, 0.6 mg, 0.7 mg, and 0.8 mg
Lincomycin HCl	Lincocin: Pharmacia & Upjohn; Kala-mazoo, MI	Tablets (scored): 100 mg, 200 mg and 500 mg Oral solution: 50 mg/ml in 20 ml bottles Injectable solution: 100 mg/ml in 20 ml vials
Loratadine	Claritin: Schering-Plough; Liberty Cor-ner, NJ	Tablets: 10 mg Oral syrup: 1 mg/ml in 480 ml bottles
Lufenuron	Program: Ciba; Greensboro, NC	Oral suspension: 135 mg and 270 mg packets Tablets: 45 mg, 90 mg, 204.9 mg, and 409.8 mg Injectable suspension: 40 mg (0.4 ml) and 80 mg (0.8 ml) in preloaded sy-ringes

Appendix D continued on following page

Drug Name	Brand Name	How Supplied
Lufenuron-milbemy-cin oxime	Sentinel: Novartis; Greensboro, NC	Tablets: 46 mg lufenuron/2.3 mg milbemycin oxime 115 mg lufenuron/5.75 mg milbemycin oxime 230 mg lufenuron/115 mg milbemycin oxime 460 mg lufenuron/230 mg milbemycin oxime
Marbofloxacin	Zeniquin: Pfizer Animal Health; Exton, PA	Tablets (scored): 25 mg, 50 mg, 100 mg, and 200 mg
Menbendazole	Vermox: Janssen; Titusville, NJ Menbendazole: Copley; Canton, MA Many other generics	Tablets: 100 mg
Methylprednisolone	Medrol: Pharmacia & Upjohn; Kalamazoo, MI	Tablets (double scored): 4 mg
	Methylprednisolone Tablets: Boehringer Ingelheim; Sioux City, IA	Tablets: 2 mg
	Methylprednisolone Tablets, Vedco; St. Joseph, MO	Tablets: 2 mg
	Depo-Medrol: Pharmacia & Upjohn; Kalamazoo, MI	Injectable suspension: 20 mg/ml in 10 ml and 20 ml vials
	Methylprednisolone Acetate Injection: Boehringer Ingelheim; Sioux Center, IA	Injectable suspension: 40 mg/ml in 5 ml and 30 ml vials
Methyltestosterone	Android: ICN Pharma; Costa Mesa, CA	Tablets: 10 mg and 25 mg
	Oreton Methyltestosterone: Schering-Plough; Liberty Corner, NJ	Tablets: 10 mg
	Testred: ICN Pharma; Costa Mesa, CA	Capsules: 10 mg
	Methyltestosterone: various manufacturers Many other generics	Tablets: 10 mg and 25 mg
Metronidazole	Flagyl: Searle; Chicago, IL	Tablets: 250 mg and 500 mg Capsules: 375 mg
	Metronidazone: Geneva Pharmaceuticals, Inc.; Broomfield, CO	Tablets (scored): 250 mg and 500 mg
Metyrapone	Metopirone: Novartis; East Hanover, NJ	Gelatin capsules: 250 mg

Drug Name	Brand Name	How Supplied
Milbemycin oxime	Interceptor: Novartis; Greensboro, NC	Tablets: 2.3 mg, 5.75 mg, 11.5 mg, and 23.0 mg
		Sentinel: same color coding as above plus lufenuron at 10 mg/kg (46 mg, 115 mg, 230 mg, 460 mg of lufenuron, respectively)
Minocycline	Minocin: Lederle; Pearl River, NY	Capsules: 50 mg and 100 mg Oral suspension: 10 mg/ml in 60 ml bottles
	Dynacin: Medicus Dermatologics; Phoenix, AZ	Capsules: 50 mg and 100 mg
	Minocycline HCl: Warner Chilcott; Rockaway, NJ	Capsules: 50 mg and 100 mg
	Many other generics	
Misoprostol	Cytotec: Searle; Chicago, IL	Tablets: 100 mg Tablets (scored): 200 mg
Mitotane	Lysodren: Bristol-Myers Squibb; Princeton, NJ	Tablets (scored): 500 mg
Naltrexone	ReVia: DuPont; Wilmington, DE	Tablets (scored): 50 mg
	Depade: Mallinckrodt: St. Louis, MO	
Niacinamide	OTC (Many manufacturers)	Tablets: 100 mg and 500 mg
Orbifloxacin	Orbax: Schering-Plough; Union, NJ	Tablets: 5.7 mg Tablets (scored): 22.7 mg and 68 mg
Ormetoprim/sulfadimethoxime	Primor: Pfizer Animal Health; Exton, PA	Tablets (scored): 120 mg, 240 mg, 600 mg, and 1200 mg
Oxacillin	Oxacillin Sodium: Teva Pharmaceuticals; Montgomeryville, PA	Capsules: 250 mg and 500 mg
Pentoxifylline	Trental: Hoescht Marion Russell; Kansas City, MO	Tablets: 400 mg
	Pentoxifylline: Copley; Canton, MA	
	Many other generics	
Phenobarbital	Many manufacturers	Tablets: 15 mg, 30 mg, 60 mg, and 100 mg
		Oral elixir: 3–4 mg/ml
		Injectable solution: 130 mg/ml
Potassium iodide	Potassium iodide: Roxane; Columbus, OH	Oral solution: 1 g/ml in 30 ml and 240 ml bottles
	PIMA: Fleming; Fenton, MO	Oral solution: 65 mg/ml
	Many other generics	

Appendix D continued on following page

Drug Name	Brand Name	How Supplied
Prednisone	Prednisone: Geneva Pharmaceuticals, Inc.; Broomfield, CO	Tablets: 5 mg, 10 mg, 20 mg, and 50 mg
	Prednisone: Roxane Laboratories; Columbus, OH	Tablets: 1 mg Oral solution: 1 mg/ml in 5 ml and 500 ml bottles
	Many other generics	
Prednisolone	Prednistabs: Vedco; St. Joseph, MO	Tablets: 5 mg
	Prednistabs: Vet-A-Mix; Shenandoah, IA	Tablets: 5 mg and 20 mg
	Predate 50: Legere; Scottsdale, AZ	Oral suspension (prednisolone acetate): 50 mg/ml in 10 ml vials
	Sterisol-20: Anthony; Arcadia, CA	Injectable solution (prednisolone sodium phosphate): 20 mg/ml in 50 ml vials
	Solu-Delta-Cortef: Pharmacia & Upjohn; Kalamazoo, MI	Powder for injection (prednisolone sodium succinate): 100 mg/ml and 500 mg/ml in 10 ml vials
	Many other generics	
Pyrantel pamoate	Nemex: Pfizer; Exton, PA	Tablets: 22.7 mg and 113.5 mg Oral suspension: 4.54 mg/ml in 2 fl oz bottles
	Many other generics	
Pyrazinamide	Pyrazinamide: Lederle; Pearl River, NY	Tablets (scored): 500 mg
Rifampin	Rifadin: Hoechst Marion Russell; Kansas City, MO	Capsules: 150 mg and 300 mg
	Rimactane: Ciba; Duluth, GA	Capsules: 300 mg
	Many other generics	
Selegiline HCl (L-deprenyl)	Anipryl: Pfizer; Exton, PA	Tablets: 2 mg, 5 mg, 10 mg, 15 mg, and 30 mg
	Carbex: DuPont Pharma; Wilmington, DE	Tablets: 5 mg
	Eldepryl: Somerset; Tampa, FL	Capsules: 5 mg
	Selegiline HCl: Apothecon; Princeton, NJ	Tablets: 5 mg
Sulfadiazine	Sulfadiazine: Eon; Laurelton, NY Sulfadiazine: Major; Livonia, MI	Tablets: 500 mg
	Many other generics	
Sulfamethizole	Thiosulfil Forte: Wyeth-Ayerst; Philadelphia, PA	Tablets (scored): 500 mg
Sulfisoxazole	Sulfisoxazole: Moore; New Britain, CT Sulfisoxazole: Geneva; Broomfield, CO	Tablets: 500 mg
	Many other generics	

Drug Name	Brand Name	How Supplied
Terbinafine HCl	Lamisil: Sandoz/Novartis; East Hanover, NJ	Tablets: 250 mg
Tetracycline HCL	Achromycin: Lederle Laboratories; Pearl River, NY	Capsules: 250 mg and 500 mg Oral suspension 25 mg/ml Injectable solution: 100 mg, 250 mg, and 500 mg vials
	Panmycin Aquadrops: Pharmacia and Upjohn; Kalamazoo, MI	Oral suspension: 100 mg/ml in 15 ml and 30 ml bottles
	Tetracycline HCL: Global; Philadelphia, PA	Capsules: 250 mg
Thiabendazole	Mintezol: Merck; West Point, PA	Tablets (scored): 500 mg Oral solution: 50 mg/ml in 120 ml bottles
Ticarcillin	Ticar: SmithKline Beecham; Philadelphia, PA	Powder for injection: 1 g, 3 g, 6 g, 20 g, and 30 g vials
Ticarcillin-clavulanate potassium	Timentin: SmithKline Beecham; Philadelphia, PA	Powder for injection: 3 g ticarcillin, 0.1 g clavulanic acid in 3.1 g vials 3 g ticarcillin, 0.1 g clavulanic acid per 100 ml in 100 ml premixed vials
Triamcinolone acetonide	Vetalog: Fort Dodge; Fort Dodge, IA	Tablets: 0.5 mg and 1.5 mg Injectable suspension: 2 mg and 6 mg in 5 ml and 25 ml vials
	Cortalone Tablets: Vedco; St. Joseph, MO	Tablets: 0.5 mg and 1.5 mg
	Triamcinolone Acetonide Tablets: Boehringer-Ingelheim; Sioux City, IA	Tablets: 0.5 mg and 1.5 mg
	Triamtabs: Vetus; Farmer's Branch, TX	Tablets: 0.5 mg and 1.5 mg
Trimeprazine-prednisolone	Temeril-P: Pfizer; Exton, PA	Tablets: 5 mg trimeprazine/2 mg prednisolone
Trimethoprim-sulfadiazine	Tribrissen: Schering-Plough; Union, NJ	Tablets: 30 mg and 120 mg Tablets (scored): 480 mg and 960 mg
Trimethoprim-sulfamethoxazole	Bactrim: Roche Laboratories, Inc; Nutley, NJ	Tablets (scored): 480 mg and 960 mg Oral suspension: 48 mg/ml in 16 oz bottles Injectable solution: 96 mg/ml in 10 ml and 30 ml vials
	Septra: Monarch Pharmaceuticals; Bristol, TN	Tablets (scored): 480 mg and 960 mg Oral suspension: 48 mg/ml in 16 oz bottles Injectable solution: 96 mg/ml in 5 ml, 10 ml, and 20 ml vials
	Many other generics	
Vincristine sulfate	Oncovin: Lily; Indianapolis, IN	Injectable solution: 1 mg/ml in 1 ml, 2 ml, and 5 ml vials
	Vincristine Sulfate: various manufacturers	
	Vincasar: Pharmacia & Upjohn; Peapack, NJ	

Index

Note: Page numbers in *italics* indicate figures; those followed by t indicate tables.